2011
YEAR BOOK OF
GASTROENTEROLOGY™

The 2011 Year Book Series

Year Book of Anesthesiology and Pain Management™: Drs Chestnut, Abram, Black, Gravlee, Lien, Mathru, and Roizen

Year Book of Cardiology®: Drs Gersh, Cheitlin, Elliott, Gold, Graham, and Thourani

Year Book of Critical Care Medicine®: Drs Dellinger, Parrillo, Balk, Dorman, Dries, and Zanotti-Cavazzoni

Year Book of Dermatology and Dermatologic Surgery™: Dr Del Rosso

Year Book of Diagnostic Radiology®: Drs Osborn, Abbara, Elster, Manaster, Oestreich, Offiah, Rosado de Christenson, Stephens, and Walker

Year Book of Emergency Medicine®: Drs Hamilton, Bruno, Handly, Mullin, Quintana, and Ramoska

Year Book of Endocrinology®: Drs Schott, Apovian, Clarke, Eugster, Ludlam, Meikle, Schinner, Schteingart, and Toth

Year Book of Gastroenterology™: Drs Talley, DeVault, Harnois, Murray, Pearson, Philcox, Picco, and Smith

Year Book of Hand and Upper Limb Surgery®: Drs Yao and Steinmann

Year Book of Medicine®: Drs Barker, Garrick, Gersh, Khardori, LeRoith, Panush, Talley, and Thigpen

Year Book of Neonatal and Perinatal Medicine®: Drs Fanaroff, Benitz, Donn, Neu, Papile, Polin, and Van Marter

Year Book of Neurology and Neurosurgery®: Drs Klimo and Rabinstein

Year Book of Obstetrics, Gynecology, and Women's Health®: Drs Dungan and Shulman

Year Book of Oncology®: Drs Arceci, Bauer, Chiorean, Gordon, Lawton, Murphy, Thigpen, and Tsao

Year Book of Ophthalmology®: Drs Rapuano, Cohen, Flanders, Fudemberg, Hammersmith, Milman, Myers, Nagra, Nelson, Penne, Pyfer, Sergott, Shields, Talekar, and Vander

Year Book of Orthopedics®: Drs Morrey, Beauchamp, Huddleston, Swiontkowski, and Trigg

Year Book of Otolaryngology-Head and Neck Surgery®: Drs Sindwani, Balough, Franco, Gapany, and Mitchell

Year Book of Pathology and Laboratory Medicine®: Drs Raab, Parwani, Bejarano, and Bissell

Year Book of Pediatrics®: Dr Stockman

Year Book of Plastic and Aesthetic Surgery™: Drs Miller, Gosain, Gurtner, Gutowski, Ruberg, Salisbury, and Smith

2011

The Year Book of
GASTROENTEROLOGY™

Editor-in-Chief
Nicholas J. Talley, MD, PhD
Pro Vice-Chancellor, Dean of Health, and Professor of Medicine, University of Newcastle, Callaghan, New South Wales, Australia; Adjunct Professor, Mayo Clinic Florida, Jacksonville, Florida; Adjunct Professor, University of North Carolina, Chapel Hill, North Carolina

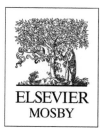

ELSEVIER
MOSBY

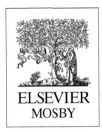

ELSEVIER
MOSBY

Vice President, Continuity: Kimberly Murphy
Senior Editor: Kerry Holland
Production Supervisor, Electronic Year Books: Donna M. Skelton
Electronic Article Manager: Mike Sheets
Illustrations and Permissions Coordinator: Dawn Vohsen

2011 EDITION

Composition by TNQ Books and Journals Pvt Ltd, India

Editorial Office:
Elsevier
1600 John F. Kennedy Blvd.
Suite 1800
Philadelphia, PA 19103-2899

International Standard Serial Number: 0739-5930
International Standard Book Number: 978-0-323-08414-7

Printed and bound by CPI Group (UK) Ltd, Croydon, CR0 4YY

Transferred to Digital Print 2011

Associate Editors

Kenneth R. DeVault, MD
Professor and Chair, Department of Medicine, Mayo Clinic Florida, Jacksonville, Florida

Denise M. Harnois, DO
Associate Professor, Department of Medicine, Mayo Clinic Florida, Jacksonville, Florida

Joseph A. Murray, MD
Professor of Medicine; Consultant, Division of Gastroenterology and Hepatology and Department of Immunology, The Mayo Clinic Rochester, Rochester, Minnesota

Randall K. Pearson, MD
Associate Professor of Medicine, Division of Gastroenterology and Hepatology, The Mayo Clinic Rochester, Rochester, Minnesota

Stephen M. Philcox, FRACP, MBBS (Hons), BMedSc
Department of Gastroenterology, John Hunter Hospital, New Lambton Heights, New South Wales, Australia

Michael F. Picco, MD, PhD
Assistant Professor of Medicine, Department of Gastroenterology and Hepatology, Mayo Clinic Florida, Jacksonville, Florida

C. Daniel Smith, MD
Professor and Chair, Department of Surgery, and Surgeon-in-Chief, Mayo Clinic Florida, Jacksonville, Florida

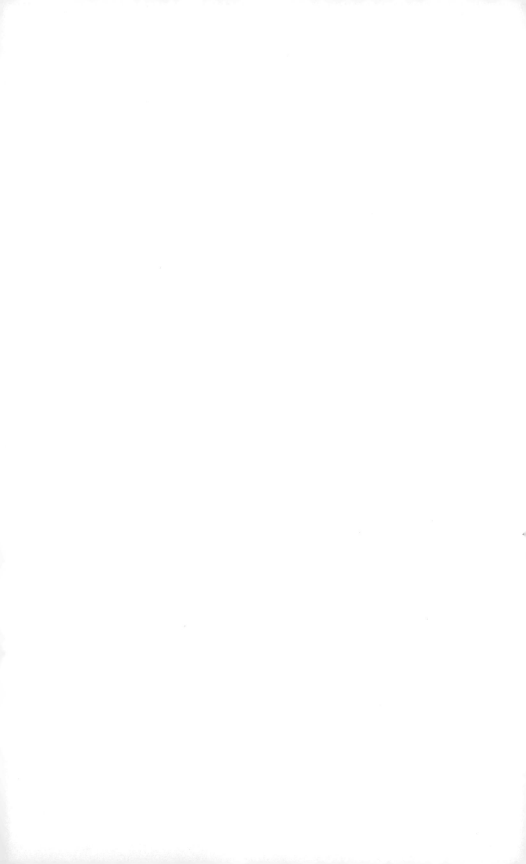

Table of Contents

Journals Represented

Journals represented in this YEAR BOOK are listed below.

AJR American Journal of Roentgenology
Alimentary Pharmacology & Therapeutics
American Journal of Gastroenterology
American Journal of Medicine
American Journal of Surgery
American Surgeon
Anesthesia & Analgesia
Annals of Medicine
Annals of Surgery
Annals of Surgical Oncology
Archives of Surgery
British Journal of Cancer
British Journal of Surgery
British Journal of Urology International
Clinical Gastroenterology and Hepatology
Clinical Pharmacology & Therapeutics
Cochrane Database of Systematic Reviews
Digestive Diseases and Sciences
Diseases of the Colon and Rectum
European Journal of Clinical Investigation
Gastroenterology
Gastrointestinal Endoscopy
Gut
Heart
Heart Rhythm
Hepatology
International Journal of Colorectal Disease
Interactive CardioVascular and Thoracic Surgery
Journal of Clinical Gastroenterology
Journal of Gastroenterology
Journal of Hepatology
Journal of Parenteral and Enteral Nutrition
Journal of Pediatric Gastroenterology and Nutrition
Journal of the American College of Surgeons
Journal of the American Medical Association
Lancet
Lancet Neurology
Liver Transplantation
Neurogastroenterology and Motility
New England Journal of Medicine
Obstetrics & Gynecology
Pediatrics
Proceedings of the National Academy of Sciences of the United States of America
Public Library of Science One

Surgery
Surgical Endoscopy
World Journal of Surgery

STANDARD ABBREVIATIONS

The following terms are abbreviated in this edition: acquired immunodeficiency syndrome (AIDS), cardiopulmonary resuscitation (CPR), central nervous system (CNS), cerebrospinal fluid (CSF), computed tomography (CT), deoxyribonucleic acid (DNA), electrocardiography (ECG), health maintenance organization (HMO), human immunodeficiency virus (HIV), intensive care unit (ICU), intramuscular (IM), intravenous (IV), magnetic resonance (MR) imaging (MRI), ribonucleic acid (RNA), and ultrasound (US).

NOTE

The YEAR BOOK OF GASTROENTEROLOGY is a literature survey service providing abstracts of articles published in the professional literature. Every effort is made to assure the accuracy of the information presented in these pages. Neither the editors nor the publisher of the YEAR BOOK OF GASTROENTEROLOGY can be responsible for errors in the original materials. The editors' comments are their own opinions. Mention of specific products within this publication does not constitute endorsement.

To facilitate the use of the YEAR BOOK OF GASTROENTEROLOGY as a reference tool, all illustrations and tables included in this publication are now identified as they appear in the original article. This change is meant to help the reader recognize that any illustration or table appearing in the YEAR BOOK OF GASTROENTEROLOGY may be only one of many in the original article. For this reason, figure and table numbers will often appear to be out of sequence within the YEAR BOOK OF GASTROENTEROLOGY.

Introduction

We wish our readers a very warm welcome to the new edition of the YEAR BOOK OF GASTROENTEROLOGY. We appreciate how difficult it is to keep up-to-date in an environment in which clinicians are busier than ever, the medical literature continues to expand rapidly, and new journals in our field seem to spring up almost monthly. To select the topics included in the YEAR BOOK OF GASTROENTEROLOGY, a rigorous selection process has been put in place. An international team of expert editors has been assembled to bring you this year's most important developments in clinical gastroenterology and hepatology. After an independent reviewer screens and provides abstracts of the world's literature, the editors pick out the best and most important articles for inclusion. Expert commentaries are developed to follow each abstracted article, with a goal of placing the information in context and helping guide your practice.

In this edition, the topics vary broadly but the new information is at times breathtaking. What is the must-know information this year? Let me present a few examples that will likely inform clinical practice going forward.

In the esophagus section, you'll read that budesonide has been confirmed to be efficacious in eosinophilic esophagitis. Did you know achalasia probably increases the risk of not just squamous cell but also adenocarcinoma of the esophagus? New data fuel the ongoing controversy surrounding endoscopic screening of patients who have gastroesophageal reflux disease (GERD) symptoms for Barrett's esophagus (probably screening can be restricted to those with frequent reflux symptoms over the age of 60). Radiofrequency catheter ablation of atrial fibrillation and celiac disease may be new causes of GERD. Self-expandable metal stents can be safely and effectively applied for benign esophageal perforations. A localized esophageal squamous cell carcinoma less than 3 cm can be effectively managed by endoscopic mucosal resection rather than surgery. Guidance on safely prescribing proton pump inhibitors (PPIs) with the antiplatelet agent clopidogrel is provided.

Neurogastroenterology is undergoing a reformation. A clinical trial indicates that pneumatic dilatation is as good as myotomy for achalasia. PPIs may predispose to bacterial overgrowth and precipitating irritable bowel syndrome (IBS), although this remains controversial. On the other hand, there is now no doubt a non-absorbable antibiotic changes the natural history of diarrhea-predominant IBS, improving symptoms in a subset. Those whose intestinal flora produces methane are more likely to develop constipation. Cow's milk allergy and intestinal inflammation are both risk factors for functional gut disorders.

Management of inflammatory bowel disease (IBD) continues to evolve. Important new clinical trials evaluating treatment modalities in Crohn's disease and ulcerative colitis in the past year are presented in this volume. Real-world experience with the biologics is also summarized. Local injection of mesenchymal stem cells holds promise for refractory fistulizing Crohn's disease. Should you prescribe adjunctive therapy with probiotics for your outpatients with ulcerative colitis, because new evidence supports this idea? Can you recognize segmental colitis associated with diverticulosis (SCAD), which presents like IBD? Don't be fooled: IBS often causes symptoms in patients with IBD and, here, increasing immunosuppression won't help. Thiopurines seem safe in pregnancy, but decisions on their use then still need to be individualized. Duodenal lymphocytosis on biopsy (Marsh grade 1) is not always due to celiac disease, and other causes are uncovered in a new population-based study. Gluten is also an apparent cause of gastrointestinal symptoms in the absence of celiac disease.

In the colon, cancer screening by colonoscopy is king, but problems remain with adenoma and cancer detection, particularly in the right colon. Chromoendoscopy may help, enhancing adenoma detection rates in an average-risk population. Non-alcoholic steatohepatitis is associated with a high prevalence of advanced colonic lesions, while in IBS there is a lower risk! Peutz-Jeghers syndrome is associated with an increased cancer risk, and more aggressive screening is justified on the basis of new observations (including colonoscopy from age 30). More good data have emerged on aspirin; taking it long term at doses of at least 75 mg daily reduces colon cancer incidence and mortality.

In the pancreas, screening at-risk relatives from familial pancreatic cancer families has utility, particularly in relatives over age 65 years, but screening is still controversial. More insights into autoimmune pancreatitis are presented; although a rare condition, it can be mistaken for pancreatic cancer. Pancreatic stent placement appears to decrease the risk of pancreatitis after endoscopic retrograde cholangiopancreatography (ERCP).

There is important news in liver disease. Did you know constipation may precipitate the rupture of esophageal varices? Patients with minimal hepatic encephalopathy appear to be safer drivers on rifaximin compared with placebo. Long-term tenofovir looks safe and efficacious for patients with chronic hepatitis B. It may be possible to prescribe an efficacious interferon-free hepatitis C therapy using a nucleoside analogue polymerase inhibitor and protease inhibitor. Up-to-date recommendations on how to best manage hepatitis C genotype 4 are summarized. New insights into the classification and management of liver adenomas are welcome. Advice on the diagnosis and treatment of drug-induced cholestasis is presented. Budesonide may be a better alternative to prednisone in autoimmune hepatitis.

Did you know that after gastric bypass surgery for obesity, alcohol handling can be very problematic? More information on those who do poorly after anti-obesity surgery is now available. Procalcitonin levels may predict intestinal ischemia and help determine who should go to earlier surgery.

This is just a taste of what awaits you inside the book. We hope you will enjoy reading the YEAR BOOK OF GASTROENTEROLOGY as much as we have enjoyed preparing this new edition for you and the field.

Nicholas J. Talley, MD, PhD

1 Esophagus

Achalasia

13-Year Follow-Up of a Prospective Comparison of the Long-Term Clinical Efficacy of Temporary Self-Expanding Metallic Stents and Pneumatic Dilatation for the Treatment of Achalasia in 120 Patients
Li Y-D, Tang G-Y, Cheng Y-S, et al (Shanghai Jiao Tong Univ, People's Republic of China; Shanghai Tong Ji Univ, People's Republic of China)
AJR Am J Roentgenol 195:1429-1437, 2010

Objective.—The purpose of this article is to compare the efficacy of self-expanding metallic stents and pneumatic dilation for the long-term clinical treatment of achalasia.

Subjects and Methods.—Patients diagnosed with achalasia ($n = 120$) were allocated for treatment with pneumatic dilation ($n = 30$; group A) or a temporary self-expanding metallic stent with a diameter of 20 mm ($n = 30$; group B), 25 mm ($n = 30$; group C), or 30 mm ($n = 30$; group D). Data on clinical symptoms, complications, and long-term clinical outcomes were collected, and follow-up was performed at 6 months and at 1, 3–5, 5–8, 8–10, and more than 10 years after surgery.

Results.—Pneumatic dilation and stent placement were technically successful in all patients. The follow-up at more than 10 years revealed that the clinical remission rate in group D (83.3%) was higher than that in groups A (0%), B (0%), and C (28.6%), and the overall cumulative clinical failure rate in group D (13%) was lower than that in groups A (76.7%), B (53.3%), and C (26.7%). Patients in group D exhibited reduced dysphagia scores and lower esophageal sphincter pressures and had normal levels of barium height and width during the follow-up periods, whereas these markers increased with time in the other groups. The duration of primary patency in group D was also longer than that in groups A, B, and C.

Conclusion.—A temporary self-expanding metallic stent with a diameter of 30 mm has superior clinical efficacy for the treatment of achalasia compared with pneumatic dilation or self-expanding metallic stents with diameters of 20 or 25 mm.

► Previous studies have reported conflicting data on the outcome of endoscopically placed stents in achalasia, with some series suggesting poor efficacy and high complication rates. The patients in this large series were randomly assigned to balloon dilation versus 3 different stent sizes. They demonstrated that the largest stent (30 mm) was superior to balloon dilation or the 2 smaller stents (20 and 25 mm). In addition to poorer outcomes, the smaller stents were much more likely to migrate. This was a self-designed, covered stent and was used over a 13-year period (1994 to 2007). The stent was only left in place for 3 to 7 days and then removed. Follow-up included both radiographic and clinical endpoints. Importantly, there were no perforations in any of the treatment groups. One issue with the study is the method of balloon dilation. They performed progressive dilation with a 28-, 30-, and 32-mm self-constructed balloon on a weekly basis with inflation to 8 to 10 psi. The standard approach in the West is to begin with a 30-mm commercially available balloon and progress to a 35- or 40-mm balloon if the patient does not respond clinically or, in some centers, if there is no improvement in esophageal emptying. Based on these data, I would assume the 30-mm stent is functioning much like a 30-mm pneumatic balloon and has the potential to offer a reasonable alternative in achalasia. Concerns about wider application mainly surround the commercial availability of a similarly functioning stent and whether these results are transferable outside of these investigators' experiences.

K. R. DeVault, MD

Pneumatic Dilation versus Laparoscopic Heller's Myotomy for Idiopathic Achalasia

Boeckxstaens GE, for the European Achalasia Trial Investigators (Academic Med Ctr, Amsterdam, The Netherlands; et al)
N Engl J Med 364:1807-1816, 2011

Background.—Many experts consider laparoscopic Heller's myotomy (LHM) to be superior to pneumatic dilation for the treatment of achalasia, and LHM is increasingly considered to be the treatment of choice for this disorder.

Methods.—We randomly assigned patients with newly diagnosed achalasia to pneumatic dilation or LHM with Dor's fundoplication. Symptoms, including weight loss, dysphagia, retrosternal pain, and regurgitation, were assessed with the use of the Eckardt score (which ranges from 0 to 12, with higher scores indicating more pronounced symptoms). The primary outcome was therapeutic success (a drop in the Eckardt score to ≤3) at the yearly follow-up assessment. The secondary outcomes included the need for retreatment, pressure at the lower esophageal sphincter, esophageal emptying on a timed barium esophagogram, quality of life, and the rate of complications.

Results.—A total of 201 patients were randomly assigned to pneumatic dilation (95 patients) or LHM (106). The mean follow-up time was 43 months (95% confidence interval [CI], 40 to 47). In an intention-to-treat analysis, there was no significant difference between the two groups in the primary outcome; the rate of therapeutic success with pneumatic dilation was 90% after 1 year of follow-up and 86% after 2 years, as compared with a rate with LHM of 93% after 1 year and 90% after 2 years (P = 0.46). After 2 years of follow-up, there was no significant between-group difference in the pressure at the lower esophageal sphincter (LHM, 10 mm Hg [95% CI, 8.7 to 12]; pneumatic dilation, 12 mm Hg [95% CI, 9.7 to 14]; P = 0.27); esophageal emptying, as assessed by the height of barium-contrast column (LHM, 1.9 cm [95% CI, 0 to 6.8]; pneumatic dilation, 3.7 cm [95% CI, 0 to 8.8]; P = 0.21); or quality of life. Similar results were obtained in the per-protocol analysis. Perforation of the esophagus occurred in 4% of the patients during pneumatic dilation, whereas mucosal tears occurred in 12% during LHM. Abnormal exposure to esophageal acid was observed in 15% and 23% of the patients in the pneumatic-dilation and LHM groups, respectively (P = 0.28).

Conclusions.—After 2 years of follow-up, LHM, as compared with pneumatic dilation, was not associated with superior rates of therapeutic success. (European Achalasia Trial Netherlands Trial Register number, NTR37, and Current Controlled Trials number, ISRCTN56304564.)

▶ The treatment options for achalasia include oral medications to decrease lower esophageal sphincter (LES) pressure, botulinum toxin injection of the LES, forceful pneumatic dilation (PD), and surgical myotomy. The first 2 approaches rarely result in long-term remission, so most patients fit for endoscopy or surgery end up choosing between the last 2 approaches. When the myotomy required a transthoracic approach, many experts leaned strongly toward PD as the preferred treatment. The advent of a laparoscopic approach to myotomy has changed that equation in many centers, with more patients undergoing primary surgery. This study randomized more than 200 patients to either myotomy or PD. After 2 years of follow-up, there were no differences between the outcomes in the 2 groups. Esophageal perforation occurred in 4% of the patients with PD (2 were managed conservatively and 2 required surgery); and mucosal lacerations occurred in 12% of those undergoing myotomy, all of which were closed during the surgery.

In addition to the primary finding of a similar outcome between the groups, there were some additional lessons from this study. Early on, the investigators used a 35-mm balloon as the initial size, but they altered their protocol because of an unacceptably high rate of perforation: starting with a 30-mm balloon and only progressing if the patient had an unacceptable outcome. Five of the PD patients eventually had surgery, and 15 of the myotomy patients had enough postsurgical symptoms to eventually require a postoperative attempt at PD.

These data would suggest that many of us might have been premature to move away from PD toward myotomy. The choice can continue to be guided by patient preference and local expertise. It is important to remember that these results came from expert centers, and it is not clear if similar results are obtained at lower-volume community practices.

K. R. DeVault, MD

Risk of Esophageal Adenocarcinoma in Achalasia Patients, a Retrospective Cohort Study in Sweden

Zendehdel K, Nyrén O, Edberg A, et al (Karolinska Institutet, Stockholm, Sweden; The Natl Board of Health and Welfare, Stockholm, Sweden)

Am J Gastroenterol 106:57-61, 2011

Objectives.—Achalasia is a motor disorder of the lower esophageal sphincter, which fails to relax on swallowing. Although a greater risk of esophageal squamous cell carcinoma among achalasia patients is fairly well established, no epidemiological study has evaluated the risk of esophageal adenocarcinoma in these patients.

Methods.—We compiled a cohort of 2,896 patients recorded with a discharge diagnosis of achalasia between 1965 and 2003 in the Swedish Inpatient Register. The cohort was followed through 2003 via record linkages with essentially complete registers of cancer, causes of death, and migration. Standardized incidence ratios (SIRs) were used to estimate the relative risk of esophageal cancer in achalasia patients compared to the age-, sex-, and calendar period-matched Swedish population. We further estimated SIRs for esophageal cancer among patients treated with esophagomyotomy.

Results.—After excluding the first year of follow-up, we observed excess risks for both squamous cell carcinoma (SIR 11.0, 95% confidence interval [CI] 6.0–18.4) and adenocarcinoma (SIR 10.4, 95% CI 3.8–22.6) of the esophagus. Notwithstanding similar numbers of men and women in our achalasia cohort, 20 of 22 esophageal cancers developed in men (SIRs for adenocarcinoma and squamous cell carcinoma were 8.4 and 13.1, respectively). Increased SIRs among operated patients pertained mainly to esophageal squamous cell carcinoma. We found no evidence that surgical esophagomyotomy increases the risk of esophageal adenocarcinoma.

Conclusions.—Male achalasia patients have substantially greater risks for both squamous cell carcinoma and adenocarcinoma of the esophagus. Small numbers preclude a firm conclusion about the risk among women.

▶ It has been suggested that patients with achalasia, whether treated or not, are at an increased risk of esophageal squamous cell carcinoma (ESCC), although the magnitude of that risk is not known, and specific screening programs are not generally advocated. In addition, there have been isolated reports of esophageal adenocarcinoma (EAC) developing in patients with achalasia. It has been assumed that this might be because of the development of reflux and Barrett's esophagus in treated patients with achalasia. This study examined a large number of patients in a Swedish database and found that both ESCC and EAC were increased in male patients. The risk for cancer was increased in both patients who had and who had not undergone esophagomyotomy. They did not find the same association in women for unclear reasons. Data such as these may make the idea of an endoscopic surveillance program after the diagnosis of achalasia attractive to some. On the other hand, with a cancer incidence rate of only 145 out of 100 000 patient-years and no clear method to stratify that risk (particularly of ESCC), there is little likelihood that an endoscopic screening program could be proven to be beneficial in achalasia.

K. R. DeVault, MD

Barrett's Esophagus

Endoscopic radiofrequency ablation combined with endoscopic resection for early neoplasia in Barrett's esophagus longer than 10 cm
Herrero LA, van Vilsteren FGI, Pouw RE, et al (Academic Med Ctr, Amsterdam, The Netherlands; et al)
Gastrointest Endosc 73:682-690, 2011

Background.—Radiofrequency ablation (RFA) is safe and effective for eradicating Barrett's esophagus (BE) and BE-associated early neoplasia. Most RFA studies have limited the baseline length of BE (<10 cm), and therefore little is known about RFA for longer BE.

Objective.—To assess the safety and efficacy of RFA with or without prior endoscopic resection (ER) for BE ≥10 cm containing neoplasia.

Design.—Prospective trial.

Setting.—Two tertiary-care centers.

Patients.—This study involved consecutive patients with BE ≥10 cm with early neoplasia.

Intervention.—Focal ER for visible abnormalities, followed by a maximum of 2 circumferential and 3 focal RFA procedures every 2 to 3 months until complete remission.

Main Outcome Measurements.—Complete remission, defined as endoscopic resolution of BE and no intestinal metaplasia (CR-IM) or neoplasia (CR-neoplasia) in biopsy specimens.

Results.—Of the 26 patients included, 18 underwent ER for visible abnormalities before RFA. The ER specimens showed early cancer in 11, high-grade intraepithelial neoplasia (HGIN) in 6, and low-grade intraepithelial neoplasia (LGIN) in 1. The worst residual histology, before RFA and after any ER, was HGIN in 16 patients and LGIN in 10 patients. CR-neoplasia and CR-IM were achieved in 83% (95% confidence interval [CI], 63%-95%) and 79% (95% CI, 58%-93%), respectively. None of the patients had fatal or severe complications and 15% (95% CI, 4%-35%) had moderate complications. During a mean (± standard deviation) follow-up of 29 (± 9.1) months, no neoplasia recurred.

Limitations.—Tertiary-care center, short follow-up.

Conclusion.—ER for visible abnormalities, followed by RFA of residual BE is a safe and effective treatment for BE ≥10 cm containing neoplasia, with a low chance of recurrence of neoplasia or BE during follow-up.

▶ The optimal treatment for patients who have developed high-grade dysplasia or limited cancers in a segment of Barrett's esophagus (BE) continues to evolve.

Several years ago, the only options were esophagectomy or continued surveillance. The advent of photodynamic therapy changed this equation, as did the more recent development of radiofrequency ablation. Many centers have begun to endoscopically resect any visible abnormalities in segments of dysplastic BE to provide larger histologic samples as well as actually to provide total resection and cure of some lesions. It is common practice to allow those resections to heal and then have the patient return for further efforts at ablation of all of the visible Barrett's epithelium. This article provides data on the outcome of patients treated in this manner.

These patients had very long segments (>10 cm of BE) with advanced dysplasia or early cancers. Any visible lesions were resected followed by sequential ablation until there was no evidence of residual BE. They were then followed up at 3, 6, and 12 months and annually there afterward. There were no perforations and only a few procedure-related adverse events. Twenty of 24 patients had complete resolution of neoplasia (one of these did have some residual metaplasia). At a mean follow-up of 29 months, BE was seen to recur in 5 patients (2 with visible BE and 3 with intestinal metaplasia distal to their new squamocolumnar junction). There was no recurrence of neoplasia. This study supports an endoscopically based approach to dysplasia and early neoplasia in patients with BE. It particularly highlights the combined approach of endoscopic mucosal resection followed by radiofrequency ablation.

K. R. DeVault, MD

Prevalence of Esophageal Eosinophils in Patients With Barrett's Esophagus
Ravi K, Katzka DA, Smyrk TC, et al (Mayo Clinic College of Medicine, Rochester, MN)
Am J Gastroenterol 106:851-857, 2011

Objectives.—Recent studies have demonstrated high esophageal eosinophil counts in patients with GERD similar to eosinophilic esophagitis (EoE) yet the frequency of esophageal eosinophilia in GERD is unknown. Our aim was to determine the prevalence of dense esophageal eosinophilia in patients with Barrett's esophagus as a manifestation of GERD.

Methods.—The Mayo Clinic pathology database was reviewed for patients diagnosed with Barrett's esophagus from January to December 2008 with squamous mucosa obtained during endoscopic surveillance. Clinical, endoscopic, and histologic findings were reviewed. Patients with ≥15 eosinophils per high powered field were identified and compared to those without esophageal eosinophilia.

Results.—Two hundred patients with Barrett's esophagus and squamous tissue obtained at the time of biopsy were identified. Fourteen of the 200 patients (7%) had ≥15 eosinophils per high powered field. Demographics, symptoms, and proton pump inhibitor therapies were similar between those with and without esophageal eosinophilia. Endoscopic features suggestive of EoE were found in the squamous mucosa of 2 patients with and 7 patients without esophageal eosinophilia. Use of photodynamic, radiofrequency ablation, or monopolar electrocoagulation therapy for ablation of Barrett's mucosa was not associated with a higher rate of esophageal eosinophilia. Basal cell hyperplasia, papillary elongation, and spongiosis occurred frequently in association with esophageal eosinophilic infiltration.

Conclusions.—High esophageal eosinophil counts were found in 7% of this cohort of 200 patients with Barrett's esophagus and likely underestimates prevalence. The finding of esophageal eosinophilia in this cohort was independent of proton pump inhibitor use, features of EoE, or endoscopic therapy for Barrett's esophagus. Further studies are needed to assess if these findings are applicable to all patients with GERD.

▶ Eosinophilic esophagitis (EoE) is a common finding in patients with esophageal symptoms. The classic presentation is of dysphagia with a stenosis in the esophagus and a ringed or furrowed mucosal appearance at endoscopy. Some guidelines have suggested biopsies of normal-appearing esophagus in patients with unexplained dysphagia and perhaps in those with other difficult-to-explain symptoms. The findings that gastroesophageal reflux (GER) can result in an increase in esophageal eosinophils and that treatment with a proton pump inhibitor may decrease the eosinophil count and resolve symptoms in patients with EoE adds to the confusion. In this study, random biopsies of the squamous mucosa in patients with Barrett's esophagus (BE) met diagnostic criteria for EoE in 7% of cases. A few of the patients had an appearance consistent with both BE and EoE, but it appears the majority had a fairly normal appearance to the squamous mucosa.

Is there an association between BE and EoE? Is that association simply part of the overlap between GER and EoE, or are these 2 common conditions that simply overlap? EoE does not actually appear to be overly common in normal populations, with a rate of 23 per 100 000 in a recent population-based study from Switzerland[1] and 1% in a study from Sweden,[2] so there must be something more than chance in this relationship. In a study of patients presenting with noncardiac chest pain, eosinophil counts of > 21 per high-power field were found in 6%, a very similar number.[3] It seems most likely that this association represents an overlap between a complication of GER (BE) and EoE. Because initial proton pump inhibitor therapy remains a mainstay of the treatment of BE, GER, and EoE, these data should not change our approach to patients with BE. The bigger, unanswered question is whether one should search for and treat EoE in patients without classical presentations and findings who are not responding to conventional GER disease therapy, before considering them as having "refractory GER disease."

K. R. DeVault, MD

References

1. Straumann A, Simon HU. Eosinophilic esophagitis: escalating epidemiology? *J Allergy Clin Immunol.* 2005;115:418-419.

2. Potter JW, Saeian K, Staff D, et al. Prevalence of oesophageal eosinophils and eosinophilic oesophagitis in adults: the population-based Kalixanda study. *Gut.* 2007;56:615-620.

3. Achem SR, Almansa C, Krishna M, et al. Oesophageal eosinophilic infiltration in patients with noncardiac chest pain. *Aliment Pharmacol Ther.* 2011;33:1194-1201.

Esophageal Adenocarcinoma Incidence in Individuals With Gastroesophageal Reflux: Synthesis and Estimates From Population Studies

Rubenstein JH, Scheiman JM, Sadeghi S, et al (Veterans Affairs Ctr of Excellence for Clinical Management Res, Ann Arbor, MI; Univ of Michigan Med School, Ann Arbor; Queensland Inst of Med Res, Brisbane, Australia; et al)
Am J Gastroenterol 106:254-260, 2011

Objectives.—Recent advances in the management of Barrett's esophagus may kindle enthusiasm for screening for esophageal adenocarcinoma (EAC). Symptoms of gastroesophageal reflux disease (GERD) are recognized as *relative* risks for EAC. However, the *absolute* incidence of EAC in specific populations with GERD is unknown. We aimed to estimate the symptom-, age-, and sex-specific incidences of EAC, and place these incidences in the perspective of other cancers for which screening is endorsed.

Methods.—A Markov computer model utilizing published and publicly available data was created to estimate the age- and sex-specific incidences of EAC in American white non-Hispanics with GERD symptoms.

Results.—The incidence of EAC in men younger than 50 years with GERD symptoms is very low (for instance, at the age of 35 years, incidence = 1.0/100,000), and their incidence of colorectal cancer is relatively much higher (for instance, at the age of 35 years, incidence of colorectal cancer is 6.7-fold greater). The incidence of EAC in older men with weekly GERD symptoms is substantial (for instance, at the age of 70 years, incidence = 60.8/100,000 person-years), but their incidence of colorectal cancer is at least threefold greater. The incidence of EAC in women with GERD is extremely low, and similar to that of breast cancer in men (for instance, 3.9/100,000 person-years at the age of 60 years).

Conclusions.—Screening for EAC should not be performed in men younger than 50 years or in women because of very low incidences of cancer, regardless of the frequency of GERD symptoms. In white men with weekly GERD over the age of 60 years, the incidence of EAC is substantial, and might warrant screening if that practice is particularly accurate, safe, effective, and inexpensive.

▶ Screening for Barrett's esophagus (BE) in patients with symptoms consistent with gastroesophageal reflux disease (GERD) has been widely adopted despite limited data supporting it as a cancer preventative or mortality improving strategy. This article examines the practice using a Markov computer model and suggests that screening for BE should be limited to white males older than 60 years with weekly symptoms (perhaps at age 55 with daily symptoms) and that it is not effective in other groups. For example, the incidence of esophageal adenocarcinoma in women is similar to the incidence of breast cancer in men! Should we change our practice based on these data? BE may be equivalent to a genie who has been let out of the bottle (now that it is open, we have to deal with it). The authors quote a recent study suggesting that 70% of gastroenterologists would screen a 35-year-old male and 42% would screen a 55-year-old woman, neither of which is supported by these data. Insurance plans seem to be willing to pay for this practice, and occasional lawsuits are successful, claiming that physicians should have screened a patient who presents with a history of GERD and advanced cancer. In addition to providers, it is clear that patients significantly overestimate their risk of cancer before and after the diagnosis of BE. Care should be taken in using a model to change practice, but long-term studies with real end points (cancer or death) are unlikely to be performed, and these data may be all that we will have for the foreseeable future. It therefore seems appropriate to begin to educate both patients and physicians about the low risk of this cancer and perhaps not offer screening to every patient with GERD symptoms.

K. R. DeVault, MD

American Gastroenterological Association Medical Position Statement on the Management of Barrett's Esophagus
American Gastroenterological Association
Gastroenterology 140:1084-1091, 2011

Background.—A medical position statement issued by the American Gastroenterological Association Institute addresses the major clinical issues of treating patients with Barrett's esophagus. The condition was defined and recommendations for diagnosis and treatment offered.

Definition.—Barrett's esophagus is a condition in which any extent of metaplastic columnar epithelium that predisposes to the development of cancer replaces the stratified squamous epithelium naturally found lining the distal esophagus. Intestinal metaplasia is included in the definition, but cardia-type epithelium in the esophagus, while abnormal, is not because the degree of risk for malignancy with this type of epithelium is unknown. The traditional and still accepted endoscopic landmark that best identifies the level at which the esophagus ends and the stomach begins is the proximal extent of the gastric folds. Measuring and recording the extent of Barrett's metaplasia seen endoscopically is recommended and has clinical value. A diagnosis of Barrett's esophagus has marked influences on individual patients. The annual incidence of esophageal cancer is about 0.5%, but cardiovascular associations increase mortality, poor quality of life is common, and patients often suffer psychological stress and higher life and health insurance costs.

Recommendations.—Screening for Barrett's esophagus is recommended for patients with multiple risk factors related to esophageal adenocarcinoma but not for the general population with gastroesophageal reflux disease (GERD). Such factors include age 50 years or older, male gender, white race, chronic GERD, hiatal hernia, elevated body mass index, and intra-abdominal distribution of body fat. The diagnosis of dysplasia in Barrett's esophagus should be confirmed by two pathologists, at least one of whom is an expert in esophageal histopathology. For patients diagnosed with Barrett's esophagus, endoscopic surveillance is recommended every 3 to 5 years if there is no dysplasia, every 6 to 12 months if there is low-grade dysplasia, and every 3 months if there is high-grade dysplasia and no eradication therapy is performed. No molecular biomarkers provide sufficient predictive value to justify their use to either confirm the histologic diagnosis of dysplasia or contribute to risk stratification.

The biopsy protocol recommended for endoscopic surveillance of Barrett's esophagus should employ white light endoscopy and obtain four-quadrant biopsy specimens every 2 cm, except for patients with known or suspected dysplasia, whose specimens should be taken every 1 cm. Specific biopsy specimens of any mucosal irregularities should be submitted separately to the pathologist. Chromoendoscopy and advanced imaging techniques are not required for routine surveillance.

Measures not recommended for cancer prevention include eliminating esophageal acid exposure using proton pump inhibitors (PPIs) in doses exceeding once daily, esophageal pH monitoring to titrate PPI dosing, and antireflux surgery. Patients should be screened for cardiovascular risk factors treatable by aspirin therapy, but the use of aspirin solely to prevent esophageal adenocarcinoma with no other indications is not recommended. Endoscopic eradication therapy with radiofrequency ablation (RFA), photodynamic therapy (PDT), or endoscopic mucosal resection (EMR) is preferred to surveillance in patients with confirmed high-grade dysplasia in Barrett's esophagus. To determine the T stage of the neoplasia in patients with dysplasia in Barrett's esophagus and a visible mucosal irregularity, EMR is recommended, proving valuable as a diagnostic/staging procedure and a potentially therapeutic procedure.

Evidence indicates that complete eradication of all Barrett's epithelium is more effective therapeutically than removal of a localized area of dysplasia only. RFA and PDT achieve comparable efficacy, but RFA has fewer serious adverse effects. Treatment with eradication therapy is designed to achieve reversion to normal-appearing squamous epithelium throughout the length of the esophagus with no islands of buried intestinal metaplasia. RFA can produce this reversion in a high proportion of subjects at any stage of disease; the reversion lasts for up to 5 years. RFA therapy also reduces the progression to esophageal cancer in patients with high-grade dysplasia. If the patient has no dysplasia, endoscopic eradication therapy may be no more effective at reducing cancer risk and no more cost-effective than long-term endoscopic surveillance.

Conclusions.—The recommendations for clinical management of Barrett's esophagus are founded on the assumption that the diagnosis and the absence of low-grade and high-grade dysplasia are accurate to the highest degree possible according to the best current standards of practice. Over

90% of patients with low-grade dysplasia and 70% to 80% of patients who have high-grade dysplasia are successfully managed with endoscopic eradication therapy. Esophagectomy is another option, but should only be done at surgical centers that specialize in treating foregut cancers and high-grade dysplasia.

▶ A great deal of effort goes into the prevention of adenocarcinoma of the esophagus through the identification and surveillance of Barrett's esophagus (BE). The American Gastroenterological Association recently published these guidelines and a technical review article.[1] There were many consistencies and a few changes in the suggested approach to this condition compared with other recent statements. Endoscopic screening was suggested for gastroesophageal reflux disease (GERD) populations at increased risk for BE (particularly older white males with long-term GERD) but not the general population with GERD (other risk factors include elevated body mass index/abdominal obesity and hiatal hernia). Confirmation of dysplasia by expert pathologists was a recommendation. Suggested surveillance intervals for nondysplastic BE were expanded to 3 to 5 years, and low-grade intervals remained at 6 to 12 months. If surveillance was elected for high-grade dysplasia, it was suggested to be repeated on a 3-month interval. The standard 4-quadrant biopsy protocol obtained every 2 cm was advocated for nondysplastic BE with an increase to every 1 cm for dysplastic BE. In addition, any mucosal irregularity should be sampled separately. The Association did not feel that the data were strong enough to recommend routine high-dose proton pump inhibitor therapy or aspirin as chemopreventatives. Endoscopic mucosal resection was advocated for dysplastic lesions associated with a visible abnormality in a segment of BE. They suggested endoscopic ablation as the treatment of choice for high-grade dysplasia and a preferred approach compared with watchful waiting and esophagectomy.

K. R. DeVault, MD

Reference

1. Spechler SJ, Sharma P, Souza RF, Inadomi JM, Shaheen NJ. American Gastroenterological Association technical review on the management of Barrett's esophagus. *Gastroenterology.* 2011;140:e18-e52.

Patients With Nondysplastic Barrett's Esophagus Have Low Risks for Developing Dysplasia or Esophageal Adenocarcinoma
Wani S, Falk G, Hall M, et al (Veterans Affairs Med Ctr and Univ of Kansas School of Medicine, MO; Cleveland Clinic Foundation, OH; et al)
Clin Gastroenterol Hepatol 9:220-227, 2011

Background & Aims.—The risks of dysplasia and esophageal adenocarcinoma (EAC) are not clear for patients with nondysplastic Barrett's esophagus (NDBE); the rate of progression has been overestimated in previous studies. We studied the incidences of dysplasia and EAC and investigated factors associated with progression of BE.

Methods.—The BE study is a multicenter outcomes project of a large cohort of patients with BE. Neoplasia was graded as low-grade dysplasia, high-grade dysplasia (HGD), or EAC. Patients followed up for at least 1 year after the index endoscopy examination were included, whereas those diagnosed with dysplasia and EAC within 1 year of diagnosis with BE (prevalent cases) were excluded. Of 3334 patients with BE, 1204 met the inclusion criteria (93.7% Caucasian; 88% male; mean age, 59.3 y) and were followed up for a mean of 5.52 years (6644.5 patient-years).

Results.—Eighteen patients developed EAC (incidence, 0.27%/y; 95% confidence interval [CI], 0.17–0.43) and 32 developed HGD (incidence, 0.48%/y; 95% CI, 0.34–0.68). The incidence of HGD and EAC was 0.63%/y (95% CI, 0.47–0.86). There were 217 cases of low-grade dysplasia (incidence, 3.6%/y; 95% CI, 3.2–4.1). Five and 10 years after diagnosis, 98.6% (n = 540) and 97.1% (n = 155) of patients with NDBE were cancer free, respectively. The length of the BE was associated significantly with progression (EAC <6 cm, 0.09%/y vs EAC ≥6 cm, 0.65%/y; $P = 0.001$).

Conclusions.—There is a lower incidence of dysplasia and EAC among patients with NDBE than previously reported. Because most patients are cancer free after a long-term follow-up period, surveillance intervals might be lengthened, especially for patients with shorter segments of BE (Fig 3).

▶ A great deal of effort goes into the prevention of adenocarcinoma of the esophagus through the identification and surveillance of Barrett's esophagus (BE), yet the true rate of progression to dysplasia and cancer varies greatly from study to study. This article is one of the more comprehensive perspective reports of a large group of patients (more than 1000) in a surveillance program. Important findings from the study were a low rate of progression to cancer (0.27%/y) and high-grade dysplasia (0.48%/y). Cancer-free rates were high at 5 (98.6%) and 10 years (97.1%) after initial diagnosis of BE. In contrast to some other studies,[1] there was a clear relationship between length of BE and risk of progression (risk was only 0.09%/y in segments less than 6 cm). It is important to note that only 18 patients developed cancer.

This is the lowest rate of progression yet reported (see Fig 3 for comparison of several large series). The study was of mostly male veterans and military personnel, which would seem to be a group at high risk. One would assume that a study including women (who have a documented lower risk) would demonstrate even lower rates of progression. The cost of screening for and surveillance of BE has always been difficult to justify, but the process has been embraced by primary care providers, specialists, and, perhaps most important, third-party payers. From a public health prospective, these data make that approach even more problematic. That having been said, this article and the accompanying editorial did not call for an immediate change in our approach but did call for better predictors of progression such as molecular markers.

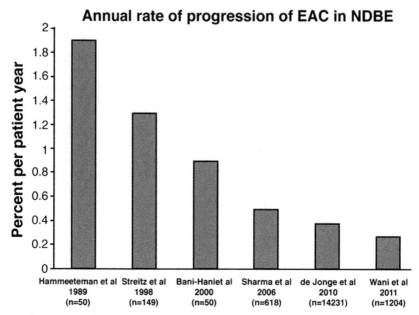

FIGURE 3.—Bar diagram highlighting a lower incidence of EAC in larger contemporary studies and a higher incidence in smaller and older cohort studies. (Reprinted from Wani S, Falk G, Hall M, et al. Patients with nondysplastic Barrett's esophagus have low risks for developing dysplasia or esophageal adenocarcinoma. *Clin Gastroenterol Hepatol.* 2011;9:220-227, with permission from the AGA Institute.)

I would caution that the only way such markers will be of benefit is when a simple, relatively inexpensive test can identify a subset of patients with BE who are at minimal risk so that their BE can simply be ignored.

K. R. DeVault, MD

Reference

1. Lewis JJ, Rubenstein JH. Barrett's esophagus progressing to cancer: a needle in a haystack? *Clin Gastroenterol Hepatol.* 2011;9:194-195.

Esophageal Motility Disorders

Esophageal Dysmotility Disorders After Laparoscopic Gastric Banding—An Underestimated Complication

Naef M, Mouton WG, Naef U, et al (Spital STS AG Thun, Switzerland; et al)
Ann Surg 253:285-290, 2011

Objective.—To evaluate the effects of laparoscopic adjustable gastric banding (LAGB) on esophageal dysfunction over the long term in a prospective study, based on a 12-year experience.

Background.—Esophageal motility disorders and dilatation after LAGB have been reported. However, only a few studies present long-term follow-up data.

Methods.—Between June 1998 and June 2009, all patients with implantation of a LAGB were enrolled in a prospective clinical trial including a yearly barium swallow. Esophageal motility disorders were recorded and classified over the period. An esophageal diameter of 35 mm or greater was considered dilated.

Results.—Laparoscopic adjustable gastric banding was performed in 167 patients (120 females and 47males) with a mean age of 40.1 ± 5.2 years. Overall patient follow-up was 94%. Esophageal dysmotility disorders were found in 108 patients (68.8% of patients followed). Esophageal dilatation occurred in 40 patients (25.5%)with a mean esophageal diameter of 47.3 ± 6.9 mm (35.0—94.6) after a follow-up of 73.8 ± 6.8 months (36—120) compared with 26.2 ± 2.8 mm (18.3—34.2) in patients without dilatation (diameter of <35 mm) ($P < 0.01$). Thirty-four patients suffered from stage III dilatation (band deflation necessary) and 6 from stage IV (major achalasia-like dilatation, band removal mandatory). In 29 patients, upper endoscopy was carried out because of heartburn/dysphagia. In 18 patients, the endoscopy was normal; 9 patients suffered from gastroesophageal reflux disease, 1 from a stenosis, and 1 from a hiatus hernia.

Conclusions.—This study demonstrates that esophageal motility disorders after LAGB are frequent, poorly appreciated complications. Despite adequate excess weight loss, LAGB should probably not be considered the procedure of first choice and should be performed only in selected cases until reliable criteria for patients with a low risk for the procedures long-term complications are developed.

▶ There has been at least a 10-fold increase in the use of surgery to control obesity. Laparoscopic gastric banding (LGAB) is one of the more common procedures. This is a purely restrictive procedure that places an inflatable band around the proximal stomach. Postoperative symptoms are common and may include dysphagia and unacceptable early satiety, although it is often difficult to determine if the symptoms are simply part of the restrictive nature of the surgery or if they are because of a complication. This study looks at problems related to dysphagia and esophageal dysfunction in these patients. The study is limited by its use of barium testing rather than tube-based pressure measurements, but it is an important cautionary report. Through barium testing, they found evidence of esophageal dysfunction in more than half of their patients with severe disorders that required band deflation in 34 out of 167 (20.4%) and removal of the band in 6 out of 167 (3.6%).

Are the authors' conclusions that "LAGB should probably not be considered the procedure of first choice" and that manometry should be considered prior to the surgery warranted? The advantages of LAGB remain and include the ability to adjust the degree of restriction and the less-invasive initial surgery that maintains integrity of the gastrointestinal tract. It seems that appropriate positioning of the band is crucial but somewhat difficult to define. If the band is too proximal, then secondary achalasia is more likely; and if it is too distal, severe reflux and lack of appropriate weight loss seem more likely. This would indicate that the procedure should be carried out carefully and only in centers of excellence.

If patients have dysphagia prior to surgery, it should be evaluated; but it appears that many of the patients in this report had no preoperative symptoms. It is tempting to suggest an esophageal manometry prior to surgery, but we have no data to suggest that an abnormal baseline manometry is predictive of a negative outcome. Additional study of this topic is certainly needed.

K. R. DeVault, MD

Gastroesophageal Reflux

ACCF/ACG/AHA 2010 Expert Consensus Document on the Concomitant Use of Proton Pump Inhibitors and Thienopyridines: A Focused Update of the ACCF/ACG/AHA 2008 Expert Consensus Document on Reducing the Gastrointestinal Risks of Antiplatelet Therapy and NSAID Use

Abraham NS, American College of Gastroenterology Representative, American College of Cardiology Foundation Representative, American Heart Association Representative (American College of Gastroenterology Representative, Bethesda, MD; et al)

Am J Gastroenterol 105:2533-2549, 2010

Background.—Expert consensus documents inform practitioners, payers, and other parties about changing areas of clinical practice or technological advances. Often the evidence base, experience with technology, or clinical practice has not yet developed to the point that a formal American College of Cardiology Foundation (ACCF) and American Heart Association (AHA) practice guideline can be formulated. These documents seek to inform clinical practice in the absence of rigorous evidence. The ACCF, AHA, and American College of Gastroenterology (ACG) issued an expert consensus document concerning the use of a proton pump inhibitor (PPI) in patients with risk factors for upper gastrointestinal (GI) bleeding who are receiving dual antiplatelet therapy, specifically thienopyridines and aspirin.

Major Findings and Recommendations.—Dual antiplatelet therapy with clopidogrel and aspirin reduces the number of major cardiovascular (CV) events compared to placebo or aspirin alone in patients who have established ischemic heart disease. This therapy also reduces coronary stent thrombosis. However, it is not recommended routinely for patients who have had an ischemic stroke because of the increased bleeding risk. Clopidogrel, aspirin, and the combination of the two are all associated with an increased risk of GI bleeding. Patients who have had GI bleeding previously and are taking antiplatelet therapy are at the highest risk for recurrent bleeding. Higher risk is also associated with advanced age; concurrent use of anticoagulants, steroids, or nonsteroidal anti-inflammatory drugs (NSAIDs), including aspirin; and infection with *Helicobacter pylori*.

As the number of risk factors increases, so does the risk of GI bleeding. The risk of upper GI bleeding can be lowered from by adding a PPI or a histamine H_2 receptor antagonist (H2RA). A comparison of PPIs and H2RAs shows that PPIs reduce upper GI bleeding more than H2RAs. PPIs are recommended for patients who have a history of upper GI bleeding and appropriate for those with multiple risk factors for GI bleeding who are taking antiplatelet therapy. The risk of complications must be weighed against the overall benefits of the PPI or H2RA treatment. Patients at lower risk for upper GI bleeding should not routinely receive a PPI or an H2RA because the potential for benefit is greatly reduced. The potential for both CV and GI complications must be considered. In addition, pharmacokinetic and pharmacodynamics studies using platelet assays as surrogate endpoints indicate that using clopidogrel and a PPI reduces the effectiveness of clopidogrel as an antiplatelet agent. Omeprazole and clopidogrel demonstrated the strongest interaction. The effect of using different surrogate endpoints is unknown. In addition, the effects on CV outcomes of concomitant use of thienopyridines and PPIs have been inconsistent in the available observational studies and single randomized clinical trial. Data are insufficient to rule out a clinically important interaction, especially in certain subgroups. Basing management decisions on either pharmacogenomic testing or platelet function testing is not currently feasible.

Conclusions.—PPIs and antiplatelet drugs are used together to reduce the higher risk of GI complications caused by the antiplatelet agents. GI protection is especially needed as the number of risk factors increases. Many gaps exist in the current knowledge about these agents and their interactions, so further research is needed.

▶ A potential negative interaction between proton pump inhibitors (PPIs) and activation of the antiplatelet agent clopidogrel has recently been reported and has led to a Food and Drug Administration black box warning on clopidogrel packaging. This is felt to be because of competitive inhibition of cytochrome CYP2C19, which is responsible for the metabolism of some PPIs and also for the activation of clopidogrel. This field is rapidly evolving, but the summary recommendations of this article are important for all physicians using these agents.

Summary of findings and consensus recommendations:

1. Clopidogrel reduces major cardiovascular (CV) events compared with placebo or aspirin.

2. Dual antiplatelet therapy with clopidogrel and aspirin, compared with aspirin alone, reduces major CV events in patients with established ischemic heart disease, and it reduces coronary stent thrombosis but is not routinely recommended for patients with prior ischemic stroke because of the risk of bleeding.

3. Clopidogrel alone, aspirin alone, and their combination are all associated with increased risk of gastrointestinal (GI) bleeding.

4. Patients with prior GI bleeding are at highest risk for recurrent bleeding on antiplatelet therapy. Other clinical characteristics that increase the risk of GI bleeding include advanced age, concurrent use of anticoagulants, steroids, or nonsteroidal anti-inflammatory drugs, including aspirin and *Helicobacter pylori* infection. The risk of GI bleeding increases as the number of risk factors increases.

5. Use of a PPI or histamine H_2 receptor antagonist (H2RA) reduces the risk of upper GI bleeding compared with no therapy. PPIs reduce upper GI bleeding to a greater degree than do H2RAs.

6. PPIs are recommended to reduce GI bleeding among patients with a history of upper GI bleeding. PPIs are appropriate in patients with multiple risk factors for GI bleeding who require antiplatelet therapy.

7. Routine use of either a PPI or an H2RA is not recommended for patients at lower risk of upper GI bleeding, who have much less potential to benefit from prophylactic therapy.

8. Clinical decisions regarding concomitant use of PPIs and thienopyridines must balance overall risks and benefits, considering both CV and GI complications.

9. Pharmacokinetic and pharmacodynamic studies, using platelet assays as surrogate end points, suggest that concomitant use of clopidogrel and a PPI reduces the antiplatelet effects of clopidogrel. The strongest evidence for an interaction is between omeprazole and clopidogrel. It is not established that changes in these surrogate end points translate into clinically meaningful differences.

10. Observational studies and a single randomized clinical trial have shown inconsistent effects on CV outcomes of concomitant use of thienopyridines and PPIs. A clinically important interaction cannot be excluded, particularly in certain subgroups, such as poor metabolizers of clopidogrel.

11. The role of either pharmacogenomic testing or platelet function testing in managing therapy with thienopyridines and PPIs has not yet been established.

Based on this article and others, the prudent approach is to avoid PPI in patients who really do not need them and use the PPI carefully in those who require them for symptomatic control after an open discussion of the risks and benefits with the patient involved.

K. R. DeVault, MD

Morbidity and mortality associated with antireflux surgery with or without paraesophogeal hernia: a large ACS NSQIP analysis
Lidor AO, Chang DC, Feinberg RL, et al (Johns Hopkins Univ School of Medicine, Baltimore, MD; Univ of California San Diego)
Surg Endosc 2011 [Epub ahead of print]

Background.—Surgical repair of paraesophageal hernias (PEH) represents a considerable technical challenge in patients who are older and have multiple comorbidities. We sought to identify factors associated with increased rates of mortality and morbidity in these patients.

Methods.—We performed a retrospective analysis of the National Surgical Quality Improvement Program from 2005 through 2007. Patients who underwent an antireflux operation or repair of PEH and with a primary diagnosis of PEH or GERD were included. Primary outcome was 30-day mortality. Secondary outcomes included intraoperative blood transfusion (BT) and standard comorbidities. Multivariate analyses were performed, adjusting for factors of age and BMI.

Results.—A total of 3518 patients were identified, including 1290 PEH patients. Compared to GERD patients, PEH patients were significantly older and had more comorbidities. On adjusted analysis for PEH patients only, BT and age ≥70 years were significantly associated with multiple outcome variables, including pulmonary complications and venous thromboembolism (VTE), but had no association with mortality. BMI was not found to be associated with any of our outcome measures.

Conclusion.—Despite higher rates of complications, notably pulmonary and VTE, PEH can be repaired in the elderly with mortality rates comparable to those in younger populations. BMI does not adversely impact any short-term outcome measures in patients undergoing PEH repair (Table 3).

▶ Laparoscopic antireflux surgery (LARS) is commonly performed in patients with symptomatic gastroesophageal reflux disease (GERD) and also in patients presenting with symptomatic or complicated paraesophageal hernias (PEH). This large database of more than 3500 patients reports the morbidity and mortality associated with LARS in patients with and without a PEH. The PEH patients were older and more likely to be female. The initial surgeries were longer, required more transfusions, were more likely to have to return to the OR, were more likely to be converted to an open procedure, and in general had multiple other complications (see Table 3). Most important, the 30-day mortality was 0.9% in the PEH patients and 0.2% in the patients without a PEH, but it is important to note that these percentages were based on only a few deaths (11 and 4, respectively). These data come from a variety of

TABLE 3.—Unadjusted Comparison Between GERD and PEH Patients

	GERD ($n = 2228$) n	%	PEH ($n = 1290$) n	%	p Value
Age (mean)	50.1		62.4		<0.001
Female gender	1,351	60.6	898	69.6	<0.001
Race, white	1,810	81.2	1,055	81.8	n.s.
Race, other	199	8.9	131	10.2	
BMI (mean)	29.3		29.80		0.029
Laparoscopic cases	2,098	94.2	933	72.3	<0.001
Operative time (mean) (min)	123		165		<0.001
30-day mortality	4	0.2	11	0.9	0.003
Intraoperative transfusion	13	0.6	42	3.3	<0.001
Return to OR	28	1.3	52	4.0	<0.001
Splenectomy	3	0.1	10	0.8	0.003
Esophageal laceration	0	0.0	4	0.3	0.009
Pneumonia	19	0.9	44	3.4	<0.001
Respiratory complications[a]	13	0.6	46	3.6	<0.001
VTE[b]	3	0.1	27	2.1	<0.001
Length of stay (mean)	2.2		4.6		<0.001

[a]Respiratory complications include reintubation and failure to wean.
[b]VTE includes deep vein thrombosis and pulmonary embolism.

practices that choose to report to this database, so unlike many studies, these were not selected patients from high-volume academic centers.

LARS is a generally safe procedure, but older, sicker patients, particularly those with PEH, are at increased risk of complications and death. The risk of death in this study for those with standard hernias was 1 in 500, whereas it was almost 1 in 100 in those with a PEH. Providers must understand these risks and weigh them against the morbidity of continued medical therapy. It is important also to note that success in completing the PEH repair laparoscopically was associated with an improved outcome. When the potential benefit of repair outweighs the risks, it would seem prudent to seek out an experienced surgeon, because other data have clearly suggested an increased risk of both complications and need for early conversion to an open procedure (first 50 cases) in a surgeon's experience.[1]

K. R. DeVault, MD

Reference

1. Flum DR, Koepsell T, Heagerty P, Pellegrini CA. The nationwide frequency of major adverse outcomes in antireflux surgery and the role of surgeon experience, 1992-1997. *J Am Coll Surg.* 2002;195:611-618.

The Effect of Dexlansoprazole MR on Nocturnal Heartburn and GERD-Related Sleep Disturbances in Patients With Symptomatic GERD

Fass R, Johnson DA, Orr WC, et al (Southern Arizona VA Health Care System, Tucson, AZ; Eastern Virginia Med School, Norfolk, VR; The Lynn Health Science Inst, OK; et al)
Am J Gastroenterol 106:421-431, 2011

Objectives.—Nocturnal heartburn and related sleep disturbances are common among patients with gastroesophageal reflux disease (GERD). This study evaluated the efficacy of dexlansoprazole MR 30 mg in relieving nocturnal heartburn and GERD-related sleep disturbances, improving work productivity, and decreasing nocturnal symptom severity in patients with symptomatic GERD.

Methods.—Patients ($N = 305$) with frequent, moderate-to-very severe nocturnal heartburn and associated sleep disturbances were randomized 1:1 in a double-blind fashion to receive dexlansoprazole MR or placebo once daily for 4 weeks. The primary end point was the percentage of nights without heartburn. Secondary end points were the percentage of patients with relief of nocturnal heartburn and of GERD-related sleep disturbances over the last 7 days of treatment. At baseline and week 4 final visit, patients completed questionnaires that assessed sleep quality, work productivity, and the severity and impact of nocturnal GERD symptoms.

Results.—Dexlansoprazole MR 30 mg ($n = 152$) was superior to placebo ($n = 153$) in median percentage of nights without heartburn (73.1 vs. 35.7%, respectively; $P < 0.001$). Dexlansoprazole MR was significantly better than placebo in percentage of patients with relief of nocturnal heartburn and GERD-related sleep disturbances (47.5 vs. 19.6%, 69.7 vs. 47.9%, respectively; $P < 0.001$), and led to significantly greater improvements in sleep quality and work productivity and decreased nocturnal symptom severity. Adverse events were similar across treatment groups.

Conclusions.—In patients with symptomatic GERD, dexlansoprazole MR 30 mg is significantly more efficacious than placebo in providing relief from nocturnal heartburn, in reducing GERD-related sleep disturbances and the consequent impairments in work productivity, and in improving sleep quality quality of life.

▶ This is an industry-sponsored, placebo-controlled trial of a new proton pump inhibitor (PPI) formulation evaluating nocturnal heartburn and gastroesophageal reflux disease (GERD)-related sleep disturbances. The medication (dexlansoprazole MR 30 mg) or placebo was given as a morning dose. Active treatment was superior to placebo in all measures. Dexlansoprazole MR is a new agent that uses R-lansoprazole (the slower metabolized enatiomer of lansoprazole) in which a portion of the granules inside the capsule are engineered with a delayed release, resulting in absorption further along the small intestine. This results in a longer duration of effective serum concentration and some increased efficacy in acid control compared with standard lansoprazole.

It is clear that a good deal of the impairment in quality of life (QOL) associated with GERD is related to nocturnal symptoms and sleep disturbance. Several PPIs have been suggested to improve those symptoms as well as QOL. One would assume that dexlansoprazole MR would be at least as effective and perhaps more so than standard-release PPIs. These data suggest morning PPI as a reasonable initial treatment even in patients with predominantly nighttime symptoms. Because placebo was the only control in this article, the study does not determine whether longer-acting PPIs are superior to standard formulations or how this approach compares with PPIs taken later in the day or twice daily. Another factor that could weigh in favor of dexlansoprazole MR is the concept that the extended serum concentrations offered by this formulation allow the medication to be taken regardless of food intake, which is not the case for most PPIs.

K. R. DeVault, MD

Impact of ineffective oesophageal motility and wrap type on dysphagia after laparoscopic fundoplication
Broeders JA, Sportel IG, Jamieson GG, et al (Royal Adelaide Hosp, South Australia, Australia)
Br J Surg 2011 [Epub ahead of print]

Background.—Laparoscopic 360° fundoplication is the most common operation for gastro-oesophageal reflux disease, but is associated with postoperative dysphagia in some patients. Patients with ineffective oesophageal motility may have a higher risk of developing postoperative dysphagia, but this remains unclear.

Methods.—From 1991 to 2010, 2040 patients underwent primary laparoscopic fundoplication for gastro-oesophageal reflux disease and met the study inclusion criteria; 343 had a 90°, 498 a 180° and 1199 a 360° fundoplication. Primary peristalsis and distal contraction amplitude during oesophageal manometry were determined for 1354 patients. Postoperative dysphagia scores (range 0—45) were recorded at 3 and 12 months, then annually. Oesophageal dilatations and/or reoperations for dysphagia were recorded.

Results.—Preoperative oesophageal motility did not influence postoperative dysphagia scores, the need for dilatation and/or reoperation up to 6 years. Three-month dysphagia scores were lower after 90° and 180° compared with 360° fundoplication (mean(s.e.m.) 8·0(0·6) and 9·8(0·5) respectively *versus* 11·9(0·4); $P < 0·001$ and $P = 0·003$), but these differences diminished after 6 years of follow-up. The incidence of dilatation and reoperation for dysphagia was lower after 90° (2·6 and 0·6 per cent respectively) and 180° (4·4 and 1·0 per cent) fundoplications than with a 360° wrap (9·8 and 6·8 per cent; both $P < 0·001$ *versus* 90° and 180° groups).

Conclusion.—Tailoring the degree of fundoplication according to preoperative oesophageal motility by standard manometric parameters has no long-term impact on postoperative dysphagia. There is, however, a proportionate increase in short-term dysphagia scores with increasing degree of wrap, and a corresponding proportionate increase in dilatations and reoperations for dysphagia. These differences in dysphagia scores diminish with time.

▶ It is common practice to perform esophageal manometry prior to laparoscopic antireflux surgery to both exclude severe loss of peristalsis (ie, achalasia presenting as gastroesophageal reflux disease) and to allow a tailored approach to surgery (loose or partial fundoplication in those who have poor peristalsis). This concept has been challenged in several publications, including this article. They found that the preoperative motility did not predict postoperative dysphagia scores, the need for dilation, or the need for reoperation, but that all of these were more common with full rather than partial fundoplications. This study did not evaluate reflux control with the various types of surgery.

Should we stop doing manometry prior to fundoplications? Based on these data, it seems that manometry is optional, particularly prior to partial fundoplications. I would only temper that finding with the concept that patients with achalasia occasionally present with refluxlike symptoms, which can result in a poor outcome if they are not identified prior to fundoplication. It is possible that a careful barium study and endoscopy could be used to screen, and then only proceed to manometry if there are suggestive findings on 1 or both of those tests. It is clear from these data and others that full fundoplications are more likely to produce dysphagia. What is not clear is the relative efficacy of reflux control with partial versus total fundoplication. Some studies have suggested equivalent control,[1] whereas others suggest better control with the full fundoplication.[2] It is likely that a well-performed fundoplication by an experienced operator in appropriately selected patients should provide reflux control with minimal postoperative dysphagia.

K. R. DeVault, MD

References

1. Nijjar RS, Watson DI, Jamieson GG, et al. Five-year follow-up of a multicenter, double-blind randomized clinical trial of laparoscopic Nissen vs anterior 90 degrees partial fundoplication. *Arch Surg.* 2010;145:552-557.
2. Cai W, Watson DI, Lally CJ, Devitt PG, Game PA, Jamieson GG. Ten-year clinical outcome of a prospective randomized clinical trial of laparoscopic Nissen versus anterior 180° partial fundoplication. *Br J Surg.* 2008;95:1501-1505.

Laparoscopic Antireflux Surgery in Patients with Throat Symptoms: A Word of Caution
Ratnasingam D, Irvine T, Thompson SK, et al (Flinders Univ, South Australia, Australia; Univ of Adelaide, South Australia, Australia)
World J Surg 35:342-348, 2011

Background.—A subset of patients undergoing laparoscopic fundoplication presents with atypical throat symptoms, and the benefit of surgery in these patients is debated. These patients can present with throat symptoms alone or in combination with typical reflux symptoms. We evaluated the clinical outcome in these patients and compared their outcomes with a larger group of patients who did not have throat symptoms before fundoplication.

Methods.—Outcome data for 893 consecutive patients who underwent a laparoscopic fundoplication from January 2002 to June 2008 were collected prospectively and managed on a database. Ninety-three patients with atypical throat symptoms were identified, and divided into subgroups with ($n = 66$) and without ($n = 27$) typical reflux symptoms (heartburn and/or regurgitation), and outcomes were compared with patients ($n = 800$) who didn't have throat symptoms. Symptoms were assessed with analog symptom scores for heartburn and dysphagia, as well as satisfaction with the surgical outcome. Case records for patients with throat symptoms were also reviewed to obtain more detail about specific throat symptoms and their resolution.

Results.—Cough was the commonest atypical symptom, followed by sore throat. Heartburn scores improved following surgery in all patient groups. Dysphagia was more common 3 months after surgery in patients without throat symptoms, although there were no differences for dysphagia at later follow-up. Following surgery satisfaction scores were highest in patients with atypical throat symptoms who also had typical reflux symptoms, and the scores were lowest in patients who only had atypical throat symptoms. Nearly twice as many patients who had throat and reflux symptoms reported improvement or resolution of symptoms, compared to patients who only had throat symptoms.

Conclusions.—Fundoplication achieves a good outcome in patients with atypical throat symptoms who also report typical symptoms of reflux. However, surgeons should be cautious about operating on the subgroup of patients with objective evidence of gastroesophageal reflux who describe throat symptoms but do not report heartburn or regurgitation. In this subgroup, expectations of a good outcome should be minimized.

▶ Several throat symptoms have been attributed to gastroesophageal reflux (GER), most commonly including cough, sore throat, or hoarseness. Reflux extending into this area has been labeled laryngopharyngeal reflux (LPR). The response of patients with possible LPR to medical therapy is variable; therefore, refractory LPR is a common reason patients are referred for antireflux surgery. This article looked at the surgical outcome in patients with throat symptoms who either did or did not also have typical reflux symptoms (heartburn, regurgitation, or both). Patients who had throat symptoms and typical reflux symptoms were much more likely to respond to surgery than those with throat symptoms alone. It is important to note that all of the patients in this study had objective evidence of GER (ulcerative esophagitis, abnormal pH monitoring, or both). The pH studies were considered positive if there was more than 7% acid exposure or if there was 4% to 7% exposure with a positive symptom index. Patients with normal acid exposure but a positive symptom index and those with normal amounts of distal acid but increased proximal acid were not included.

These data suggest that it is reasonable to offer surgery to patients with throat symptoms who also have typical symptoms and who have objective evidence of reflux. On the other hand, patients with isolated throat symptoms, even with positive pH tests, are much less likely to respond. Although not addressed in this study, it is likely that patients with normal acid exposure and isolated throat symptoms (even with a positive symptom index) would have less response than either of the groups in this study and that surgery should be avoided in that group.

K. R. DeVault, MD

Gastroesophageal Reflux Symptoms in Patients With Celiac Disease and the Effects of a Gluten-Free Diet
Nachman F, Vázquez H, González A, et al (Dr C. Bonorino Udaondo Gastroenterology Hosp, Buenos Aires, Argentina)
Clin Gastroenterol Hepatol 9:214-219, 2011

Background & Aims.—Celiac disease (CD) patients often complain of symptoms consistent with gastroesophageal reflux disease (GERD). We aimed to assess the prevalence of GERD symptoms at diagnosis and to determine the impact of the gluten-free diet (GFD).

Methods.—We evaluated 133 adult CD patients at diagnosis and 70 healthy controls. Fifty three patients completed questionnaires every

3 months during the first year and more than 4 years after diagnosis. GERD symptoms were evaluated using a subdimension of the Gastrointestinal Symptoms Rating Scale for heartburn and regurgitation domains.

Results.—At diagnosis, celiac patients had a significantly higher reflux symptom mean score than healthy controls ($P < .001$). At baseline, 30.1% of CD patients had moderate to severe GERD (score >3) compared with 5.7% of controls ($P < .01$). Moderate to severe symptoms were significantly associated with the classical clinical presentation of CD (35.0%) compared with atypical/silent cases (15.2%; $P < .03$). A rapid improvement was evidenced at 3 months after initial treatment with a GFD ($P < .0001$) with reflux scores comparable to healthy controls from this time point onward.

Conclusions.—GERD symptoms are common in classically symptomatic untreated CD patients. The GFD is associated with a rapid and persistent improvement in reflux symptoms that resembles the healthy population.

▶ Symptoms from the upper gastrointestinal tract are often nonspecific. Gastroesophageal reflux disease (GERD), dyspepsia, gall bladder disease, and other disorders may present with similar and often overlapping presentations. This article provides further evidence for symptom overlap, this time between GERD and celiac disease (CD). They were able to demonstrate an increased prevalence of GERD symptoms in patients with CD compared with the control and, most importantly, demonstrated an impressive improvement in GERD symptoms once the patient was placed on a gluten-free diet.

How should we use these data? The data confirm that all heartburn is not caused by GERD. I suspect many of these patients could have been labeled refractory GERD and perhaps undergone additional tests and procedures had their CD not been diagnosed and treated. The mechanism of this association is not clear. It is possible that the GERD symptoms are nonspecific, but it is also possible that something related to the CD treatment is resulting in an actual decrease in gastroesophageal reflux. CD could adversely affect motility of the upper gastrointestinal tract either directly or perhaps because of some neurohumoral feedback mechanism. It is important to remember that these patients all had established CD and not to extrapolate into a routine search for CD in patients with reflux symptoms, although selective testing is certainly reasonable.

K. R. DeVault, MD

The effects of itopride on oesophageal motility and lower oesophageal sphincter function in man
Scarpellini E, Vos R, Blondeau K, et al (Catholic Univ of Leuven, Belgium)
Aliment Pharmacol Ther 33:99-105, 2011

Background.—Itopride is a new prokinetic agent that combines antidopaminergic and cholinesterase inhibitory actions. Previous studies suggested that itopride improves heartburn in functional dyspepsia, and decreases oesophageal acid exposure in gastro-oesophageal reflux disease. It remains unclear whether this effect is due to effects of itopride on the lower oesophageal sphincter (LES).

Aims.—To study the effects of itopride on fasting and postprandial LES function in healthy subjects.

Methods.—Twelve healthy volunteers (five men; 32.6 ± 2.0 years) underwent three oesophageal sleeve manometry studies after 3 days pre-medication with itopride 50 mg, itopride 100 mg or placebo t.d.s. Drug was administered after 30 min and a standardized meal was administered after 90 min, with measurements continuing to 120 min postprandially. Throughout the study, 10 wet swallows were administered at 30-min intervals, and gastrointestinal symptoms were scored on 100 mm visual analogue scales at 15-min intervals.

Results.—Lower oesophageal sphincter resting pressures, swallow-induced relaxations and the amplitude or duration of peristaltic contractions were not altered by both doses of itopride, at all time points. Itopride pre-treatment inhibited the meal-induced rise of transient LES relaxations (TLESRs).

Conclusions.—Itopride inhibits TLESRs without significantly affecting oesophageal peristaltic function or LES pressure. These observations support further studies with itopride in gastro-oesophageal reflux disease.

▶ Available prokinetic medications have poor efficacy and poor side effect profiles and, therefore, are used on a very limited basis. Despite this, considerable effort continues toward development of prokinetic agents to treat the motility aspects of gastroesophageal reflux disease (GERD) and other disorders affecting the gastrointestinal tract. This is a small study in healthy volunteers but still deserves attention. Itopride is a mixed antidopaminergic and anticholinesterase agent that has been shown to improve functional dyspepsia, accelerate gastric emptying, and decrease esophageal acid exposure in patients with GERD. In this study, the agent did not change baseline motility parameters but did inhibit meal-induced, transient relaxations of the lower esophageal sphincter (TLESRs).

GERD is actually a disease of impaired motility at the esophagogastric junction. A portion of patients will have a very low pressure, ineffective, lower esophageal sphincter, but it appears that more symptoms are related to TLESRs than to baseline sphincter dysfunction, and vigorous research is being devoted to the development of agents that inhibit these relaxations. Itopride appears to be an agent whose antireflux effect is related to inhibition of TLESRs. It is not clear if this agent or other similar agents will reach the market, but this field should be watched because it is almost inevitable that some agent of this type will be approved and marketed in the next few years.

K. R. DeVault, MD

Laparoscopic Antireflux Surgery vs Esomeprazole Treatment for Chronic GERD: The LOTUS Randomized Clinical Trial

Galmiche J-P, for the LOTUS Trial Collaborators (Nantes Univ, France; et al)
JAMA 305:1969-1977, 2011

Context.—Gastroesophageal reflux disease (GERD) is a chronic, relapsing disease with symptoms that have negative effects on daily life. Two treatment options are long-term medication or surgery.

Objective.—To evaluate optimized esomeprazole therapy vs standardized laparoscopic antireflux surgery (LARS) in patients with GERD.

Design, Setting, and Participants.—The LOTUS trial, a 5-year exploratory randomized, open, parallel-group trial conducted in academic hospitals in 11 European countries between October 2001 and April 2009 among 554 patients with well-established chronic GERD who initially responded to acid suppression. A total of 372 patients (esomeprazole, n=192; LARS, n=180) completed 5-year follow-up.

Interventions.—Two hundred sixty-six patients were randomly assigned to receive esomeprazole, 20 to 40 mg/d, allowing for dose adjustments; 288 were randomly assigned to undergo LARS, of whom 248 actually underwent the operation.

Main Outcome Measure.—Time to treatment failure (for LARS, defined as need for acid suppressive therapy; for esomeprazole, inadequate symptom control after dose adjustment), expressed as estimated remission rates and analyzed using the Kaplan-Meier method.

Results.—Estimated remission rates at 5 years were 92% (95% confidence interval [CI], 89%-96%) in the esomeprazole group and 85% (95% CI, 81%-90%) in the LARS group (log-rank $P=.048$). The difference between groups was no longer statistically significant following best-case scenario modeling of the effects of study dropout. The prevalence and severity of symptoms at 5 years in the esomeprazole and LARS groups, respectively, were 16% and 8% for heartburn ($P=.14$), 13% and 2% for acid regurgitation ($P<.001$), 5% and 11% for dysphagia ($P<.001$), 28% and 40% for bloating ($P<.001$), and 40% and 57% for flatulence ($P<.001$). Mortality during the study was low (4 deaths in the esomeprazole group and 1 death in the LARS group) and not attributed to treatment, and the percentages of patients reporting serious adverse events were similar in the esomeprazole group (24.1%) and in the LARS group (28.6%).

Conclusion.—This multicenter clinical trial demonstrated that with contemporary antireflux therapy for GERD, either by drug-induced acid suppression with esomeprazole or by LARS, most patients achieve and remain in remission at 5 years.

Trial Registration.—clinicaltrials.gov Identifier: NCT00251927.

▶ When patients have well-documented chronic gastroesophageal reflux disease (GERD), management options include long-term proton pump inhibitor (PPI) therapy or surgical intervention. The advent of a laparoscopic approach to GERD has resulted in an increase in the use of this therapy. This article reports on more than 370 patients who were randomized to undergo laparoscopic anti-reflux surgery (LARS) or maintained on chronic esomeprazole (ESO) therapy. The remission rates between the groups were not statistically different (LARS 85%, ESO 92%), but there were other trends in the data. LARS was superior at controlling acid regurgitation at the cost of an increased rate of dyspahgia, bloating, and flatulence. Serious adverse events and mortality were no different.

How should we use these data? First, this study was actually not powered to find a difference and was labeled as "exploratory." That being said, the study does provide important, suggestive data. Second, these are clearly optimally treated patients. LARS was carried out by expert surgeons, and the medication was managed by study coordinators; both of these practices do not reflect the typical practice (at least in the United States), where the majority of surgeries are carried out by low-volume, less-experienced surgeons and it has been documented that a significant percentage of patients do not take their medications optimally. In any trial of this type, the endpoints for medical and surgical treatment are, by nature, different. Patients in the ESO group were started on 20 mg daily; but if they had breakthrough symptoms, they were escalated to 40 mg daily followed by 20 mg twice daily prior to being considered a failure. To fail in the LARS group, you had to either be restarted on PPI therapy or have unacceptable side effects (none of the ESO patients failed because of side effects). Where do these data leave us? First, patients should understand that either treatment is generally effective. If acid regurgitation is the major symptom, then surgery may be superior. What is also clear from this study, and other studies, is that the side-effect profile of surgery is inferior to medical therapy, and patients must understand this going into this procedure or any other invasive procedure for which there is a similarly effective medical option.

K. R. DeVault, MD

Concomitant irritable bowel syndrome is associated with failure of step-down on-demand proton pump inhibitor treatment in patients with gastro-esophageal reflux disease
Wu JCY, Lai LH, Chow DKL, et al (The Chinese Univ of Hong Kong, Shatin)
Neurogastroenterol Motil 23:155-160, e31, 2011

Background.—The predictors for treatment failure of on-demand proton pump inhibitor (PPI) therapy in gastro-esophageal reflux disease (GERD) patients are unclear. We studied the efficacy and predictors for treatment failure of step-down on-demand PPI therapy in patients with non-erosive reflux disease (NERD) and those with low grade erosive esophagitis.

Methods.—Consecutive symptomatic GERD patients who had positive esophageal pH studies and complete symptom resolution with initial treatment of esomeprazole were given step-down on-demand esomeprazole for 26 weeks. Patients with esophagitis of Los Angeles (LA) grade C or above and recent use of PPI were excluded. Treatment failure was defined as an inadequate relief of reflux symptoms using global symptom assessment.

Potential predictors of treatment failure were determined using multivariate analysis.

Key Results.—One hundred and sixty three NERD and 102 esophagitis patients were studied. The 26-week probability of treatment failure was 36.2% (95% CI: 23.9−46.5%) in NERD group and 20.1% (95% CI: 10.9−28.3%) in esophagitis group, respectively (P = 0.021). Irritable bowel syndrome (adjusted HR: 2.1, 95% CI: 1.5−3.8, P = 0.01), in addition to daily reflux symptom (adjusted hazard ratio: 2.7, 95% CI: 1.9−4.2, P = 0.001) and concomitant dyspepsia (adjusted hazard ratio: 1.7, 95% CI: 1.1−2.8, P = 0.04), were independent predictors for treatment failure.

Conclusions & Inferences.—Compared to patients with esophagitis, NERD patients have higher failure rate of on-demand PPI therapy. Concomitant irritable bowel syndrome, in addition to daily reflux symptom and dyspepsia, is associated with the failure of on-demand PPI in these patients.

▶ Several studies have suggested that many patients with gastroesophageal reflux disease (GERD) who have their symptoms controlled on a proton pump inhibitor (PPI) do not need daily PPI and could be managed with on-demand therapy. This study took patients with either low-grade (Los Angeles A or B) esophagitis or nonerosive reflux disease (NERD) who had their symptoms controlled on esomeprazole and placed them on a regimen of on-demand esomeprazole for up to 6 months. A total of 63.8% of the patients with NERD and 79.9% of the patients with esophagitis were successfully treated. Independent predictors of failure included preexisting irritable bowel syndrome (IBS), daily symptoms, and coexisting dyspepsia.

This study demonstrates that many patients, including those with mild esophagitis, can be well managed with on-demand therapy for GERD. I suspect a significant subset of patients will prefer this strategy from both a cost and convenience perspective. The data on dyspepsia and IBS suggest that some of these patients may have a disorder of visceral sensation that could affect more than one area of the gastrointestinal tract. It is interesting that these difficult-to-step-down patients with other functional complaints are also patients that may not respond to antireflux surgery and those without other functional complaints. It was also demonstrated that on-demand therapy was more successful with patients with esophagitis than patients with NERD. Data on complications of PPI therapy associate an increased risk of complication with higher-dose therapy, so these data provide additional support for attempting to step down patients who are on daily PPI therapy. An increased likelihood of success is expected in patients with less frequent symptoms and who do not have coexisting IBS or dyspepsia.

K. R. DeVault, MD

Comparison of the Impact of Wireless Versus Catheter-based pH-metry on Daily Activities and Study-related Symptoms

Bradley AG, Crowell MD, DiBaise JK, et al (Mayo Clinic, Scottsdale, AZ)
J Clin Gastroenterol 45:100-106, 2011

Aims.—To evaluate the variation in tolerance to wireless pH-metry compared with catheter-based pH-metry, and to determine clinical characteristics that might predict reduced tolerance to wireless pH-metry.

Methods.—Consecutive outpatients (n = 341) completing wireless (n = 234) or catheter-based pH-metry (n = 106) were evaluated. All patients completed the pH-Metry Impact Scale and the pH-Metry Symptoms Scale to assess the impact of the pH-metry on activities of daily living and pH-metry associated changes in study-related symptoms. All data are presented as mean (SD) or odds ratios (95% confidence interval).

Results.—The impact of pH-metry on activities of daily living were modest, but wireless pH-metry had less impact than catheter-based pH-metry ($P = 0.01$). A sense of foreign body in the chest, chest discomfort, and chest pain were reported more frequently during wireless pH-metry. Difficulty swallowing and painful swallowing were more common during catheter-based pH-metry. Noncardiac chest pain was associated with increased symptom severity. Patients with poor tolerance were twice as likely to have a diagnosis of noncardiac chest pain (odds ratio = 2. 53; 95% confidence interval, 1.4-4.6).

Conclusions.—Wireless pH-metry has less of an impact on activities of daily living but is not associated with fewer study-related symptoms compared with catheter-based pH-metry. The prevalence of specific study-related symptoms does differ between the 2 groups and noncardiac chest pain seems to be the primary risk factor for more severe study-related symptoms and reduced tolerance for wireless pH-metry. This information may be useful in helping to decide which patients should undergo the wireless pHmetry or receive additional counseling on procedural expectations.

▶ Ambulatory reflux monitoring can be performed in one of several ways. Catheter-based testing can monitor acid at 1 or more locations in the upper gastrointestinal tract and can, when designed properly, also look for nonacid reflux using impedance technology. Wireless testing uses a temporary implantable capsule that transmits data through radiotelemetry to an external data collector. In general, the wireless systems provide longer term testing, while the catheter-based systems may provide additional data. It has been suggested that patients undergoing catheter-based testing often limit their activities because of the discomfort and social stigma associated with a transnasal tube, but this was based more on conjecture than solid data. This study provides a more objective look at those issues. Interestingly, it was true that catheter-based testing had a great impact on daily activity, but somewhat surprisingly, there was a similar amount of study-related symptoms in the 2 groups (although the specific symptoms did vary between the groups). Patients with noncardiac chest pain were particularly bothered by symptoms produced by the wireless capsule. These data suggest that either technique is acceptable to most patients and that the information needed from the study and individual patient preference should drive the decision on which type of system to use rather than an overall superiority of tolerability of one over the other.

K. R. DeVault, MD

Effects of long-term PPI treatment on producing bowel symptoms and SIBO

Compare D, Pica L, Rocco A, et al (Univ of Naples "Federico II", Italy; et al)
Eur J Clin Invest 41:380-386, 2011

Background.—Gastroesophageal reflux disease (GERD), including erosive reflux disease and non-erosive reflux disease (NERD), is a chronic disease with a significant negative effect on quality of life. State-of-the-art treatment involves proton pump inhibitors (PPIs). However, relapse of symptoms occurs in the majority of the patients who require recurrent or continuous therapy. Although PPIs are well tolerated, little information is available about gastrointestinal side effects.

Aim.—To evaluate the effects of long-term PPI treatment on development of bowel symptoms and/or small intestinal bacterial overgrowth (SIBO).

Methods.—Patients with NERD not complaining of bowel symptoms were selected by upper endoscopy, 24-h pH-metry and a structured questionnaire concerning severity and frequency of bloating, flatulence, abdominal pain, diarrhoea and constipation. Patients were treated with esomeprazole 20 mg bid for 6 months. Prior to and after 8 weeks and 6 months of therapy, patients received the structured questionnaire and underwent evaluation of SIBO by glucose hydrogen breath test (GHBT).

Results.—Forty-two patients with NERD were selected out of 554 eligible patients. After 8 weeks of PPI treatment, patients complained of bloating, flatulence, abdominal pain and diarrhoea in 43%, 17%, 7% and 2%, respectively. After 6 months, the incidence of bowel symptoms further increased and GHBT was found positive in 11/42 (26%) patients. By a post hoc analysis, a significant ($P < 0.05$) percentage of patients (8/42) met Rome III criteria for irritable bowel syndrome.

Conclusions.—Prolonged PPI treatment may produce bowel symptoms and SIBO; therefore, the strategy of step-down or on-demand PPI therapy should be encouraged in GERD.

▶ Proton pump inhibitors (PPI) are the mainstay for treatment of acid peptic diseases. Recently, potential side effects have been suggested, including vitamin and mineral malabsorption, loss of bone density, and several infectious complications. It is also well known that there is at least some overlap between nonerosive gastroesophageal reflux disease (NERD) and other functional gastrointestinal (GI) conditions, such as dyspepsia and irritable bowel syndrome.[1] This article found that a subset of patients with NERD treated with twice-daily PPI go on to develop new GI symptoms, including bloating, flatulence, abdominal pain, and diarrhea (Fig 2 in the original article). At 6 months, they found that 11 out of 42 (26%) patients had developed breath-test evidence of bacterial overgrowth and that bacterial overgrowth was more common in the patients who were experiencing new GI symptoms and who met the diagnostic criteria for irritable bowel syndrome (Fig 3 in the original article).

It seems that this may be yet another complication of PPI therapy, although I am a bit surprised that more data of this type would have come out of the large maintenance trials required for registration of each of the marketed PPI. The authors propose that the symptoms and breath-test changes are related and caused by the lack of the antibacterial effects of gastric acid, which is at least partially supported from other trials.[2] Interestingly, a similar increase in symptoms of this type was noted after fundoplication for GERD.[3] This was initially blamed on either vagal changes or perhaps changes in gastric emptying brought about by the surgery, either of which could also predispose to bacterial overgrowth. Prospective trials are needed to see if stopping the PPI or perhaps treating with antibiotics or probiotics results in improvement in the symptoms and testing associated with bacterial overgrowth.

K. R. DeVault, MD

References

1. Locke GR III, Zinsmeister AR, Talley NJ, Fett SL, Melton LJ III. Familial association in adults with functional gastrointestinal disorders. *Mayo Clin Proc.* 2000; 75:907-912.
2. Lombardo L, Foti M, Ruggia O, Chiecchio A. Increased incidence of small intestinal bacterial overgrowth during proton pump inhibitor therapy. *Clin Gastroenterol Hepatol.* 2010;8:504-508.
3. Klaus A, Hinder RA, DeVault KR, Achem SR. Bowel dysfunction after laparoscopic antireflux surgery: incidence, severity, and clinical course. *Am J Med.* 2003;114:6-9.

Gastro-oesophageal reflux treatment for prolonged non-specific cough in children and adults

Chang AB, Lasserson TJ, Gaffney J, et al (Royal Children's Hosp, Brisbane, Australia; The Cochrane Collaboration, London, UK; et al)
Cochrane Database Syst Rev CD004823, 2011

Background.—Gastroesophageal reflux disease (GORD) is said to be the causative factor in up to 41% of adults with chronic cough. Treatment for GORD includes conservative measures (diet manipulation), pharmaceutical therapy (motility or prokinetic agents, H_2-antagonist and proton pump inhibitors (PPI)) and fundoplication.

Objectives.—To evaluate the efficacy of GORD treatment on chronic cough in children and adults with GORD and prolonged cough that is not related to an underlying respiratory disease, i.e. non-specific chronic cough.

Search Strategy.—We searched the Cochrane Airways Group Specialised Register, the Cochrane Register of Controlled Trials (CENTRAL), MED-LINE, EMBASE, review articles and reference lists of relevant articles. The date of last search was 8 April 2010.

Selection Criteria.—All randomised controlled trials (RCTs) on GORD treatment for cough in children and adults without primary lung disease.

Data Collection and Analysis.—Two review authors independently assessed trial quality and extracted data. We contacted study authors for further information.

Main Results.—We included 19 studies (six paediatric, 13 adults). None of the paediatric studies could be combined for meta-analysis. A single RCT in infants found that PPI (compared to placebo) was not efficacious for cough outcomes (favouring placebo OR 1.61; 95% CI 0.57 to 4.55) but those on PPI had significantly increased adverse events (OR 5.56; 95% CI 1.18 to 26.25) (number needed to treat for harm in four weeks was 11 (95% CI 3 to 232)). In adults, analysis of H2 antagonist, motility agents and conservative treatment for GORD was not possible (lack of data) and there were no controlled studies of fundoplication. We analysed nine adult studies comparing PPI (two to three months) to placebo for various outcomes in the meta-analysis. Using intention-to-treat, pooled data from studies resulted in no significant difference between treatment and placebo in total resolution of cough (OR 0.46; 95% CI 0.19 to 1.15). Pooled data revealed no overall significant improvement in cough outcomes (end of trial or change in cough scores). We only found significant differences in sensitivity analyses. We found a significant improvement in change of cough scores at end of intervention (two to three months) in those receiving PPI (standardised mean difference −0.41; 95% CI −0.75 to −0.07) using generic inverse variance analysis on cross-over trials. Two studies reported improvement in cough after five days to two weeks of treatment.

Authors' Conclusions.—PPI is not efficacious for cough associated with GORD symptoms in very young children (including infants) and should not be used for cough outcomes. There is insufficient data in older children to draw any valid conclusions. In adults, there is insufficient evidence to conclude definitely that GORD treatment with PPI is universally beneficial for cough associated with GORD. Clinicians should be cognisant of the period (natural resolution with time) and placebo effect in studies that utilise cough as an outcome measure. Future paediatric and adult studies should be double-blind, randomised controlled and parallel-design, using treatments for at least two months, with validated subjective and objective cough outcomes and include ascertainment of time to respond as well as assessment of acid and/or non-acid reflux.

▶ The association of chronic cough with gastroesophageal reflux disease (GERD) has been proposed and extensively debated. The Cochrane collaborative elected to evaluate this association in both children and adults. Despite a great deal of discussion on the topic, they were only able to identify 19 potential studies to include in their analysis and only 6 that could be combined in a meta-analysis. In adults, proton pump inhibitor (PPI) therapy did not seem to be beneficial for cough when compared with placebo (although there was a large treatment and placebo effect). There were not enough valuable data to address this association in children or to address the effect of surgery on reflux-associated cough.

Although it is attractive to associate cough and reflux, the data to this point have been quite variable. Some studies suggest GERD is more common in patients with cough, whereas others have not found this to be true. This article highlights the overall lack of efficacy of PPI in this symptom. There are several possible explanations. It is possible that there is no association between GERD and cough, but it is also possible that the wrong populations have been studied. Perhaps the problem in cough and GERD are related to common visceral hypersensitivity and would more likely be present in patients with minimal amounts of reflux rather than in those with esophagitis or a grossly positive ambulatory pH test. It is also possible that treating acid is not addressing other factors that might induce cough, most likely including distention-related receptors in the esophagus that may be stimulated even if acid is controlled. These data highlight the concept that providers should not be overly surprised when a patient with a cough does not respond to GERD therapy and, most importantly, that patients should not be labeled as having refractory GERD and subjected to aggressive, long-term reflux therapy (medical, endoscopic, or surgical) unless GERD is confirmed with either an abnormal endoscopy or ambulatory reflux test. Even then, it is not clear that reflux-associated cough refractory to PPI will respond to surgical or endoscopic intervention.

K. R. DeVault, MD

Miscellaneous

Feasibility of endoscopic resection in superficial esophageal squamous carcinoma

Choi JY, Park YS, Jung H-Y, et al (Asan Digestive Disease Res Inst, Seoul, South Korea)

Gastrointest Endosc 73:881-889, 2011

Background.—Endoscopic resection in patients with superficial esophageal squamous carcinoma (SESC) is limited by the presence of lymph node metastasis (LNM), highlighting the importance of determining which patients have virtually no risk of LNM.

Objective.—To investigate the clinicopathological parameters predicting LNM in patients who underwent esophagectomy for SESCs and to identify the best candidate patients for endoscopic resection.

Design.—Retrospective, single-center study.

Setting.—Tertiary-care center.

Patients.—A total of 190 patients who underwent esophagectomy for SESCs between 1991 and 2009.

Interventions.—Esophagectomy with lymph node dissection.

Main Outcome Measurements.—LNM.

Results.—Of 190 patients, 39 (20.5%) had LNM. The rates of LNM in patients with m1, m2, m3, sm1, sm2, and sm3 lesions were 0.0% (0/18), 8.7% (4/46), 25.0% (6/24), 15.0% (3/20), 26.0% (7/27), and 37.3% (19/51), respectively. On multivariate analysis, lymphovascular invasion (LVI) (P < .001), superficial tumor size (P = .004), and lower LMM (lamina muscularis mucosae) invasion width (P < .001) were independent predictors of LNM in patients with SESC invading the LMM. Among 63 patients with mucosal or sm1 cancer 3 cm or smaller, only 1 had LNM without LVI showing a lower LMM invasion width greater than 3.0 mm.

Limitations.—Retrospective analysis.

Conclusions.—Endoscopic resection should be performed for mucosal cancer of 3 cm or less without positive lymph nodes. Moreover, if pathological examination of the endoscopically resected specimens shows invasion of the sm1 layer and a lower LMM invasion width of 3.0 mm or less, indicating an absence of LVI, the patient can be carefully observed without additional treatment.

▶ Endoscopic resection of superficial carcinomas of the gastrointestinal tract has been available in Asia for several years and is being offered in more western centers. This article examined the pathology samples from 190 patients who underwent esophagectomy for superficial esophageal squamous carcinoma (SESC). The table in the original article shows their data. In patients with minimal invasion (m1 or m2) and lesion size < 3 cm, there was no lymph node or lymphovascular invasion, suggesting that a less-aggressive approach could have been curative.

Although this is a pathology study and does not provide patient outcome on this less-aggressive approach, it does support the endoscopic approach many centers are using. Based on these data, an esophageal carcinoma of < 3 cm in size should undergo endoscopic mucosal resection. The chance of lymph node involvement in these small superficial tumors is low, but most would still advocate an evaluation (likely with a combination of CT or MRI and endoscopic ultrasound scan). If the invasion is limited to m1-2 and there are no pathologic lymph nodes, then the patient is likely cured. Although these data are from patients with SESC, most would assume a similar approach to be reasonable in patients with esophageal adenocarcinoma arising in Barrett esophagus. Additional prospective data need to be collected to make sure this pathology study is predictive of long-term clinical outcomes.

K. R. DeVault, MD

Budesonide is Effective in Adolescent and Adult Patients With Active Eosinophilic Esophagitis

Straumann A, Conus S, Degen L, et al (Univ Hosp Basel, Switzerland; Univ of Bern, Switzerland; et al)
Gastroenterology 139:1526-1537, 2010

Background & Aims.—Eosinophilic esophagitis (EoE) is a chronic inflammatory disease of the esophagus characterized by dense tissue eosinophilia; it is refractory to proton pump inhibitor therapy. EoE affects all age groups but most frequently individuals between 20 and 50 years of age. Topical corticosteroids are effective in pediatric patients with EoE, but no controlled studies of corticosteroids have been reported in adult patients.

Methods.—We performed a randomized, double-blind, placebo-controlled trial to evaluate the effect of oral budesonide (1 mg twice daily for 15 days) in adolescent and adult patients with active EoE. Pretreatment and posttreatment disease activity was assessed clinically, endoscopically, and histologically. The primary end point was reduced mean numbers of eosinophils in the esophageal epithelium (number per highpower field [hpf] = esophageal eosinophil load). Esophageal biopsy and blood samples were analyzed using immunofluorescence and immunoassays, respectively, for biomarkers of inflammation and treatment response.

Results.—A 15-day course of therapy significantly decreased the number of eosinophils in the esophageal epithelium in patients given budesonide (from 68.2 to 5.5 eosinophils/hpf; $P < .0001$) but not in the placebo group (from 62.3 to 56.5 eosinophils/hpf; $P = .48$). Dysphagia scores significantly improved among patients given budesonide compared with those given placebo (5.61 vs 2.22; $P < .0001$). White exudates and red furrows were reversed in patients given budesonide, based on endoscopy examination. Budesonide, but not placebo, also reduced apoptosis of epithelial cells and molecular remodeling events in the esophagus; no serious adverse events were observed.

Conclusions.—A 15-day course of treatment with budesonide is well tolerated and highly effective in inducing a histologic and clinical remission in adolescent and adult patients with active EoE.

▶ Eosinophilic esophagitis (EOE) is a commonly diagnosed condition in both children and adults. Treatment options include proton pump inhibitors (PPI), topical steroids, and esophageal dilation (if dysphagia is the predominant symptom). Budesonide is a poorly absorbed steroid with limited side effects, which is readily available in a liquid formulation and would seem to be an ideal candidate for treating EOE topically. This agent produced both a decrease in esophageal eosinophils and an improvement in dysphagia when compared with placebo.[1]

If topical steroids are to be used in EOE, they could be used as a first-line therapy, as a second-line therapy for patients who fail a trial of PPI, or either before or after the planned esophageal dilation. Unfortunately, both the exact role for topical steroids and the dosage and duration of EOE therapy is not clear. This study used 1 mg of budesonide twice daily for 15 days, whereas some others have used a lower dosage (500 µg) twice daily for 4 to 6 weeks. It is clear that the available data are not strong enough to make a strong recommendation either on dosage or duration. On the other hand, if topical steroids are to be used, budesonide seems to be a logical and reasonable agent for this indication. Although these authors used this agent in its liquid form, others have combined it with a sucralose-based product (Splenda in the United

States) and have patients swallow this to possibly help with adherence to the esophageal mucosa.

K. R. DeVault, MD

Reference

1. Dohil R, Newbury R, Fox L, Bastian J, Aceves S. Oral viscous budesonide is effective in children with eosinophilic esophagitis in a randomized, placebo-controlled trial. *Gastroenterology.* 2010;139:418-429.

Esophageal Eosinophilic Infiltration Responds to Proton Pump Inhibition in Most Adults

Molina-Infante J, Ferrando-Lamana L, Ripoll C, et al (Hosp San Pedro de Alcantara, Caceres, Spain; Hosp Gregorio Marañon, Madrid, Spain)
Clin Gastroenterol Hepatol 9:110-117, 2011

Background & Aims.—Despite consensus recommendations, eosinophilic esophagitis (EoE) is commonly diagnosed upon esophageal eosinophilic infiltration (EEI; based on ≥15 eosinophils per high power field; eo/HPF). We evaluated the prevalence of EEI before and after proton pump inhibitor (PPI) therapy and assessed the accuracy of EEI and pH monitoring analyses.

Methods.—Biopsies were taken from the upper-middle esophagus of 712 adults with upper gastrointestinal symptoms who were referred for endoscopy due to upper gastrointestinal symptoms. Patients with EEI were treated with rabeprazole (20 mg, twice daily) for 2 months. EoE was defined by persistent symptoms and >15 eo/HPF following PPI therapy.

Results.—Thirty-five patients (4.9%) had EEI, of whom 55% had a history of allergies, and 70% had food impaction or dysphagia as their primary complaint. Twenty-six EEI patients (75%) achieved clinicopathological remission with PPI therapy; of these, 17 had GERD-like profile (EEI <35 eo/HPF and objective evidence of reflux, based on endoscopy or pH monitoring), and 9 had EoE-like profile (EEI 35−165 eo/HPF, typical EoE symptoms and endoscopic findings). The PPI response was 50% in the EoE-like profile patients. The PPI-response was 50% in EoE-like profile patients. Likewise, PPI-responsive EEI occurred with normal (33%) and pathologic (80%) pH monitoring. Higher histologic cut-off values improved specificity and positive predictive for EoE (35%−35% for >20 eo/HPF; 46%−39% for >24 eo/HPF; 65%−50% for 35 eo/HPF).

Conclusions.—In adults with EEI, 75% of unselected patients and 50% with an EoE phenotype respond to PPI therapy; pH monitoring is poorly predictive of response. Patients with PPI-responsive EEI >35 eo/HPF are phenotypically undistinguishable from EoE patients. EoE might be overestimated without clinical and pathologic follow-up of patient response to PPI.

▶ Eosinophilic esophagitis (EOE) is a commonly diagnosed condition in both children and adults, which is diagnosed based on eosinophilic infiltration (EEI) on examination of esophageal biopsies. There is considerable controversy about the best initial treatment of these patients; some experts suggest a trial of proton pump inhibitors (PPI) and others suggest topical steroids. This study found that most patients with EOE respond to a course of PPI. They also divided their patients into those whose symptoms and endoscopic findings were more GERD-like and those with a more typical EOE symptom (usually dysphagia) and endoscopic presentation. Both groups had at least a 50% response, but the response rate was higher in those who were more GERD-like. Interestingly, ambulatory pH testing did not predict whether the patients were going to respond to PPI treatment.

In this important study, the authors attempt to make a case that patients with EEI who respond to PPI do not have EOE. I do not think that can be clearly inferred from this study, and there are some emerging data that PPI may actually downregulate some inflammatory markers seen in EOE independent of their affect on gastric acid.[1] The best we can say is that EOE symptoms (both typical and atypical) may respond to PPI. The fact that pH results did not predict the response to PPI is both surprising and troubling. It is possible that the pH test is not sufficiently sensitive in this population or that reflux amounts less than those usually considered abnormal might influence this particular population. Future studies are needed to confirm and expand these findings. The take-home message is that a reinforcement of the concept of a trial of PPI is an acceptable and perhaps preferred initial approach to most patients with EOE.

K. R. DeVault, MD

Reference

1. Cortes JR, Rivas MD, Molina-Infante J, et al. Omeprazole inhibits IL-4 and IL-13 signaling signal transducer and activator of transcription 6 activation and reduces lung inflammation in murine asthma. *J Allergy Clin Immunol.* 2009;124:607-610.

Comparison Between Definitive Chemoradiotherapy and Esophagectomy in Patients With Clinical Stage I Esophageal Squamous Cell Carcinoma
Yamamoto S, Ishihara R, Motoori M, et al (Osaka Med Center for Cancer and Cardiovascular Diseases, Japan)
Am J Gastroenterol 106:1048-1054, 2011

Objectives.—Chemoradiotherapy (CRT) has been proposed as an alternative therapy to esophagectomy for esophageal cancer, because of its favorable survival rate and mild toxicity. However, no comparative studies of esophagectomy and CRT have been reported in patients with clinical stage I esophageal squamous cell carcinoma.

Methods.—A total of 54 patients with clinical stage I esophageal squamous cell carcinoma were treated with definitive CRT and 116 patients with esophagectomy at Osaka Medical Center for Cancer and Cardiovascular Diseases between 1995 and 2008, and were included in the analysis. Overall survival and recurrence rates were evaluated.

Results.—Complete follow-up data were available for 169 of the 170 patients (99%). The median (range) observation period was 67 (10–171) months in the esophagectomy group and 30 (4–77) months in the CRT group ($P < 0.0001$). The 1- and 3-year overall survival rates were 97.4 % and 85.5 %, respectively, in the esophagectomy group and 98.1% and 88.7%, respectively, in the CRT group ($P = 0.78$). Cox proportional hazards modeling showed that the overall survival was comparable between the two groups after adjusting for age, sex, and tumor size. The hazard ratio of CRT for overall survival was 0.95 (95% confidence interval 0.37–2.47). The incidence of local recurrence, including metachronous esophageal cancer, was significantly higher in the CRT group than in the esophagectomy group ($P < 0.0001$). Most local recurrences in the CRT group were intramucosal carcinomas, and were cured after salvage treatment, mainly using endoscopy.

Conclusions.—The overall survival rate of patients with clinical stage I esophageal cancer treated with CRT was comparable to that in those treated with esophagectomy, despite a high local recurrence rate. Locally recurrent carcinoma was endoscopically treatable in most patients, with no effect on overall survival. CRT seems to be a viable alternative to esophagectomy in patients with clinical stage I esophageal cancer.

▶ The approach to patients with esophageal carcinoma continues to evolve. Some of the greatest degree of controversy surrounds those with limited disease. This was a retrospective evaluation of patients with limited esophageal squamous cell cancer (stage I-T1N0M0) who either underwent an esophagectomy or chemoradiation and found no difference in survival. The chemoradiation group had more recurrent disease, but this was usually amiable to local therapy at the time of recurrence. It is important to understand how this group in Japan approaches lesions of this type. It sounds as if patients with smaller stage I tumors were offered endoscopic resection, so the patients in this report were likely to have larger tumors. Because this was a nonrandomized allocation, the patients offered chemoradiation were older and had larger tumors, and they may have also had more comorbidities. These factors would bias toward a better outcome with surgery, which was not seen in this study. These important data suggest that it is reasonable to offer both alternatives (immediate surgery versus chemoradiation with intensive follow-up) to patients with early esophageal squamous cancer. It is not clear if similar results would occur in adenocarcinoma, which is the much more common type in Western countries.

K. R. DeVault, MD

Potential Precipitating Factors of Esophageal Variceal Bleeding: A Case—Control Study
Liao W-C, Hou M-C, Chang C-J, et al (Natl Yang Ming Univ, Taipei, Taiwan; Taipei Veterans General Hosp, Taiwan)
Am J Gastroenterol 106:96-103, 2011

Objectives.—Valsalva maneuver-associated activities such as straining during defecation, vomiting, and cough are believed to cause abrupt increase in variceal pressure. Whether these actions can precipitate rupture of esophageal varices (EV) is unknown. The association of EV bleeding with these activities and other potential risk factors such as ingestion of alcohol and non-steroidal anti-inflammatory drugs was investigated.

Methods.—Between January 2003 and May 2009, 240 patients with liver cirrhosis and acute EV bleeding (group A) and 240 matched patients with Child-Pughs class and moderate size EV without bleeding (group B) were included. Each patient was questioned regarding constipation, vomiting, cough, and other potential risk factors in the week prior to index bleeding (group A) or endoscopy (group B) using a standard questionnaire.

Results.—Group A had more patients with constipation ($n = 44$ vs. $n = 16$, $P < 0.001$) and higher constipation scores (0.791.67 vs. 0.25 ± 0.92, $P < 0.001$) than group B. Group A also had more patients with vomiting ($n = 60$ vs. $n = 33$, $P = 0.002$) and higher vomiting scores (3.0 ± 0.86 vs. 1.85 ± 0.87, $P < 0.001$). No difference in cough existed between the two groups ($n = 77$ group A vs. $n = 73$ group B); however, group A had higher cough scores (5.08 ± 2.70 vs. 3.19 ± 2.23, $P < 0.001$). Group A had more patients with excessive alcohol consumption in the week preceding inclusion in the study ($n = 58$ vs. $n = 5$, $P < 0.001$). On multivariate analysis, constipation score and vomiting score and alcohol consumption were independent determinants of first EV bleeding.

Conclusions.—Constipation, vomiting, severe coughing, and excessive consumption of alcohol may precipitate rupture of EV. A prospective cohort study is required to clarify the causal relationship between potential precipitating factors and EV bleeding.

▶ Predicting which patient with liver disease and esophageal varices (EV) will experience a first bleed remains an imprecise science. Previous bleeding, size of the varices, and certain superficial stigmata are currently used to decide when banding should be initiated. This study looked at multiple clinical factors to attempt to create a phenotype of the patient with an increased risk of EV bleeding, particularly focusing on symptoms and activities that result in Valsalva, which has been associated with bleeding in previous studies. Clinically, the bleeding patients were more likely to have experienced portal vein thrombosis, a higher Model for End-Stage Liver Disease score, lower serum albumin, lower hemoglobin, and higher creatinine. EV size did not correlate well with bleeding, but a superficial red-color sign did. Constipation, vomiting, severity of coughing, and recent alcohol consumption were all increased in the patients with EV bleeding. In contrast to conventional teaching, the use of nonsteroidal antiinflammatory drugs or aspirin did not increase the risk of bleeding.

Most of the findings in this study were somewhat expected, but constipation is an overlooked risk factor for EV bleeding. Although there are no data to suggest that decreased straining and Valsalva with relief of constipation decreases bleeding risk, it would seem prudent to make sure liver patients with EV have their constipation controlled as a potential preventative measure. Severe coughing and vomiting should also be sought out during history taking and addressed if present.

K. R. DeVault, MD

Coffee intake and oral–oesophageal cancer: follow-up of 389 624 Norwegian men and women 40–45 years
Tverdal A, Hjellvik V, Selmer R (Norwegian Inst of Public Health, Nydalen, Oslo, Norway)
Br J Cancer 105:157-161, 2011

Background.—The evidence on the relationship between coffee intake and cancer of the oral cavity and oesophagus is conflicting and few follow-up studies have been done.

Methods.—A total of 389 624 men and women 40–45 years who participated in a national survey programme were followed with respect to cancer for an average of 14.4 years by linkage to the Cancer Registry of Norway. Coffee consumption at baseline was reported as a categorical variable (0 or <1 cup, 1–4, 5–8, 9+ cups per day).

Results.—Altogether 450 squamous oral or oesophageal cancers were registered during follow-up. The adjusted hazard ratios with 1–4 cups per day as reference were 1.01 (95% confidence interval: 0.70, 1.47), 1.16 (0.93, 1.45) and 0.96 (0.71, 1.14) for 0 or <1 cup, 5–8 and 9+ cups per day, respectively. Stratification by sex, type of coffee, smoking status and dividing the end point into oral and oesophageal cancers gave heterogeneous and non-significant estimates.

Conclusion.—This study does not support an inverse relationship between coffee intake and incidence of cancer in the mouth or oesophagus, but cannot exclude a weak inverse relationship.

▶ The affects of coffee consumption on the gastrointestinal tract have been long debated. Coffee and caffeine intake are thought to be risk factors for gastroesophageal reflux disease (GERD), and, therefore, one might assume that they would increase the risk of esophageal adenocarcinoma. In addition, some studies have suggested that high-temperature drinks may increase the risk of esophageal cancer. On the other hand, there are some data suggesting a protective effect against cancer of the esophagus and other organs in patients with moderate amounts of coffee intake. This large registry from Scandinavia was able to address this issue and found that coffee intake had no affect (positive or negative) on the risk of esophageal and oral carcinomas. There were some other interesting associations in the study. Heavy coffee users were more likely to be men, smokers, and heavier alcohol users, but they were less likely to be highly educated or physically active. Based on these data and others, we should continue to suggest moderation in coffee and caffeine intake in our patients with symptomatic GERD, but we should also counsel that there is little chance that this beverage changes the risk for esophageal cancer.

K. R. DeVault, MD

Stents for proximal esophageal cancer: a case-control study
Parker RK, White RE, Topazian M, et al (Rhode Island Hosp and The Warren Alpert Med School of Brown Univ, Providence; Mayo Clinic, Rochester, MN)
Gastrointest Endosc 73:1098-1105, 2011

Background.—Self-expandable metal stents (SEMSs) are an established palliative therapy for esophageal cancer. SEMS placement for cancers near the upper esophageal sphincter (UES) is controversial because of a perceived increased risk of complications.

Objective.—To compare outcomes after patients stented for proximal esophageal cancer (PC) and distal esophageal cancer (DC).

Design.—Matched case-control study from a prospective database.

Setting.—Tertiary referral center, Tenwek Hospital, Bomet, Kenya.

Patients.—All patients with PC located within 6 cm of the UES were matched with randomly selected controls with DC.

Interventions.—Outcomes of PC cases were compared with those of DC controls.

Main Outcome Measurements.—Dysphagia score, complications, median survival.

Results.—A total of 151 patients with PC were identified and were randomly matched with DC controls. Ninety-three case-control pairs had adequate follow-up information available. Mean dysphagia scores (scale 0-4) improved from 3.4 and 3.3 before stenting for PC and DC, respectively, to 1.5 after stenting for both groups ($P = .93$). Early complications occurred in 6.5% of PC cases and 9.7% of DC controls ($P = .44$). Late complications occurred in 20.4% of PC cases and 15.1% of DC controls ($P = .25$). Median survival was 210 days for PC cases and 272 days for DC controls ($P = .25$). Outcomes were similar for the subgroup of PC cases whose cancer extended to within 2 cm of the UES.

Limitation.—An important limitation is the absence of adequate follow-up data for 58 of the 151 case-control pairs.

Conclusions.—SEMSs effectively palliate dysphagia in PC cases, whereas complication and survival rates are not statistically different from those of DC controls.

▶ Esophageal cancer (EC) is a common problem that often is not amenable to cure. Many patients develop severe stenosis in their esophagus that limits their nutrition and contributes markedly to their general decline during the process of their disease. Self-expandable metal stents (SEMS) have the ability to palliate dysphagia in many patients with advanced EC. These were initially deployed more commonly for distal cancer, particularly those at the esophagogastric junction. Proximal stents were often avoided because many providers assumed that the stent would produce unacceptable symptoms if located too far proximal. This study suggests that stents can be used pretty much anywhere within the esophagus. Complications, response to dysphagia, and survival were similar whether the stent was placed in the proximal or distal esophagus. Most impressive was their group with very proximal cancers (< 2 cm distal to upper esophageal sphincter), where the stents were quite effective and well tolerated. It is important to note that these patients received radiation or chemotherapy, which have been associated with stent complications in other studies.

It appears that SEMS are a viable option for any cancer localized to the esophagus. In the article and accompanying editorial,[1] important points to help optimize the success of the procedure were discussed. Operator experience is very important, and experienced interventional endoscopists should deploy SEMS. Despite the good results from this study, the endoscopist will likely have to remove some stents because of unacceptable symptoms and needs to be comfortable with those techniques. The authors also customized their stent technique depending on the level of stenosis, using smaller-diameter stents for proximal lesions and making intraprocedural decisions on which stent to use from one of several manufacturers. The editorial makes the point that this is one time when a standardized "one tool fits all" approach is inappropriate.

K. R. DeVault, MD

Reference

1. Weston AP. Stents in the proximal esophagus: tailoring the stent to the patient to achieve success. *Gastrointest Endosc.* 2011;73:1106-1108.

Acute development of gastroesophageal reflux after radiofrequency catheter ablation of atrial fibrillation

Martinek M, Hassanein S, Bencsik G, et al (Elisabethinen Univ Teaching Hosp, Linz, Austria; Univ of Szeged, Hungary)
Heart Rhythm 6:1457-1462, 2009

Background.—Induction of gastroesophageal reflux after radiofrequency catheter ablation (RFCA) of atrial fibrillation (AF) may have an impact on the progression of esophageal injury.

Objective.—The purpose of this study was to assess the acute effect of RFCA on distal esophageal acidity using leadless pH-metry capsules.

Methods.—A total of 31 patients (27 male and 4 female; 25 with paroxysmal AF) who underwent RFCA and esophagoscopy 24 hours before and after ablation were assessed for reflux and esophageal lesions. A leadless pH-metry capsule was inserted into the lower esophagus to screen for pH changes, number and duration of refluxes, and the DeMeester score (a standardized measure of acidity and reflux). No patient had a history of reflux or was taking proton pump inhibitors within 4 weeks before and 24 hours after ablation.

Results.—Five patients (16.1%) who presented with asymptomatic reflux prior to ablation were excluded from further examination. Of the remaining 26 patients, 5 (19.2%) demonstrated a significant pathologic increase in DeMeester score after ablation. No statistical differences in baseline parameters, method of sedation, ablation approach, and total energy delivered on the posterior wall were observed between patients with and those without a pathologic DeMeester score. One patient with asymptomatic reflux prior to ablation developed esophageal ulceration.

Conclusion.—A significant number of patients undergoing RFCA of AF develop pathologic acid reflux after ablation. In addition, a subgroup of patients has a preexisting condition of asymptomatic reflux prior to ablation. This finding may explain a potential mechanism for progression of esophageal injury to atrio-esophageal fistulas in patients undergoing RFCA.

▶ This small study performed ambulatory pH testing before and after radiofrequency ablation of atrial fibrillation. Approximately 20% of the patients demonstrated a significant increase in reflux as measured by the DeMeester score.

The esophagus and the heart are anatomically and embryologically connected. It is clear that chest pain may be produced by both organs and that stimulation of the organs produce similar symptoms. Catheter-based radiofrequency ablation of aberrant cardiac pathways has become commonly used. There have been reported gastrointestinal (GI) complications, including atrio-esophageal fistulae and esophageal ulceration. These effects are local and likely related to direct trauma. Another possible mechanism of GI injury is inadvertent damage to esophageal nerves, either intramural or via vagal pathways. Gastroesophageal reflux (GER) is one possible complication of this therapy. While this study suggests a worsening in GER disease measurements after therapy in a small number of patients, one needs to consider the possibility that these changes are related to poor day-to-day reproducibility of pH monitoring, although if that were the case, then one would expect to see some patients actually get better on the second test. It would seem reasonable to consider proton pump inhibitor therapy after ablation and to be watchful for any new or worsened GI symptoms that may develop.

K. R. DeVault, MD

Comparison of open three-field and minimally-invasive esophagectomy for esophageal cancer
Gao Y, Wang Y, Chen L, et al (West China Hosp of Sichuan Univ, Chengdu, China)
Interact Cardiovasc Thorac Surg 12:366-369, 2011

The aim was to compare the early outcomes between thoracoscopic and laparoscopic esophagectomy (TLE) and open three-field esophagectomy for esophageal cancer. We retrospectively analyzed clinical data from 96 patients with esophageal cancer who underwent TLE, and 78 patients who underwent open three-field esophagectomy from March 2008 to September 2010. All the operations were successful. There was no significant difference between TLE and open three-field esophagectomy with regard to the number of lymph nodes procured (17.75 ± 5.56 vs. 18.03 ± 6.20, $P>0.05$), complications (32.3% vs. 46.2%, $P>0.05$), and operative mortality (2.1% vs. 3.8%, $P>0.05$). However, hospital stay was significantly shorter in the TLE group than the open esophagectomy group (12.64 ± 8.82 vs. 17.53 ± 6.40 days, $P<0.01$), and the TLE group had significantly less blood loss (346.68 ± 41.13 vs. 519.26 ± 47.74 ml, $P<0.01$). This showed that TLE for esophageal cancer offers results as good as or better than those with open three-field esophagectomy (Table 3).

▶ Esophageal cancer is a devastating illness with a very high rate of mortality and almost universal morbidity. Esophagectomy can offer the highest chance of long-term survival in selected patients but has a high rate of immediate and late complications. A less invasive approach to esophagectomy has been developed and is being used in several centers. This retrospective study compared the early outcome in patients who had undergone either a minimally invasive esophagectomy (MIE) or an open esophagectomy (OE). The number of lymph nodes obtained, complications, and mortality were the same in both groups. There was a shorter length of stay and less blood loss in the MIE group, although the MIE studies did require, on average, an additional 46 minutes of operative time.

This was not a randomized study, and it is not clear from the methods how patients were allocated, although in contrast to some other reports the patients were collected over roughly the same time periods. The complications were no different in the 2 groups, but they were substantial and are presented in Table 3. It is important to understand that these data come from a high-volume expert center and that several studies have suggested that optimal outcomes are only available at such centers.[1] It would be prudent for these patients to all be referred to such centers and for those centers to continue to work toward optimizing the outcomes of these difficult procedures. A randomized trial

TABLE 3.—Postoperative Morbidity and Mortality

Parameters	TLE ($n = 96$)	Open ($n = 78$)	P-Value
Complications	31 (32.3%)	36 (46.2%)	>0.05
Pulmonary complications	13 (13.5%)	11 (14.1%)	>0.05
Anastomotic leakage	7 (7.3%)	6 (7.7%)	>0.05
RLN-injury*	2 (2.1%)	4 (5.1%)	>0.05
Delayed gastric emptying	2 (2.1%)	5 (6.4%)	>0.05
Chylothorax	1 (1.05%)	2 (2.6%)	>0.05
Diaphragmatocele	1 (1.05%)	1 (1.3%)	>0.05
Anastomotic stricture	5 (5.2%)	7 (9.0%)	>0.05
Operative mortality†	2 (2.1%)	3 (3.8%)	>0.05

TLE, Thoracoscopic and laparoscopic esophagectomy.
*Recurrent laryngeal nerve injury.
†Death within 30 days following the operation.

comparing MIE with OE apparently has been initiated and should help to clarify questions related to which procedure is optimal.[2]

K. R. DeVault, MD

References

1. Flum DR, Koepsell T, Heagerty P, Pellegrini CA. The nationwide frequency of major adverse outcomes in antireflux surgery and the role of surgeon experience, 1992—1997. *J Am Coll Surg.* 2002;195:611-618.
2. Biere SS, Maas KW, Bonavina L, et al. Traditional invasive vs. minimally invasive esophagectomy: a multi-center, randomized trial (TIME-trial). *BMC Surg.* 2011; 11:2.

Self-expandable metal stents for the treatment of benign upper GI leaks and perforations

Swinnen J, Eisendrath P, Rigaux J, et al (Université Libre de Bruxelles, Belgium)

Gastrointest Endosc 73:890-899, 2011

Background.—Self-expandable metal stents (SEMSs) have been suggested for the treatment of benign upper GI leaks and perforations. Nevertheless, uncomplicated removal remains difficult. Placement of a self-expandable plastic stent (SEPS) into an SEMS can facilitate retrieval.

Objectives.—This study reviews our experience with sequential SEMS/SEPS placement in patients with benign upper GI leaks or perforations.

Design.—A retrospective review of the chart of each patient who underwent SEMS placement for benign upper GI leaks or perforations, including (1) fistula after bariatric surgery, (2) other postoperative fistulae, (3) Boerhaave syndrome, (4) iatrogenic perforations, and (5) other perforations.

Setting.—Single, tertiary center.

Patients.—Eighty-eight patients (37 male, average age 51.6 years, range 18-89 years).

Interventions.—SEMS placement and removal, with or without SEPS placement.

Main Outcome Measurements.—Feasibility of SEMS removal and successful treatment of lesions and short-term and long-term complications.

Results.—A total of 153 SEMSs were placed in 88 patients; all placements were successful. Six patients died (not SEMS-related deaths) and 6 patients were lost to follow-up with SEMSs still in place. Seventy-three of the remaining 76 patients had successful SEMS removal (96.1%). The rate of successful SEMS removal per stent was 97.8% (132/135). Resolution of leaks and perforations was achieved in 59 patients (77.6%) with standard endoscopic treatment, and in 64 patients (84.2%) after prolonged, repeated endoscopic treatment. Spontaneous migration occurred in 11.1% of stents, and there were minor complications (dysphagia, hyperplasia, rupture of coating) in 20.9% and major complications (bleeding, perforation, tracheal compression) in 5.9%.

Limitations.—Retrospective design and highly selected patient population.
Conclusions.—Use of SEMSs for the treatment of benign upper GI leaks
and perforations is feasible, relatively safe, and effective, and SEMSs can
be easily removed 1 to 3 weeks after SEPS insertion. Leaks and perforations were closed in 77.6% of cases (Fig 5).

▶ Endoscopic intervention and surgery of the upper gastrointestinal (GI) tract
carry a risk of perforation that is variable depending on the procedure performed. In the past, most patients with a perforation were managed with
surgery, but recently reports have suggested that some perforations can be
managed expectantly. Attempts to improve the likelihood of the perforation
healing have included the placement of endoscopic clips and stents. This article

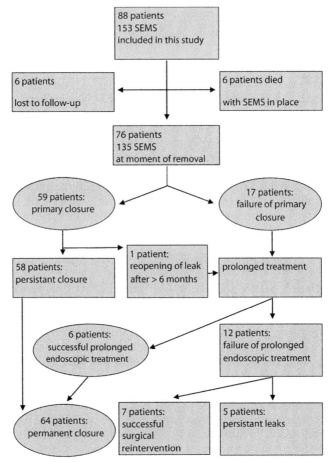

FIGURE 5.—Flowchart of results and patient outcomes. (Reprinted from Swinnen J, Eisendrath P,
Rigaux J, et al. Self-expandable metal stents for the treatment of benign upper GI leaks and perforations.
Gastrointest Endosc. 2011;73:890-899, Copyright 2011, with permission from the American Society for
Gastrointestinal Endoscopy.)

focuses on the use of stents. This report found outstanding safety and efficacy for this approach. Fig 5 illustrates the results where the bottom line was closure in 64 out of 76, eventual surgical reintervention in 7, and persistent leaks in 5.

How should these data change our approach? It would seem prudent to do only high-risk procedures, such as pneumatic dilation for achalasia or endoscopic mucosal resection, in centers where the possibility of stent placement exists. The other large indication in this series was postoperative leaks. Again, centers that perform upper GI surgery should have the option of stenting available. A word of caution: We have seen several cases of multiple stents being used in patients who were fit for surgery with the persistence of leaks, [1] so if the leak does not close after a few attempts, referral for surgery should be strongly considered.

K. R. DeVault, MD

Reference

1. Odell JA, DeVault KR. Extended stent usage for persistent esophageal leak: should there be limits? *Ann Thorac Surg.* 2010;90:1707-1708.

Adherence and Adequacy of Therapy for Esophageal Varices Prophylaxis
Maddur H, Naik S, Siddiqui AA, et al (Univ of Texas Southwestern Med Ctr, Dallas)
Dig Dis Sci 2011 [Epub ahead of print]

Aims.—Esophageal varices (EVs) are prevalent among cirrhotics and their bleeding leads to substantial morbidity and mortality. Management guidelines available during this study recommended beta-blocker therapy for primary prophylaxis and beta-blocker or band ligation (EVL) for secondary prophylaxis. We evaluated prophylaxis practice patterns.

Methods.—We performed a retrospective cohort study of in and outpatient cirrhotics with known EVs at two University of Texas Southwestern teaching institutions. Use of prophylactic therapy and its adequacy (defined using published guidelines) was measured.

Results.—A total of 419 patients with cirrhosis and EVs warranting prophylaxis were identified, including 276 inpatients and 143 outpatients. Of those admitted with a first bleed (i.e. eligible for primary prophylactic therapy), 30/104 (29%) were on beta blocker. In this group, only 3/104 (3%) received optimal therapy (heart rate <55). Among inpatients with a previous EV bleed, 120/172 (70%) were on a beta blocker or had undergone EVL, although only 66/172 (38%) received optimal therapy. In the inpatient cohort, ten patients died of gastrointestinal hemorrhage, three of whom were receiving optimal therapy. Among outpatients, 94/121 (78%) without previous bleeding received primary prophylaxis and 20/22 (91%) of those with previous bleeding received some form of secondary prophylaxis. However, only 11 (9%) received adequate primary prophylaxis therapy, while 9 (41%) received appropriate secondary prophylaxis.

Conclusions.—Prophylaxis intent appears to be greatly improved compared to previous reports. However, implementation of optimal therapy appeared to be suboptimal. We conclude that efforts need to be made to ensure optimal treatment.

▶ Esophageal variceal hemorrhage remains a substantial cause of morbidity and mortality in patients with chronic liver disease. Current guidelines support the use of β-blockers to prevent bleeding. Although not addressed by this article and not part of current guidelines, there is also a growing body of evidence to support primary prophylaxis using esophageal variceal banding. Once a patient has bled, it has also been suggested that the majority of eligible patients gets either no or insufficient prophylaxis (secondary). This study examined a large cohort of patients at a major teaching institution and found that there has been improvement in the proportion of patients getting primary or secondary prophylaxis (when compared with historical controls), but that the majority was not being optimally treated.

The authors suggest that the dissemination of treatment guidelines has resulted in the improvement seen in this study, although one cannot discount the fact that these data come from a major teaching institution and that internal education may be the real factor. While any treatment is superior to no treatment, very few of their patients were optimally treated. The most common issues were lack of follow-up after variceal banding and inadequate β-blocker therapy. Additional data should be obtained from community practices, and, if those results are similar or inferior to these, then additional education efforts are appropriate. The target is to obtain sufficient heart rate reduction (< 55) in all patients who tolerate β-blockers and to make sure that all patients who bled have at least 2 sessions of variceal banding (ideally banding continues until the varices are obliterated). It is likely that adherence to these guidelines will improve outcomes in this difficult-to-manage population.

K. R. DeVault, MD

2 Gastrointestinal Motility Disorders/ Neurogastroenterology

Gastric Motility

Domperidone Treatment for Gastroparesis: Demographic and Pharmacogenetic Characterization of Clinical Efficacy and Side-Effects

Parkman HP, Jacobs MR, Mishra A, et al (Temple Univ School of Medicine, Philadelphia, PA; Temple Univ School of Pharmacy, Philadelphia, PA)
Dig Dis Sci 56:115-124, 2011

Background.—Domperidone is a useful alternative to metoclopramide for treatment of gastroparesis due to better tolerability. Effectiveness and side-effects from domperidone may be influenced by patient-related factors including polymorphisms in genes encoding drug-metabolizing enzymes, drug transporters, and domperidone targets.

Aims.—The aim of this study was to determine if demographic and pharmacogenetic parameters of patients receiving domperidone are associated with response to treatment or side-effects.

Methods.—Patients treated with domperidone for gastroparesis provided saliva samples from which DNA was extracted. Fourteen single-nucleotide polymorphisms (SNPs) in seven candidate genes (*ABCB1, CYP2D6, DRD2, KCNE1, KCNE2, KCNH2, KCNQ1*) were used for genotyping. SNP microarrays were used to assess single-nucleotide polymorphisms in the *ADRA1A, ADRA1B,* and *ADRA1D* loci.

Results.—Forty-eight patients treated with domperidone participated in the study. DNA was successfully obtained from each patient. Age was associated with effectiveness of domperidone ($p = 0.0088$). Genetic polymorphism in KCNH2 was associated with effectiveness of domperidone ($p = 0.041$). The efficacious dose was associated with polymorphism in ABCB1 gene ($p = 0.0277$). The side-effects of domperidone were significantly associated with the SNPs in the promoter region of *ADRA1D* gene.

Conclusions.—Genetic characteristics associated with response to domperidone therapy included polymorphisms in the drug transporter gene

ABCB1, the potassium channel *KCNH2* gene, and α_{1D}—adrenoceptor *ADRA1D* gene. Age was associated with a beneficial response to domperidone. If verified in a larger population, this information might be used to help determine which patients with gastroparesis might respond to domperidone and avoid treatment in those who might develop side-effects (Fig 1).

▶ Domperidone is an old drug but remains widely used as a prokinetic (in part because there are relatively few alternatives). It is a dopamine receptor antagonist; dopamine inhibits gut motility. Although not approved in the United States by the Food and Drug Administration, under an Investigational New Drug program, the drug can be prescribed through compounding pharmacies. Some patients obtain the drug from Canada and Mexico. However, domperidone has potential side effects such as increased prolactin secretion (causing galactorrhea), and it may rarely prolong the QT interval causing serious arrhythmias. Interestingly, in this study older age was significantly associated with a better treatment response, which the authors speculate might be explained by dopamine receptors decreasing with age, so domperidone may be more efficient in the elderly. A goal of personalized medicine is to improve the benefit to risk ratio with drug therapy, and for this reason this study is worth reading.

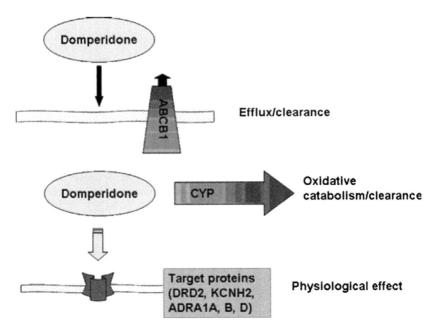

FIGURE 1.—Modulators of domperidone physiological activity. Modulators of domperidone physiological activity include the drug transporter ABCB1, the drug-metabolizing enzyme CYP2D6, and targets of domperidone (dopamine receptor D2, DRD2, α1-adrenergic receptors ADRA1A-D, and myocardial ion channels KCNE1/2, KCNH2, and KCNQ1). (Reprinted from Parkman HP, Jacobs MR, Mishra A, et al. Domperidone treatment for gastroparesis: demographic and pharmacogenetic characterization of clinical efficacy and side-effects. *Dig Dis Sci.* 2011;56:115-124, with permission from Springer Science+Business Media, LLC.)

While it represents proof of concept study and the sample size was small, the results suggest that gene testing (Fig 1) will have a role in prescribing prokinetic treatments in the near future.

N. J. Talley, MD, PhD

Clinical Features of Idiopathic Gastroparesis Vary With Sex, Body Mass, Symptom Onset, Delay in Gastric Emptying, and Gastroparesis Severity
Parkman HP, on behalf of the National Institute of Diabetes and Digestive and Kidney Diseases Gastroparesis Clinical Research Consortium (Temple Univ, Philadelphia, PA; et al)
Gastroenterology 140:101-115, 2011

Background & Aims.—Idiopathic gastroparesis (IG) is a common but poorly understood condition with significant morbidity. We studied characteristics of patients with IG enrolled in the National Institute of Diabetes and Digestive and Kidney Diseases Gastroparesis Clinical Research Consortium Registry.

Methods.—Data from medical histories, symptom questionnaires, and 4-hour gastric emptying scintigraphy studies were obtained from patients with IG.

Results.—The mean age of 243 patients with IG studied was 41 years; 88% were female, 46% were overweight, 50% had acute onset of symptoms, and 19% reported an initial infectious prodrome. Severe delay in gastric emptying (>35% retention at 4 hours) was present in 28% of patients. Predominant presenting symptoms were nausea (34%), vomiting (19%), an abdominal pain (23%). Women had more severe nausea, satiety, constipation, and overall gastroparesis symptoms. Patients who experienced acute-onset IG had worse nausea than those with insidious onset. Overweight patients had more bloating and gastric retention at 2 hours but less severe loss of appetite. Patients with severely delayed gastric emptying had worse vomiting and more severe loss of appetite and overall gastroparesis symptoms. Severe anxiety and depression were present in 36% and 18%, respectively. A total of 86% met criteria for functional dyspepsia, primarily postprandial distress syndrome.

Conclusions.—IG is a disorder that primarily affects young women, beginning acutely in 50% of cases; unexpectedly, many patients are overweight. Severe delay in gastric emptying was associated with more severe symptoms of vomiting and loss of appetite. IG is a diverse syndrome that varies by sex, body mass, symptom onset, and delay in gastric emptying.

▶ This important article raises the question, what is gastroparesis, and how is it distinguished from functional dyspepsia (FD; where about one-third of cases also have slow gastric emptying)? In the Parkman study, a group of experts in gastroparesis reviewed patients referred to a registry with a diagnosis of gastroparesis (based on upper gastrointestinal symptoms and slow gastric emptying, confirmed using the gold standard 4-hour scintigraphic test). Most of the patients were women who also fulfilled the Rome III criteria for functional (nonulcer) dyspepsia (86%), with the majority having symptoms consistent with postprandial distress syndrome (PDS; characterized by early satiety [inability to finish a normal-sized meal] and/or postprandial fullness).[1] Patients in this series with more severe delays of gastric emptying (> 35% retention at 4 hours) had more vomiting and loss of appetite. Distinguishing gastroparesis from FD is not just academic; treatment options for patients with gastroparesis (but not FD) who do not respond to standard medical therapy include nutritional support and venting where needed with a percutaneous endoscopic gastrostomy or percutaneous endoscopic jejunostomy tube, gastric electrical stimulation (which helps symptoms but not gastric emptying), possibly botulinum toxin injection into the pylorus (which is controversial), and gastric surgery as a last resort. Based on this study, it seems reasonable to restrict the term gastroparesis to those whose stomach is truly paralyzed (very slow emptying), leading to recurrent nausea and vomiting, and anorexia often with weight loss. This would reduce the number of cases labeled as gastroparesis and help clinicians to avoid confusion.

N. J. Talley, MD, PhD

Reference

1. Tack J, Talley NJ. Gastroduodenal disorders. *Am J Gastroenterol.* 2010;105: 757-763.

A 13-nation population survey of upper gastrointestinal symptoms: Prevalence of symptoms and socioeconomic factors

Haag S, Andrews JM, Gapasin J, et al (Univ Hosp Essen, Germany; Univ of Adelaide, South Australia, Australia; St Lukes Med Ctr, Quezon City, Philippines; et al)
Aliment Pharmacol Ther 33:722-729, 2011

Background.—Previous data collected in separate studies using various different survey instruments have suggested some variability in the prevalence of symptoms between nations. However, there is a lack of studies which assess and compare the prevalence of upper gastrointestinal symptoms contemporaneously in various countries using a uniform, standardised method.

Aim.—To determine the prevalence of upper gastrointestinal (UGI) symptoms in 13 European countries, and the association between socioeconomic factors and symptoms using a standardised method.

Methods.—A representative age- and gender-stratified sample of 23 163 subjects (aged 18–69 years) was surveyed.

Results.—The prevalence of UGI symptoms was 38%. UGI symptoms were most prevalent in Hungary [45%, 95% confidence interval (CI): 42.2–48.4] and lowest in the Netherlands (24%, 95% CI: 21.0–26.2). UGI symptoms were more prevalent in women (39%, 95% CI: 38.4–39.6) vs. men (37%, 95% CI: 36.4–37.6). Heartburn (24%, 95% CI:

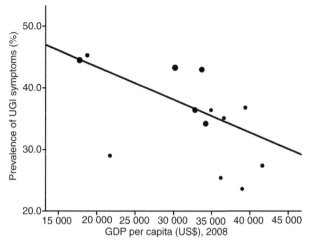

FIGURE 4.—Correlation of gross domestic productivity per capita in $ with prevalence of upper GI symptoms (● = small countries, sample size $n = 1000$; ● = large countries, sample size $n = 3000$), $r = -0.58$, $P = 0.004$. (Reprinted from Haag S, Andrews JM, Gapasin J, et al. A 13-nation population survey of upper gastrointestinal symptoms: prevalence of symptoms and socioeconomic factors. *Aliment Pharmacol Ther.* 2011;33:722-729, with permission from Blackwell Publishing Ltd.)

23.4—24.6) and acidic reflux (14%, 95% CI: 13.6—14.4) were most common. With age, the prevalence of UGI symptoms decreased (e.g. 18—29 years: 43%, 95% CI: 41.4—44.3 vs. 50—69 years: 33%, 95% CI: 32.3—34.4); in contrast, the frequency of symptom episodes/year increased with age (e.g. 18—29 years: 11.3 episodes per years, 95% CI: 10.5—12.1 vs. 50—69 years: 21.8, 95% CI: 20.7—22.9). Socioeconomic status as measured by gross domestic product was inversely associated with symptoms and in total, socioeconomic factors, gender, body mass index, smoking habits and alcohol consumption explained 83% of the variance of UGI symptoms.

Conclusions.—There are marked differences in the country specific prevalence of upper gastrointestinal complaints. Socioeconomic factors are closely associated with the prevalence of upper gastrointestinal symptoms (Fig 4).

▶ The data from this large European study suggest that dyspepsia and reflux may be determined in part by socioeconomic status (Fig 4). In particular, lower income was correlated with a higher prevalence of upper gastrointestinal (GI) symptoms. Most patients with dyspepsia in the community do not have a peptic ulcer, reflux esophagitis, or cancer as the cause and are labeled as having functional dyspepsia (FD). The dyspepsia data are consistent with other studies linking an increased risk of FD to acute GI infections (postinfectious FD), presumably because those who live in poorly hygienic or overcrowded environments would be more likely to be exposed to GI pathogens and experience acute gastroenteritis. An alternative explanation may be dietary differences in those who are less well off. Diets high in fat have been linked to dyspepsia, although this would likely be important only in a predisposed individual. Although this study is not definitive, the results suggest that more work is needed to evaluate the potential role of environmental factors in dyspepsia and reflux, including infections and diet.

N. J. Talley, MD, PhD

Dramatic Decline in Prevalence of *Helicobacter pylori* and Peptic Ulcer Disease in an Endoscopy-referral Population
McJunkin B, Sissoko M, Levien J, et al (West Virginia Univ Health Sciences Ctr, Charleston)
Am J Med 124:260-264, 2011

Purpose.—To determine if endoscopic *Helicobacter pylori* and peptic ulcer disease prevalence has changed over an 11-year period in a rural region.

Methods.—Current endoscopic records were reviewed and compared with similar data obtained over a time period 11 years earlier at the same institution with regard to *H. pylori* status, endoscopic findings, microscopic pathologic findings, and medication use.

Results.—There were 251 records reviewed in the current study group (mean age 52.8 years, 59.0% female) and 263 in the previous group (mean age 60.1 years, 56.7% female). *H. pylori* was positive in 17 (6.8%) in the current study and 173 (65.8%) in the earlier study (*P* <.0001). Peptic ulcer disease (PUD) was present in 14 (5.6%) in the current study and in 102 (38.8%) in the earlier study (*P* <.0001). *H. pylori* was positive in 1 of the 14 PUD patients (7.1%) in the current study and in 78 of 102 (76.5%) in the previous study (*P* <.0001).

Conclusions.—Endoscopic *H. pylori* prevalence in our rural locality has decreased substantially over the past decade and may reflect local overall prevalence trends, although underestimation is likely due to widespread prior noninvasive *H. pylori* diagnosis and treatment. Endoscopic PUD also has decreased precipitously, possibly related to changes in regional *H. pylori* characteristics and prolific use of antisecretory agents. Changing geographic trends regarding acid-peptic disease may prompt modification of diagnostic approach and treatment (Fig 1).

▶ The striking decline in *Helicobacter pylori* prevalence reported in this article (Fig 1) is consistent with other observations in developed countries worldwide. Most authorities believe this is largely explained by a cohort phenomenon (better hygiene in childhood leading to a substantial reduction in acquisition of *H pylori* in younger generations). Obviously, more aggressive treatment of *H pylori* infection may also contribute depending on practice patterns. Importantly, the data have implications for current management strategies for patients presenting with uninvestigated dyspepsia. The test and treat strategy has been recommended for patients presenting with previously uninvestigated dyspepsia

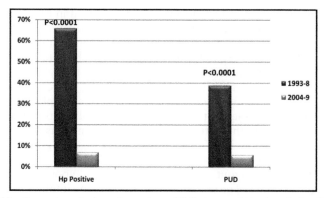

FIGURE 1.—Comparison of endoscopic prevalence of *Helicobacter pylori* and peptic ulcer disease during time periods 11 years apart. Hp = *H. pylori*; PUD = peptic ulcer disease. (Reprinted from McJunkin B, Sissoko M, Levien J, et al. Dramatic decline in prevalence of Helicobacter pylori and peptic ulcer disease in an endoscopy-referral population. *Am J Med.* 2011;124:260-264, Copyright 2011, with permission from Elsevier.)

(ie, recurrent or chronic epigastric pain or discomfort for at least a month). In this strategy, noninvasive testing for *H pylori* is performed and typically triple therapy to cure the infection is recommended for those who test *H pylori* positive rather than referral for upper endoscopy or empiric proton pump inhibitor (PPI) therapy. However, to be cost effective, the test and treat strategy requires the background *H pylori* prevalence to be at least over 10%, and this may no longer be the case in many parts of the United States. An alternative approach, namely an empiric trial of a PPI, may now become the approach of choice for uninvestigated dyspepsia; early endoscopy in the absence of alarm features (such as weight loss, bleeding, or vomiting) is not recommended, as there are robust data that this approach is just more costly and outcomes are not improved. The article does not describe whether the rates of gastroesophageal reflux disease have increased in parallel with the decline in *H pylori* prevalence in this region, but other data suggest this association is true and further support the concept of empiric PPI therapy as first line therapy for dyspepsia. If PPI fails, testing for and treating *H pylori*, and a consideration of upper endoscopy, remain the next steps.

N. J. Talley, MD, PhD

Bitter taste receptors and α-gustducin regulate the secretion of ghrelin with functional effects on food intake and gastric emptying
Janssen S, Laermans J, Verhulst P-J, et al (Catholic Univ of Leuven, Belgium)
Proc Natl Acad Sci U S A 108:2094-2099, 2011

Ghrelin is a hunger hormone with gastroprokinetic properties but the factors controlling ghrelin secretion from the stomach are unknown. Bitter taste receptors (T2R) and the gustatory G proteins, α-gustducin (gust) and α-transducin, are expressed in the gut and are involved in the chemosensation of nutrients. This study aimed to investigate whether T2R-agonists affect (*i*) ghrelin release via α-gustducin and (*ii*) food intake and gastric emptying via the release of ghrelin. The mouse stomach contains two ghrelin cell populations: cells containing octanoyl and desoctanoyl ghrelin, which were colocalized with α-gustducin and α-transducin, and cells staining for desoctanoyl ghrelin. Gavage of T2R-agonists increased plasma octanoyl ghrelin levels in WT mice but the effect was partially blunted in gust$^{-/-}$ mice. Intragastric administration of T2R-agonists increased food intake during the first 30 min in WT but not in gust$^{-/-}$ and ghrelin receptor knockout mice. This increase was accompanied by an increase in the mRNA expression of agouti-related peptide in the hypothalamus of WT but not of gust$^{-/-}$ mice. The temporary increase in food intake was followed by a prolonged decrease (next 4 h), which correlated with an inhibition of gastric emptying. The delay in emptying, which was partially counteracted by ghrelin, was not mediated by cholecystokinin and GLP-1 but involved a direct inhibitory effect of T2R-agonists on gastric contractility. This study is unique in providing functional evidence that activation of bitter taste receptors stimulates ghrelin secretion. Modulation of endogenous ghrelin levels by tastants may provide novel therapeutic applications for the treatment of weight -and gastrointestinal motility disorders.

▶ This is fascinating! Taste receptors are present in the tongue epithelium and consist of 2 G protein—coupled receptor families, T1R (for sweet) and T2R (for bitter). The study confirms that the luminal gut also has taste receptors. Essentially, the accumulating evidence suggests that the gut "tastes" what we eat and modifies gastrointestinal function accordingly, although the exact neural and hormonal pathways need to be defined. Here, evidence is presented that bitter taste receptors in the gut stimulate the ghrelin pathway. You may remember that when energy balance goes negative, ghrelin (a 28—amino acid peptide) is secreted by the "X/A-like" cells in the gastric oxyntic glands. Plasma ghrelin levels peak before a meal and decrease shortly after food consumption, influencing meal timing. In the fasted state via ghrelin receptors, ghrelin stimulates food intake, decreases fat utilization, induces gastric hunger contractions, and accelerates gastric emptying. Based on these results, in the future it may be possible to develop compounds that are tasted by the mucosa and lead to endogenous release of ghrelin in those with anorexia nervosa (to increase appetite) or functional dyspepsia (to reduce symptoms by accelerating gastric emptying), or formulations that are tasted and block ghrelin release (eg, to reduce appetite in obesity).

N. J. Talley, MD, PhD

Eosinophil Counts in Upper Digestive Mucosa of Western European Children: Variations With Age, Organs, Symptoms, *Helicobacter pylori* Status, and Pathological Findings

Kalach N, Huvenne H, Gosset P, et al (Catholic Univ of Lille, France; Saint Vincent de Paul Hosp, France; et al)

J Pediatr Gastroenterol Nutr 52:175-182, 2011

Aim.—The aim of the study was to measure the number of eosinophils per high-power field (eos/HPF) according to age, organs, and clinical symptoms and to compare the results to histological characteristics of the upper digestive tract mucosa in children.

Patients and Methods.—A systematic prospective assessment of 284 esophagus, 342 antrum, 453 corpus, and 167 duodenum biopsies was carried out in 316 girls and 366 boys referred for endoscopy (median age 9 months), eos/HPF, and histological analysis.

Results.—Counts (mean—max SD) were as follows: esophagus 1.73 to 50 eos/HPF (5.35), antrum 3.27 to 40 (4.7), corpus 2.11 to 38 (3.76), and duodenum 4.80 to 46 (7.7). Counts >15 eos/HPF were found in 2.8% esophagi, 3.5% corpora, 4.9% antra, and 10.7% duodena. Duodenal eos/HPF were significantly higher than those of esophageal, corporeal, and antral. Mucosal eos/HPF increased with age in esophagus and antrum. The highest esophageal eos/HPF were significantly associated with recurrent abdominal pain, and with anemia in antrum, corpus, and duodenum. Major and/or minor histological features of eosinophilic esophagitis were seen in 9 of 10 esophagi with 5 to 15 eos/HPF and 7 of 8 esophagi with >15 eos/HPF. Eosinophils per high-power field were significantly correlated with histological antral and corporeal gastric inflammation. *Helicobacter pylori*—positive children had higher eosinophils per high-power field than *H pylori* negative ones both in esophagus and in antrum.

Conclusions.—The present study shows that in a western European country mucosal hypereosinophilia is rare. Mucosal eosinophil counts increase from esophagus to duodenum, and also with age in esophagus and antrum. The highest eos/HPF in the esophagus are associated with recurrent abdominal pain and in the corpus, antrum, and duodenum with anemia. Features of eosinophilic esophagitis are rare but detectable in association with counts as low as 6 eos/HPF (Fig 1).

▶ There is increasing interest in the relationship between quantitative histological findings and unexplained gastrointestinal (GI) symptoms. Pathologists know that the gut normally is in a state of physiological inflammation, but we now know that if the pathologist takes the time to count the cells, some apparently normal biopsies from patients with functional or unexplained GI disorders actually have significantly increased cells (vs normal controls). The best example is eosinophilic esophagitis, as noted in the present pediatric article (Fig 1), but other examples are now rising to prominence. Thus, in adult and pediatric patients with functional dyspepsia, especially those who complain of early satiety, increased eosinophils have been noted to be present in the

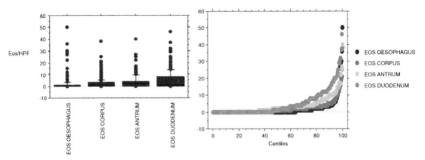

FIGURE 1.—The distribution of eos/HPF in the different parts of the upper digestive tract (esophagus, corpus, antrum, and duodenum), presented in box plot (left) and as centiles (right). eos/HPF = eosinophils per high-power field. (Reprinted from Kalach N, Huvenne H, Gosset P, et al. Eosinophil counts in upper digestive mucosa of western European children: variations with age, organs, symptoms, *Helicobacter pylori* status, and pathological findings. *J Pediatr Gastroenterol Nutr.* 2011;52:175-182, Copyright 2011 by the AAP, with permission from Journal of Pediatric Gastroenterology and Nutrition.)

duodenum (especially in the first portion). In this study, recurrent abdominal pain was linked to esophageal eosinophilia, a finding that needs to be confirmed. In contrast, increased mast cells (but not eosinophils) have been documented to be present in irritable bowel syndrome in both the small and large intestine. This pediatric study confirms other reports that eosinophils are increased in the setting of *H pylori* infection, so it is important to test for this infection in the setting of increased GI tissue eosinophilia. The rare disease eosinophilic gastroenteritis also needs to be excluded (by taking multiple biopsies from esophagus, stomach, and duodenum), but here there are typically dense sheets of eosinophils in very high numbers in some sections (unless the disease fails to involve the mucosa, which is unusual).

N. J. Talley, MD, PhD

Gastroparesis

Randomised clinical trial: ghrelin agonist TZP-101 relieves gastroparesis associated with severe nausea and vomiting - randomised clinical study subset data

Wo JM, Ejskjaer N, Hellström PM, et al (Univ of Louisville School of Medicine, KY; Aarhus Univ Hosp, DK; Uppsala Univ, Sweden; et al)
Aliment Pharmacol Ther 33:679-688, 2011

Background.—Limited therapeutic options exist for severe gastroparesis, where severe nausea and vomiting can lead to weight loss, dehydration and malnutrition due to inadequate caloric and fluid intake. TZP-101 (ulimorelin) is a ghrelin receptor agonist that accelerates gastric emptying and improves upper gastrointestinal symptoms in diabetic patients with gastroparesis.

Aim.—To assess effects of TZP-101 in diabetic gastroparesis patients with severe nausea/vomiting and baseline severity scores of ≥3.5 (range:

0—5) on the Gastroparesis Cardinal Symptom Index (GCSI) Nausea/ Vomiting subscale.

Methods.—Patients were hospitalised and received four single daily 30-min infusions of one of six TZP-101 doses (range 20—600 µg/kg) or placebo. Efficacy was assessed by symptom improvement.

Results.—At baseline, 23 patients had a mean severity score for GCSI Nausea/Vomiting of 4.45 ± 0.44. Statistically significant improvements over placebo occurred in the 80 µg/kg group for end of treatment changes from baseline in GCSI Nausea/Vomiting subscale (reduction in score of −3.82 ± 0.76, $P = 0.011$) and the GCSI Total score (−3.14 ± 0.78, $P = 0.016$) and were maintained at the 30-day follow-up assessment (−2.02 ± 1.63, $P = 0.073$ and −1.99 ± 1.33, $P = 0.032$ respectively).

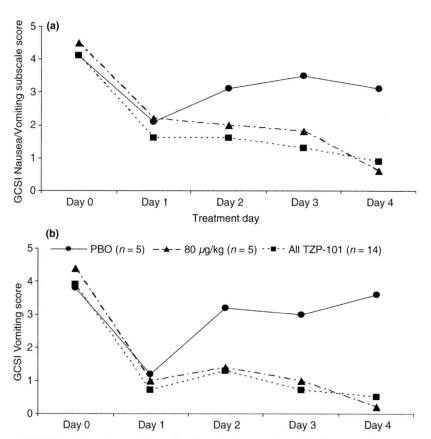

FIGURE 3.—Change in mean Nausea/Vomiting subscale scores (a) and Vomiting scores (b) over time. The slopes for days 1—4 in (a) are significantly different for the 80 µg/kg group vs. placebo ($P < 0.001$) and All TZP-101 vs. placebo ($P = 0.004$), and in (b) for 80 µg/kg group vs. placebo ($P = 0.008$) and All TZP-101 vs. placebo ($P = 0.005$). (Reprinted from Wo JM, Ejskjaer N, Hellström PM, et al. Randomised clinical trial: ghrelin agonist TZP-101 relieves gastroparesis associated with severe nausea and vomiting - randomised clinical study subset data. *Aliment Pharmacol Ther.* 2011;33:679-688, with permission from Blackwell Publishing Ltd.)

The proportion of days with vomiting was reduced significantly ($P = 0.05$) in the 80 μg/kg group (mean of 1.2 days of vomiting for four treatment days) compared with placebo (mean of 3.2 days of vomiting across 4 treatment days).

Conclusions.—TZP-101 substantially reduced the frequency and severity of nausea and vomiting as well as overall gastroparesis symptoms. The results are consistent with gastrointestinal motility effects of TZP-101, supporting further investigation of TZP-101 in the management of severe gastroparesis (Fig 3).

▶ Gastroparesis continues to be a difficult disorder to manage. Despite controlling blood sugar if diabetic and employing appropriate dietary approaches (eg, low-fat, low-fiber small meals up to 6 times a day and splitting solids and liquids, or a nutrient liquid—only diet) plus combined antiemetic (eg, promethazine) and prokinetic therapy (eg, metoclopramide or domperidone), many patients remain miserable and impaired. Metoclopramide is well known to be associated with serious side effects, including irreversible tardive dyskinesia. In those admitted for an acute exacerbation of gastroparesis with recurrent vomiting, rehydration, tight control of blood sugar if diabetic, and intravenous medical therapy are standards of care. Options then include gastric electrical stimulation or surgery, but success is limited. One new class of agents that may provide a benefit, including for acute exacerbations of gastroparesis, are the grhelin agonists. Ghrelin is a gastric peptide hormone that has prokinetic properties and coordinates motor function. This small trial in a subset of diabetic gastroparesis patients with severe nausea and vomiting suggests that 4 days of treatment with an intravenous ghrelin agonist (TZP-101) reduced symptoms (Fig 3) and was well tolerated versus placebo. More trials testing this promising line of treatment are anxiously awaited.

N. J. Talley, MD, PhD

Acupuncture in Critically Ill Patients Improves Delayed Gastric Emptying: A Randomized Controlled Trial
Pfab F, Winhard M, Nowak-Machen M, et al (Univ Hosp Regensburg, Germany; Brigham and Women's Hosp, Boston, MA; et al)
Anesth Analg 112:150-155, 2011

Background.—Malnutrition remains a severe problem in the recovery of critically ill patients and leads to increased in-hospital morbidity and in-hospital stay. Even though early enteral nutrition has been shown to improve overall patient outcomes in the intensive care unit (ICU), tubefeed administration is often complicated by delayed gastric emptying and gastroesophageal reflux. Acupuncture has been successfully used in the treatment and prevention of perioperative nausea and vomiting. In this study we evaluated whether acupuncture can improve gastric emptying in comparison with standard promotility drugs in critically ill patients receiving enteral feeding.

Methods.—Thirty mechanically ventilated neurosurgical ICU patients with delayed gastric emptying, defined as a gastric residual volume (GRV) >500 mL for ≥2 days, were prospectively and randomly assigned to either the acupoint stimulation group (ASG; bilateral transcutaneous electrical acupoint stimulation at Neiguan, PC-6) or the conventional promotility drug treatment group (DTG) over a period of 6 days (metoclopramide, cisapride, erythromycin). Patients in the ASG group did not receive any conventional promotility drugs. Successful treatment (feeding tolerance) was defined as GRV <200 mL per 24 hours.

Results.—Demographic and hemodynamic data were similar in both groups. After 5 days of treatment, 80% of patients in the ASG group successfully developed feeding tolerance versus 60% in the DTG group. On treatment day 1, GRV decreased from 970 ± 87 mL to 346 ± 71 mL with acupoint stimulation ($P = 0.003$), whereas patients in the DTG group showed a significant increase in GRV from 903 ± 60 mL to 1040 ± 211 mL ($P = 0.015$). In addition, GRV decreased and feeding balance (defined as enteral feeding volume minus GRV) increased in more patients in the ASG group (14 of 15) than in the DTG group (7 of 15; $P = 0.014$). On treatment day 1, the mean feeding balance was significantly higher in the ASG group (121 ± 128 mL) than in the DTG group (−727 ± 259 mL) ($P = 0.005$). Overall, the feeding balance improved significantly on all

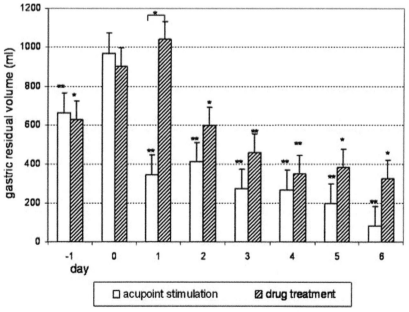

FIGURE 1.—Mean gastric residual volume per day. The asterisks indicate significant (*$P < 0.05$) or highly significant (**$P < 0.01$) differences in comparison to day 0 within each group. The brackets mark comparison between groups on day 1. (Reprinted from Pfab F, Winhard M, Nowak-Machen M, et al. Acupuncture in critically ill patients improves delayed gastric emptying: a randomized controlled trial. *Anesth Analg.* 2011;112:150-155, with permission from International Anesthesia Research Society.)

days of treatment in comparison with the DTG group. Patients in the DTG group did not show an increase in feeding balance until day 6.

Conclusions.—We introduce a new protocol for acupuncture administration in the critical care setting. We demonstrated that this protocol was more effective than standard promotility medication in the treatment of delayed gastric emptying in critically ill patients. Acupoint stimulation at Neiguan (PC-6) may be a convenient and inexpensive option (with few side effects) for the prevention and treatment of malnutrition in critically ill patients (Fig 1).

▶ The role of acupuncture in medicine remains highly controversial, but this study suggests that acupoint stimulation via transcutaneous electrical neural stimulation is feasible and equivalent to standard medical therapy in terms of increased feeding tolerance in patients with acute gastroparesis in an intensive care unit setting (Fig 1). The study had a number of limitations: no placebo control group, variable medical therapy (some received cisapride, others erythromycin in the medical therapy arm), and the fact that delayed gastric emptying was not directly measured but assessed only by gastric residual volume. Further evidence is necessary before acupuncture can be accepted as efficacious for gastroparesis, but additional, rigorously designed trials are warranted. If it does work, data on combination treatment would also be of major interest. Other data support acupressure reducing nausea and vomiting.[1]

N. J. Talley, MD, PhD

Reference

1. Lee A, Fan LT. Stimulation of the wrist acupuncture point P6 for preventing postoperative nausea and vomiting. *Cochrane Database Syst Rev.* 2009;(2). CD003281.

Irritable Bowel Syndrome

Clinical predictors of small intestinal bacterial overgrowth by duodenal aspirate culture

Choung RS, Ruff KC, Malhotra A, et al (Mayo Clinic, Rochester, MN; Mayo Clinic, Scottsdale, AZ)
Aliment Pharmacol Ther 33:1059-1067, 2011

Background.—There has been increasing interest in small intestinal bacterial overgrowth (SIBO) after reports of a link with irritable bowel syndrome (IBS), yet our understanding of this entity is limited.

Aim.—Our aim was to estimate the yield of patients undergoing duodenal aspirate culture, and to identify symptoms and features that predict SIBO.

Methods.—A medical chart review of patients who had undergone duodenal aspirate culture at an academic medical centre in 2003 was performed to record clinical characteristics and culture results. The associations between aspirate results and symptoms, medical diagnoses and medication use were assessed using logistic regression.

Results.—A total of 675 patients had available aspirate results. Mean age of the sample was 53 (s.d. 17) and 443 (66%) were female patients. Overall, 8% of aspirates were positive for SIBO; 2% of IBS patients had SIBO. Older age, steatorrhoea and narcotic use were associated with SIBO (*P* < 0.05). PPI use was not associated with SIBO, but was associated with bacterial growth not meeting criteria for SIBO (*P* < 0.05). Inflammatory bowel disease (IBD), small bowel diverticula and pancreatitis were positively associated with an abnormal duodenal aspirate (*P* < 0.05), but other conditions including IBS were not associated with SIBO.

Conclusion.—While older age, steatorrhoea, narcotic use, IBD, small bowel diverticula and pancreatitis were associated with small intestinal bacterial overgrowth based on abnormal duodenal aspirate culture results, no clear associations of true small intestinal bacterial overgrowth with IBS or PPI use were detected in contrast to recent speculation.

▶ The importance of small bowel bacterial overgrowth in irritable bowel syndrome (IBS) remains controversial. Based on glucose or lactulose hydrogen breath testing, there is good evidence that patients with IBS are more likely to have abnormal breath testing suggestive of bacterial overgrowth.[1] However, an alternative explanation for abnormal breath testing in this setting remains rapid intestinal transit with the sugar load reaching the cecum early and leading to an abnormal or early elevated peak. On the other hand, there are randomized controlled trial data that say the nonabsorbable antibiotic rifaximin does lead to an improvement of IBS symptoms in a subset of patients with nonconstipation IBS (with the number needed to treat = 10; see the article by Pimentel et al in this issue). This report by Choung and colleagues from Mayo Clinic is a large retrospective study that suggests that IBS is not associated with bacterial overgrowth. Other studies have also failed to confirm that classical bacterial overgrowth (defined as culturing from duodenal aspirates with a bacterial colony count of > 10^5) occurs in IBS, although there were increased bacterial counts of lower magnitude in IBS found in a French study.[2] Overall, while nonabsorbable antibiotic therapy may have a benefit in a subset of patients with IBS for reasons that remain to be explained, the data that link this efficacy with small bowel bacterial overgrowth are tenuous at best. The value of breath testing in IBS therefore is highly questionable and at this time should not form a part of routine management of suspected IBS.

N. J. Talley, MD, PhD

References

1. Spiegel BM. Questioning the bacterial overgrowth hypothesis of irritable bowel syndrome: an epidemiologic and evolutionary perspective. *Clin Gastroenterol Hepatol.* 2011;9:461-469.
2. Posserud I, Stotzer PO, Björnsson ES, Abrahamsson H, Simrén M. Small intestinal bacterial overgrowth in patients with irritable bowel syndrome. *Gut.* 2007;56: 802-808.

Mucosal inflammation as a potential etiological factor in irritable bowel syndrome: a systematic review

Ford AC, Talley NJ (Leeds Gastroenterology Inst, UK; Univ of Newcastle, New South Wales, Australia)
J Gastroenterol 46:421-431, 2011

Background.—The causes of irritable bowel syndrome (IBS) remain obscure. Some investigators have proposed chronic low-grade mucosal inflammation as a potential etiological factor. We performed a systematic review to examine this issue in detail.

Methods.—MEDLINE, EMBASE, and EMBASE classic were searched up to December 2010 to identify studies of case—control design applying tests for low-grade inflammation to either full-thickness intestinal or endoscopic mucosal biopsies from patients with IBS. Controls were required to be healthy individuals, or asymptomatic patients undergoing investigation for reasons other than the reporting of upper or lower gastrointestinal symptoms. Individual study results were summarized descriptively.

Results.—The literature search identified 1388 citations, of which 16 studies were eligible for inclusion. Individual study results were diverse, partly as a consequence of the different surrogate markers for inflammatory mechanisms studied. Mast cells, T lymphocytes, B lymphocytes, and mucosal cytokine production all appeared altered among cases with IBS in individual studies, while no study demonstrated a significant difference in numbers of plasma cells, neutrophils, or eosinophils. Some studies suggested a relationship between mast cell abnormalities and symptom severity and frequency, as well as co-existent fatigue and depression. Studies were limited by the lack of comparability of controls, and the fact that most were conducted in highly selected groups of patients with IBS.

Conclusions.—Low-grade mucosal inflammation, particularly mast cell activation, may be a contributory factor in the pathogenesis of IBS. Mast cell stabilizers warrant further assessment as a potential therapy in the condition.

▶ Irritable bowel syndrome (IBS) is one of the functional gastrointestinal disorders where, by definition, there is no evidence of structural or biochemical derangements. However, this definition appears to becoming rapidly outdated. Based on a careful and detailed literature review, the authors of this systematic review conclude that there is definitive evidence of an abnormal inflammatory cell infiltration in IBS, particularly by mast cells in a subset. Many of these patients do not have an obvious precipitating event such as acute bacterial gastroenteritis. There is also evidence for mucosal activation of the immune system in patients with IBS, suggesting a change to a TH2 response, akin to inflammatory bowel disease albeit much more subtle. Mast cell infiltration appears to be associated with symptoms not only in the gastrointestinal tract but also extraintestinally (eg, fatigue and depression). The data imply that a potential therapeutic approach for IBS may be anti-inflammatory or mast cell antagonists. Preliminary data suggest 5-aminosalicylic acid[1] and mast cell blocking drugs[2] could be useful, although this needs to be established by appropriately powered randomized controlled trials and exactly which population with IBS should be so treated needs to be defined. Alteration of the intestinal flora with antibiotics or probiotics might also alter the inflammatory cascade (and perhaps this is how rifaximin works?). This paradigm shift, in our understanding of IBS, is an important space for clinicians to watch because in the future it may be possible to alter the natural history of IBS by offering appropriate anti-inflammatory therapy rather than current symptom-based treatments.

N. J. Talley, MD, PhD

References

1. Corinaldesi R, Stanghellini V, Cremon C, et al. Effect of mesalazine on mucosal immune biomarkers in irritable bowel syndrome: a randomized controlled proof-of-concept study. *Aliment Pharmacol Ther.* 2009;30:245-252.
2. Klooker TK, Braak B, Koopman KE, et al. The mast cell stabilizer ketotifen visceral hypersensitivity and improves intestinal symptoms in patients with irritable bowel syndrome. *Gut.* 2010;59:1213-1220.

Combined oro-caecal scintigraphy and lactulose hydrogen breath testing demonstrate that breath testing detects oro-caecal transit, not small intestinal bacterial overgrowth in patients with IBS

Yu D, Cheeseman F, Vanner S (Queen's Univ, Kingston, Ontario, Canada)
Gut 60:334-340, 2011

Objectives.—Recent studies using the lactulose hydrogen breath test (LHBT) suggest most patients with irritable bowel syndrome (IBS) have small intestinal bacterial overgrowth (SIBO). However, the validity of the LHBT has been questioned, particularly as this test could reflect changes in oro-caecal transit. Therefore, we combined oro-caecal scintigraphy with LHBT in 40 patients who were Rome II positive for IBS to determine if the increase in hydrogen is due to the test meal reaching the caecum.

Design.—Patients ingested the test meal containing ^{99m}Tc and 10 g lactulose and simultaneous measurements of the location of the test meal using scintigraphic scanning and breath hydrogen levels were obtained every 10 min for 3 h. The LHBT was considered positive when the rise in H_2 above baseline was >20 ppm within 90 and/or 180 min. The combined test was negative for SIBO if ≥5% of the test meal was in the caecum at the time the LHBT was positive.

Results.—63% had an abnormal LHBT at 180 min and 35% at 90 min. The oro-caecal transit time based on scintigraphic scanning ranged from 10 to 220 min and correlated with IBS sub-type. At the time of increase in H_2, the % accumulation of ^{99m}Tc in the caecum was ≥5% in 88% of cases (22/25).

Conclusions.—These findings demonstrate that an abnormal rise in H_2 measured in the LHBT can be explained by variations in oro-caecal transit time in patients with IBS and therefore do not support the diagnosis of SIBO (Figs 1 and 2).

▶ The theory that small intestinal bacterial overgrowth (SIBO) explains a subset of irritable bowel syndrome (IBS) continues to be controversial. It has been speculated that intestinal dysmotility in IBS leads to pockets of stasis colonized by bacteria that ferment food substrates, releasing excess gas that distends the bowel, inducing pain and bloating. There is no doubt that a large subset of patients with IBS have abnormal lactulose hydrogen (H2) breath testing, depending on the cutoffs applied (Fig 1), as was confirmed in this study. However, this finding does not necessarily reflect small bowel bacterial breakdown of the sugar load. Importantly, this study suggests that in most cases, rapid intestinal transit is the explanation for the abnormal H2 breath testing in IBS, because the sugar load then quickly reaches the cecum where hydrogen is released and absorbed (Fig 2). Other data suggest there may be increased bacterial counts in a subset of patients with IBS based on quantitative culture of duodenal juice (although much less than is found in classical bacterial overgrowth).[1] In some cases, this finding seems to be accounted for by proton pump inhibitor use, which, because of profound acid suppression, leads to

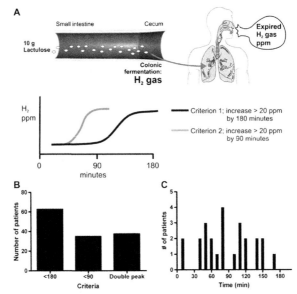

FIGURE 1.—The lactulose hydrogen breath test (LHBT). (A) Schematic drawing demonstrating the basic concept of the LHBT. Lactulose, a non-hydrolysable sugar, is ingested and transits the small intestine. It undergoes fermentation when in contact with 'colonic-type' bacteria and H_2 gas is absorbed and expired in the lungs. Sequential breath samples are analysed for the concentration of H_2, in ppm. Previous studies used two main criteria for studies of irritable bowel syndrome (IBS), outlined on bottom right. (B) Proportion of patients with IBS and with an abnormal breath test based on 180 min, 90 min and double peak criteria. (C) Time from ingestion to an abnormal H_2 level (in ppm). (Reprinted from Yu D, Cheeseman F, Vanner S. Combined oro-caecal scintigraphy and lactulose hydrogen breath testing demonstrate that breath testing detects oro-caecal transit, not small intestinal bacterial overgrowth in patients with IBS. *Gut.* 2011;60:334-340.)

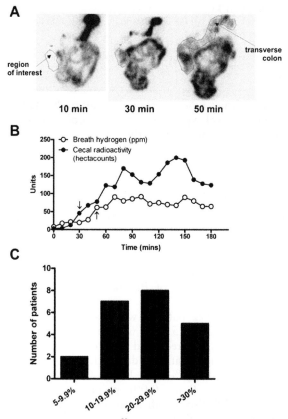

FIGURE 2.—Analysis of the combined ^{99m}Tc scintigraphic and lactulose hydrogen breath test (LHBT). (A) Representative images at times 0, 30 and 50 min from a scan of a patient with irritable bowel syndrome (IBS). (B) A plot from the same patient showing the radioactive counts in the caecum over time (from region of interest, small ellipse in A.) and the LHBT. At 30 min (downward arrow), the test meal has reached the caecum as determined by the sharp increase in radioactive counts shown in B. The breath test was positive at 50 min (upward arrow) and total colonic counts (large irregular ellipse in right scan)/total body counts is 10%. C Shows the per cent accumulation of the ^{99m}Tc signal for all patients at the time the LHBT is positive. Five per cent was the threshold for a normal test (ie, colonic vs SIBO) but most patients had >10% accumulation before the breath test was positive. (Reprinted from Yu D, Cheeseman F, Vanner S. Combined oro-caecal scintigraphy and lactulose hydrogen breath testing demonstrate that breath testing detects oro-caecal transit, not small intestinal bacterial overgrowth in patients with IBS. *Gut.* 2011;60:334-340.)

increased small bowel bacteria counts.[2] Although nonabsorbable antibiotic therapy does provide a real, albeit modest, benefit in IBS,[3] this benefit now appears unlikely to be explained by correction of SIBO in most cases.

N. J. Talley, MD, PhD

References

1. Posserud I, Stotzer PO, Björnsson ES, Abrahamsson H, Simrén M. Small intestinal bacterial overgrowth in patients with irritable bowel syndrome. *Gut.* 2007;56: 802-808.

2. Choung RS, Ruff KC, Malhotra A, et al. Clinical predictors of small intestinal bacterial overgrowth by duodenal aspirate culture. *Aliment Pharmacol Ther.* 2011;33:1059-1067.
3. Pimentel M, Lembo A, Chey WD, et al. Rifaximin therapy for patients with irritable bowel syndrome without constipation. *N Engl J Med.* 2011;364:22-32.

Randomised clinical trial: *Bifidobacterium bifidum* MIMBb75 significantly alleviates irritable bowel syndrome and improves quality of life – a double-blind, placebo-controlled study

Guglielmetti S, Mora D, Gschwender M, et al (Università degli Studi di Milano, Milan, Italy; Director of the nutritional study, Munich, Germany; et al)
Aliment Pharmacol Ther 33:1123-1132, 2011

Background.—Recent research suggests that an imbalance of the intestinal microbiota and a dysfunctional intestinal barrier might trigger irritable bowel syndrome (IBS). As probiotics have been reported to restore the intestinal microbiota and the gut barrier, the therapeutic potential of probiotics within IBS became of strong interest.

Aim.—To assess the efficacy of *Bifidobacterium bifidum* MIMBb75 in IBS.

Methods.—A total of 122 patients were randomised to receive either placebo ($N = 62$) or MIMBb75 ($N = 60$) once a day for 4 weeks. The severity of IBS symptoms was recorded daily on a 7-point Likert scale.

Results.—MIMBb75 significantly reduced the global assessment of IBS symptoms by -0.88 points (95% CI: -1.07; -0.69) when compared with only -0.16 (95% CI: -0.32; 0.00) points in the placebo group ($P < 0.0001$). MIMBb75 also significantly improved the IBS symptoms pain/discomfort, distension/bloating, urgency and digestive disorder. The evaluation of the SF12 sum scores showed a significant gain in quality of life within the bifidobacteria group. Furthermore, adequate relief was reported by 47% of the patients in the bifidobacteria and only by 11% of the patients in the placebo group ($P < 0.0001$). Overall responder rates were 57% in the bifidobacteria group but only 21% in the placebo group ($P = 0.0001$). MIMBb75 was well tolerated and adverse events were not different from placebo.

Conclusions.—*Bifidobacterium bifidum* MIMBb75 effectively alleviates global IBS and improves IBS symptoms simultaneously with an improvement of quality of life. Considering the high efficacy of MIMBb75 in IBS along with the good side-effect profile, MIMBb75 is a promising candidate for IBS therapy (Fig 3).

▶ There is increasing interest in the role of probiotics in irritable bowel syndrome (IBS), based on the simplistic concept that flooding the gut with live "good" bacteria may replace harmful species and reduce abnormal fermentation of food (reducing gas production) or modulate increased gut permeability and low-grade inflammation linked to IBS. In randomized placebo-controlled trials,

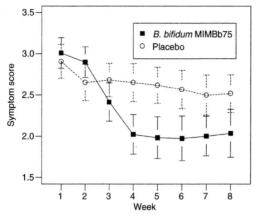

FIGURE 3.—Comparison of effects of placebo and *B. bifidum* MIMBb75 on global IBS symptoms (by SGA, recorded on a 0—6 scale) on a weekly basis. Significant improvement of global IBS symptoms in the bifidobacteria group vs. placebo. (Reprinted from Guglielmetti S, Mora D, Gschwender M, et al. Randomised clinical trial: *Bifidobacterium bifidum* MIMBb75 significantly alleviates irritable bowel syndrome and improves quality of life — a double-blind, placebo-controlled study. *Aliment Pharmacol Ther.* 2011;33:1123-1132, with permission from Blackwell Publishing Ltd.)

a specific subspecies *Bifidobacterium infantis* has been shown to be superior to placebo, but the evidence in favor of other probiotics is equivocal or negative.[1] A recent meta-analysis included 10 trials involving 918 patients and found that overall, probiotics were significantly better than placebo in IBS (with a number needed to treat of 4), but there was significant heterogeneity, suggesting more data are necessary to establish efficacy and identify optimal preparations.[2] In contrast, probiotic therapy ion appears to be safe. The present trial suggests another species of *Bifidobacterium* may have efficacy in IBS (Fig 3), although this was a relatively small study of short duration (4 weeks), and the response of IBS subtypes could not be evaluated. In my practice, I do prescribe a probiotic for my patients with IBS as adjunctive therapy, but it is costly, and we need much more information on how to optimize therapy (species, dose, duration, IBS subtypes that are likely to respond and not respond, etc).

N. J. Talley, MD, PhD

References

1. Brenner DM, Moeller MJ, Chey WD, Schoenfeld PS. The utility of probiotics in the treatment of irritable bowel syndrome: a systematic review. *Am J Gastroenterol.* 2009;104:1033-1049.
2. Moayyedi P, Ford AC, Talley NJ, et al. The efficacy of probiotics in the treatment of irritable bowel syndrome: a systematic review. *Gut.* 2010;59:325-332.

Abdomino-Phrenic Dyssynergia in Patients With Abdominal Bloating and Distension

Villoria A, Azpiroz F, Burri E, et al (Univ Hosp Vall d'Hebron, Barcelona, Spain; et al)
Am J Gastroenterol 106:815-819, 2011

Objectives.—The abdomen normally accommodates intra-abdominal volume increments. Patients complaining of abdominal distension exhibit abnormal accommodation of colonic gas loads (defective contraction and excessive protrusion of the anterior wall). However, abdominal imaging demonstrated diaphragmatic descent during spontaneous episodes of bloating in patients with functional gut disorders. We aimed to establish the role of the diaphragm in abdominal distension.

Methods.—In 20 patients complaining of abdominal bloating and 15 healthy subjects, we increased the volume of the abdominal cavity with a colonic gas load, while measuring abdominal girth and electromyographic activity of the anterior abdominal muscles and of the diaphragm.

Results.—In healthy subjects, the colonic gas load increased girth, relaxed the diaphragm, and increased anterior wall tone. With the same gas load, patients developed significantly more abdominal distension; this was associated with paradoxical contraction of the diaphragm and relaxation of the internal oblique muscle.

Conclusions.—In this experimental provocation model, abnormal accommodation of the diaphragm is involved in abdominal distension (Fig 4).

▶ Why do some patients with irritable bowel syndrome (IBS) or functional abdominal bloating have visible abdominal distention? The correct answer to this question could lead to new therapies, which is significant given that current management options are limited. Antigas therapies such as charcoal or simethicone are of unproven value. Rifaximin, a nonabsorbable antibiotic tested in IBS, may reduce bloating in a small subset, although any benefit in visible distention is uncertain and use of the drug is off label. Elegant physiological experiments in humans, including the present study, now suggest we may be closer to uncovering the truth. Visible distention is not imagined; it can be objectively demonstrated by imaging (eg, CT scan). Gas retention does occur in a subset with IBS because intestinal transit is slow. Slow transit may set the scene for bacterial overgrowth. In turn, abnormal fermentation of food because of excess small intestinal bacteria may produce a small increase in gas load with intestinal distention in a subset. And because of underlying intestinal hypersensitivity, this may be perceived as discomfort or pain. Now new observations suggest there is an abnormal abdominophrenic adaptation to increased intra-abdominal content in IBS with distention. In striking contrast to healthy control subjects, patients with unexplained distention had paradoxical contraction of their diaphragm; in addition, the anterior wall muscles failed to contract, and the internal oblique relaxed (Fig 4). Thus, abdominal distension appears to be associated with abnormal activity of the diaphragm (abnormal "accommodation" of the diaphragm). Could this in part be a learned behavioral response to

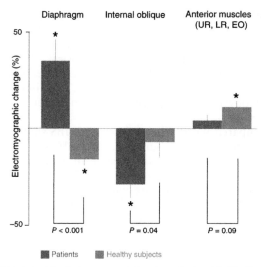

FIGURE 4.—Distorted abdominal accommodation in patients with bloating. Note paradoxical contraction of the diaphragm, relaxation of the internal oblique, and impaired contraction of the other anterior muscles (upper rectus (UR), lower rectus (LR), and external oblique (EO)). Data are mean ± s.e. of Δ values (average of last 20 minutes minus basal in each study). *P < 0.05 vs. basal. (Reprinted by permission from Macmillan Publishers Ltd: American Journal of Gastroenterology. Villoria A, Azpiroz F, Burri E, et al. Abdomino-phrenic dyssynergia in patients with abdominal bloating and distension. *Am J Gastroenterol.* 2011;106:815-819, Copyright 2011, with permission from the American College of Gastroenterology.)

discomfort, analogous to air swallowing (aerophagia) or effortless regurgitation of pleasant tasting food after meals (rumination), and could this reflex respond to specific biofeedback interventions? It is possible we will see new approaches in the future for patients with visible distention based on these novel observations.

N. J. Talley, MD, PhD

Intestinal Serotonin Release, Sensory Neuron Activation, and Abdominal Pain in Irritable Bowel Syndrome

Cremon C, Carini G, Wang B, et al (Univ of Bologna, Italy; St Joseph's Healthcare, Hamilton, Ontario, Canada; et al)
Am J Gastroenterol 106:1290-1298, 2011

Objectives.—Serotonin (5-hydroxytryptamine, 5-HT) metabolism may be altered in gut disorders, including in the irritable bowel syndrome (IBS). We assessed in patients with IBS vs. healthy controls (HCs) the number of colonic 5-HT-positive cells; the amount of mucosal 5-HT release; their correlation with mast cell counts and mediator release, as well as IBS symptoms; and the effects of mucosal 5-HT on electrophysiological responses *in vitro*.

Methods.—We enrolled 25 Rome II IBS patients and 12 HCs. IBS symptom severity and frequency were graded 0–4. 5-HT-positive enterochromaffin cells and tryptase-positive mast cells were assessed with quantitative immunohistochemistry on colonic biopsies. Mucosal 5-HT and mast cell mediators were assessed by high-performance liquid chromatography or immunoenzymatic assay, respectively. The impact of mucosal 5-HT on electrophysiological activity of rat mesenteric afferent nerves was evaluated *in vitro*.

Results.—Compared with HCs, patients with IBS showed a significant increase in 5-HT-positive cell counts ($0.37 \pm 0.16\%$ vs. $0.56 \pm 0.26\%$; $P < 0.039$), which was significantly greater in patients with diarrhea-predominant IBS vs. constipation-predominant IBS ($P < 0.035$). Compared with HCs, 5-HT release in patients with IBS was 10-fold significantly increased ($P < 0.001$), irrespective of bowel habit, and was correlated with mast cell counts. A significant correlation was found between the mucosal 5-HT release and the severity of abdominal pain ($r_s = 0.582$, $P < 0.047$). The area under the curve, but not peak sensory afferent discharge evoked by IBS samples in rat jejunum, was significantly inhibited by the 5-HT$_3$ receptor antagonist granisetron ($P < 0.005$).

Conclusions.—In patients with IBS, 5-HT spontaneous release was significantly increased irrespective of bowel habit and correlated with mast cell counts and the severity of abdominal pain. Our results suggest

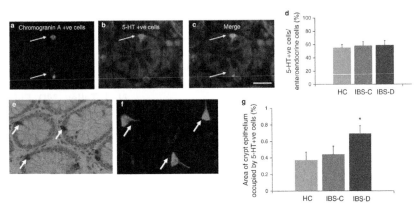

FIGURE 1.—Upper panels (a–c) show representative photomicrographs of chromogranin A-positive enteroendocrine cells (a), 5-hydroxytryptamine (5-HT)-positive enterochromaffin cells (b), and double staining (c). Note that about 50–60% of chromogranin A-positive enteroendocrine cells also expressed 5-HT immunolabelling (arrows) either in patients with irritable bowel syndrome (IBS) or in healthy controls (HC) (c, d). Lower panels show representative photomicrographs of 5-HT-positive enterochromaffin cells in an IBS patient by means of immunohistochemistry (e) and immunofluorescence (f). Overall, IBS patients showed a significant increase in the count of 5-HT-positive cells, as compared with HC (*P = 0.039; Mann–Whitney test) (g). However, the 5-HT-positive cell count was significantly greater in diarrhea-predominant IBS (IBS-D) in comparison with constipation-predominant IBS (IBS-C) (P = 0.035; Mann–Whitney test) (g). Calibration bar = 25 µm. (Reprinted by permission from Macmillan Publishers Ltd: American Journal of Gastroenterology. Cremon C, Carini G, Wang B, et al. Intestinal serotonin release, sensory neuron activation, and abdominal pain in irritable bowel syndrome. *Am J Gastroenterol.* 2011;106:1290-1298, Copyright 2011, with permission from the American College of Gastroenterology.)

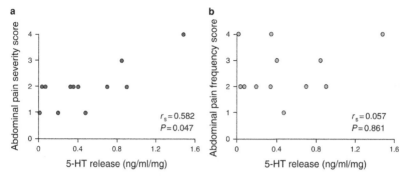

FIGURE 3.—Correlation between severity (**a**) and frequency (**b**) of abdominal pain/discomfort and the spontaneous release of 5-hydroxytryptamine (5-HT) from colonic mucosa ($r_s = 0.582$, $P = 0.047$ and $r_s = 0.057$, $P = 0.861$, respectively; Spearman's correlation). No correlation was found between sponta-neous release of 5-HT and other irritable bowel syndrome (IBS) symptoms, including bowel habit. No correlation was found between 5-HT-positive cells and IBS symptoms. (Reprinted by permission from Macmillan Publishers Ltd: *American Journal of Gastroenterology.* Cremon C, Carini G, Wang B, et al. Intestinal serotonin release, sensory neuron activation, and abdominal pain in irritable bowel syndrome. *Am J Gastroenterol.* 2011;106:1290-1298, Copyright 2011, with permission from the American College of Gastroenterology.)

that increased 5-HT release contributes to development of abdominal pain in IBS, probably through mucosal immune activation (Figs 1 and 3).

▶ Irritable bowel syndrome (IBS) is common, affecting at least 10% of Americans, and remains difficult to manage, resulting in high costs to the health care system. Accumulating evidence now implicates intestinal pathology in driving the clin-ical features of IBS. This elegant study suggests that serotonin dysregulation plays a key role in inducing abdominal pain in IBS (Fig 1) and may account in part for the clinical benefit of serotonin type 3 receptor antagonists, such as alo-setron. It also appears likely that abnormal serotonin release from the enterochro-maffin cells in IBS may occur secondary to mast cells in a subset (Fig 3), suggesting that inhibition of mast cell infiltration and/or degranulation may have therapeutic benefits. At the present time, IBS cannot be cured, but these results provide hope that by further unlocking the pathogenesis in the intestine, novel therapies will become available for this condition that result in permanent remission.

N. J. Talley, MD, PhD

A Randomized Controlled Trial of *Lactobacillus* GG in Children With Functional Abdominal Pain

Francavilla R, Miniello V, Magistà AM, et al (Univ of Bari, Italy; et al)
Pediatrics 126:e1445-e1452, 2010

Objective.—Our aim was to determine whether *Lactobacillus rhamno-sus* GG (LGG) relieves symptoms in children with recurrent abdominal pain.

Patients and Methods.—A total of 141 children with irritable bowel syndrome (IBS) or functional pain were enrolled in 9 primary care sites and a referral center. Children entered a randomized, double-blind, placebo-controlled trial and received LGG or placebo for 8 weeks and entered follow-up for 8 weeks. The primary outcome was overall pain at the end of the intervention period. At entry and at the end of the trial, children underwent a double-sugar intestinal permeability test.

Results.—Compared with baseline, LGG, but not placebo, caused a significant reduction of both frequency $(P < .01)$ and severity $(P < .01)$ of abdominal pain. These differences still were significant at the end of follow-up $(P < .02$ and $P < .001$, respectively). At week 12, treatment success was achieved in 48 children in the LGG group compared with 37 children in the placebo group $(P < .03)$; this difference still was present at the end of follow-up $(P < .03)$. At entry, 59% of the children had abnormal results from the intestinal permeability test; LGG, but not placebo, determined a significant decrease in the number of patients with abnormal results from the intestinal permeability testing $(P < .03)$. These effects mainly were in children with IBS.

Conclusions.—LGG significantly reduces the frequency and severity of abdominal pain in children with IBS; this effect is sustained and may be secondary to improvement of the gut barrier.

▶ The efficacy of probiotics in functional gastrointestinal disorders remains controversial. In particular, it remains unclear which bacteria are truly efficacious and whether the organisms must be viable to provide a benefit (many commercial shelf products after a number of weeks will have no viable organisms present); even the correct dose is uncertain, with mixed results in the literature. Arguably, the most robust data exist for *Bifidobacterium infantis* in irritable bowel syndrome (IBS), while *lactobacillus* has appeared more disappointing, but even here there is uncertainty. A meta-analysis concluded that probiotics overall were superior to placebo in adults with IBS, with a number needed to treat of 4, but there was significant heterogeneity.[1] The benefit of individual products was unable to be clarified in this review. In this randomized trial of *lactobacillus* GG in children for recurrent abdominal pain, there was an impressive reduction in pain frequency and severity on treatment that persisted for 2 months after treatment (Fig 2 in the original article). This suggests the product changes the natural history of IBS after therapy, akin to nonabsorbable antibiotic therapy (rifaximin). *Lactobacillus* treatment also improved intestinal permeability; 60% were abnormal at baseline among the subgroup that had testing, and a significant improvement in patients on *lactobacillus* but not placebo was observed (Fig 3 in the original article). Some have speculated that at least a subset of IBS is initiated by breaks in the intestinal barrier, perhaps secondary to infection, that sets up a mild but abnormal inflammatory response, inducing cytokine production and setting up a vicious cycle.[2] Healing the barrier with a probiotic approach, therefore, may be worth considering, but more studies are needed in children and adults, including head to head comparisons of promising commercially available products. Much longer follow-up is also needed to document the duration of benefit after therapy. However, based on the apparent safety of probiotic therapy, its use in IBS in clinical practice seems reasonable at this time.

N. J. Talley, MD, PhD

References

1. Moayyedi P, Ford AC, Talley NJ, et al. The efficacy of probiotics in the treatment of irritable bowel syndrome: a systematic review. *Gut.* 2010;59:325-332.
2. Walker MM, Warwick A, Ung C, Talley NJ. The role of eosinophils and mast cells in intestinal functional disease. *Curr Gastroenterol Rep.* 2011;13:323-330.

Organic colonic lesions in 3,332 patients with suspected irritable bowel syndrome and lacking warning signs, a retrospective case—control study
Gu H-X, Zhang Y-L, Zhi F-C, et al (Southern Med Univ, Guangzhou, China)
Int J Colorectal Dis 26:935-940, 2011

Purpose.—The diagnosis of irritable bowel syndrome is symptom based, and colonoscopy is the most direct way to rule out organic colonic diseases. It is controversial on the necessity of colonoscopy for patients with suspected irritable bowel syndrome and lacking alarm features. This study was designed to verify the organic lesions and discuss the value of colonoscopy in this type of patient.

Methods.—Colonoscopy of 3,332 patients with suspected irritable bowel syndrome and lacking warning signs from 2000 to 2009 were reviewed. One thousand five hundred eighty-eight patients under 50 years of age who underwent colonoscopy screening for health care in the same period were used as controls. The prevalence of different colonic organic lesions was compared between two groups.

Results.—Organic colonic lesions were found in 30.3% of the patients with suspected irritable bowel syndrome (1,010/3,332) and 39.0% of the controls (619/1,588). Compared with controls, patients with suspected irritable bowel syndrome had higher prevalence of noninflammatory bowel disease and noninfectious colitis and terminal ileitis, however, had lower prevalence of diverticular disease, adenomatous polyps, and non-adenomatous polyps (all $P<0.001$).

Conclusions.—The diagnostic sensitivity of symptom criteria on irritable bowel syndrome without colonoscopy is not more than 69.7% in patients with suspected irritable bowel syndrome lacking warning signs. Though the method of colonoscopy is hard to screen tumor in this type of patients, it is beneficial to uncover some other relevant organic lesions such as terminal ileitis. Colonoscopy should not be refused to suspected irritable bowel syndrome patients without warning signs.

▶ Many patients who present with irritable bowel syndrome (IBS)-like symptoms end up undergoing a colonoscopy despite the absence of alarm features. Gastroenterologists are trained to do procedures, and with referral filtering, they are more likely to encounter rare events (eg, colon cancer in a 20 year old); therefore, they naturally have a low threshold for doing the test. However, there remains controversy about the potential risks (which are real) versus benefits of colonoscopy in IBS. Current American College of Gastroenterology guidelines do not recommend a colonoscopy for patients under the age of 50 without warning signs or symptoms. In this Chinese study, it is particularly interesting to note that IBS appeared to be protective in terms of finding polyps, both adenomatous and nonadenomatous. The reasons why IBS may be protective are unknown, but other evidence supports these observations. As expected, patients with IBS were more likely to be found to have evidence of inflammation in the colon. Others have reported that patients with microscopic colitis were more likely to present with IBS-like symptoms. Overall, the data from this study are reassuring and support current guidelines; colonoscopy is not usually indicated for those with typical IBS symptoms unless the patient is older (50 years and more) or there are alarm features, such as rectal bleeding, unexplained weight loss, or a strong family history of colon cancer.

N. J. Talley, MD, PhD

Linaclotide Improves Abdominal Pain and Bowel Habits in a Phase IIb Study of Patients With Irritable Bowel Syndrome With Constipation

Johnston JM, Kurtz CB, MacDougall JE, et al (Ironwood Pharmaceuticals, Inc, Cambridge, MA; et al)
Gastroenterology 139:1877-1886, 2010

Background & Aims.—Linaclotide, a minimally absorbed, 14-amino acid peptide agonist of guanylate cyclase-C, has shown benefit in a proof-of-concept study for the treatment of patients with irritable bowel syndrome (IBS) with constipation (IBS-C). We assessed the efficacy and safety of linaclotide at a daily dose range of 75–600 μg in IBS-C.

Methods.—We performed a randomized, double-blind, multicenter, placebo-controlled study of 420 patients with IBS-C given oral linaclotide at doses of 75, 150, 300, or 600 μg or placebo once daily for 12 weeks. End points included change from baseline in daily bowel habits, daily abdominal symptoms, and weekly global assessments, in addition to responder criteria.

Results.—All doses of linaclotide significantly improved bowel habits, including frequency of spontaneous bowel movements and complete spontaneous bowel movements (primary end point), severity of straining, and stool consistency. Abdominal pain was significantly reduced from baseline, compared with placebo; mean changes in abdominal pain (assessed on a 5-point scale) from baseline were −0.71, −0.71, −0.90, and −0.86 for linaclotide doses of 75, 150, 300, and 600 μg, respectively, compared with −0.49 for placebo. Likewise, most doses of linaclotide significantly improved other abdominal symptoms, including discomfort and bloating, and global measures of IBS-C compared with placebo. Effects were observed within the first week and were sustained throughout 12 weeks of treatment. Except for diarrhea, the incidence of adverse events was similar between placebo and linaclotide groups.

Conclusions.—Linaclotide, across a wide range of doses, significantly improved symptoms of IBS-C, including abdominal pain and bowel symptoms. Diarrhea was the only dose-dependent adverse event and was usually of mild or moderate severity (Fig 1).

▶ Treatment options for patients with constipation-predominant irritable bowel syndrome (IBS) are limited.[1] Fiber often makes patients feel worse although psyllium may help a subset. Osmotic laxatives (eg, polyethylene glycol) can help constipation, but any benefit on the global IBS complex is uncertain. Anticholinergics are constipating. Lubiprostone, a selective chloride channel activator, is of modest benefit. Selective serotonin reuptake inhibitors theoretically may accelerate intestinal transit and do appear to have a benefit in IBS, although adequate IBS subgroup data are unavailable. Linaclotide is in a new drug class; it acts locally on the guanylate cyclase-C receptor to induce chloride, bicarbonate, and fluid secretion into the intestine. Linaclotide increases colonic transit and improves stool consistency and ease of passage; proof-of-concept randomized controlled trials such as this one (Fig 1) support its application in chronic

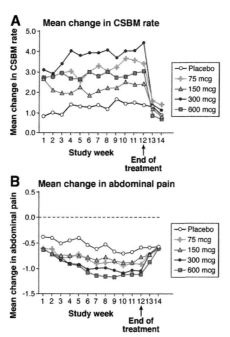

FIGURE 1.—Weekly mean change from baseline in CSBM rate (*A*) and abdominal pain (*B*) for linaclotide 75, 150, 300, and 600 μg and placebo. (Reprinted from Johnston JM, Kurtz CB, MacDougall JE, et al. Linaclotide improves abdominal pain and bowel habits in a phase IIb study of patients with irritable bowel syndrome with constipation. *Gastroenterology.* 2010;139:1877-1886 Copyright 2010, with permission from the AGA Institute.)

(functional) constipation and constipation-predominant IBS. One note of caution: This study did not screen for pelvic floor dysfunction (eg, by anorectal manometry and balloon expulsion testing) even though these patients had significant constipation. Pelvic floor dysfunction (or functional outlet obstruction) is a potentially curable condition with biofeedback (about 70% respond), usually is resistant to laxatives, and may account for some of the treatment failures.[2]

N. J. Talley, MD, PhD

References

1. American College of Gastroenterology Task Force on Irritable Bowel Syndrome, Brandt LJ, Chey WD, Foxx-Orenstein AE, et al. An evidence-based position statement on the management of irritable bowel syndrome. *Am J Gastroenterol.* 2009; 104:S1-35.
2. Chiarioni G, Whitehead WE, Pezza V, Morelli A, Bassotti G. Biofeedback is superior to laxatives for normal transit constipation due to pelvic floor dyssynergia. *Gastroenterology.* 2006;130:657-664.

Irritable bowel syndrome and risk of colorectal cancer: a Danish nationwide cohort study

Nørgaard M, Farkas DK, Pedersen L, et al (Aarhus Univ Hosp, Aalborg, Denmark)
Br J Cancer 104:1202-1206, 2011

Background.—Little is known about the risk of colorectal cancer among patients with irritable bowel syndrome (IBS).

Methods.—We conducted a nationwide cohort study using data from the Danish National Registry of Patients and the Danish Cancer Registry from 1977 to 2008. We included patients with a first-time hospital contact for IBS and followed them for colorectal cancer. We estimated the expected number of cancers by applying national rates and we computed standardised incidence ratios (SIRs) by comparing the observed number of colorectal cancers with the expected number. We stratified the SIRs according to age, gender, and time of follow-up.

Results.—Among 57 851 IBS patients, we identified 407 cases of colon cancer during a combined follow-up of 506 930 years (SIR, 1.14 (95% confidence interval (CI): 1.03–1.25) and 115 cases of rectal cancer, corresponding to a SIR of 0.67 (95% CI: 0.52–0.85). In the first 3 months after an IBS diagnosis, the SIR was 8.42 (95% CI: 6.48–10.75) for colon cancer and 4.81 (95% CI: 2.85–7.60) for rectal cancer. Thereafter, the SIRs declined and 4–10 years after an IBS diagnosis, the SIRs for both colon and rectal cancer remained below 0.95.

Conclusion.—We found a decreased risk of colorectal cancer in the period 1–10 years after an IBS diagnosis. However, in the first 3 months after an IBS diagnosis, the risk of colon cancer was more than eight-fold increased and the risk of rectal cancer was five-fold increased. These increased risks are likely to be explained by diagnostic confusion because of overlapping symptomatology.

▶ The relationship between colorectal cancer and irritable bowel syndrome (IBS) has not been carefully investigated, but this is remedied by this large high-quality epidemiological study. At first glance, the results seem to suggest that patients who have IBS-like symptoms in the population are 8-fold more likely to have colorectal cancer, a frightening observation. However, when this was looked into more carefully, it becomes clear that this apparent increased risk is all because of detection bias. Overall, the risk of colon cancer is actually decreased in patients with long-standing IBS symptoms. The conclusions seem clear; colon cancer can present with IBS-like symptoms, but those with a firm diagnosis of IBS have a lower risk than normal for colon cancer (see also the Chinese study documenting a lower risk of adenomatous polyps in IBS in this volume). Why the risk of colon cancer is decreased in IBS is unknown. The data indicate that there is no requirement to change the current American College of Gastroenterology guidelines for diagnosis of IBS that recommend colonoscopy only in patients older than 50 years with IBS-like symptoms or those who have alarm features (eg, rectal bleeding, unexplained weight loss, or a strong family history of colon cancer).

N. J. Talley, MD, PhD

Rifaximin Therapy for Patients with Irritable Bowel Syndrome without Constipation

Pimentel M, for the TARGET Study Group (Cedars—Sinai Med Ctr, Los Angeles, CA; et al)
N Engl J Med 364:22-32, 2011

Background.—Evidence suggests that gut flora may play an important role in the pathophysiology of the irritable bowel syndrome (IBS). We evaluated rifaximin, a minimally absorbed antibiotic, as treatment for IBS.

Methods.—In two identically designed, phase 3, double-blind, placebo-controlled trials (TARGET 1 and TARGET 2), patients who had IBS without constipation were randomly assigned to either rifaximin at a dose of 550 mg or placebo, three times daily for 2 weeks, and were followed for an additional 10 weeks. The primary end point, the proportion of patients who had adequate relief of global IBS symptoms, and the key secondary end point, the proportion of patients who had adequate relief of IBS-related bloating, were assessed weekly. Adequate relief was defined as self-reported relief of symptoms for at least 2 of the first 4 weeks after treatment. Other secondary end points included the percentage of patients who had a response to treatment as assessed by daily self-ratings of global IBS symptoms and individual symptoms of bloating, abdominal pain, and stool consistency during the 4 weeks after treatment and during the entire 3 months of the study.

Results.—Significantly more patients in the rifaximin group than in the placebo group had adequate relief of global IBS symptoms during the first 4 weeks after treatment (40.8% vs. 31.2%, P = 0.01, in TARGET 1; 40.6% vs. 32.2%, P = 0.03, in TARGET 2; 40.7% vs. 31.7%, P<0.001, in the two studies combined). Similarly, more patients in the rifaximin group than in the placebo group had adequate relief of bloating (39.5% vs. 28.7%, P = 0.005, in TARGET 1; 41.0% vs. 31.9%, P = 0.02, in TARGET 2; 40.2% vs. 30.3%, P<0.001, in the two studies combined). In addition, significantly more patients in the rifaximin group had a response to treatment as assessed by daily ratings of IBS symptoms, bloating, abdominal pain, and stool consistency. The incidence of adverse events was similar in the two groups.

Conclusions.—Among patients who had IBS without constipation, treatment with rifaximin for 2 weeks provided significant relief of IBS symptoms, bloating, abdominal pain, and loose or watery stools. (Funded by Salix Pharmaceuticals; ClinicalTrials.gov numbers, NCT00731679 and NCT00724126.) (Fig 4).

▶ There is accumulating evidence that antibiotic therapy temporarily improves irritable bowel syndrome (IBS) symptoms. In a previous randomized controlled trial, 87 IBS patients who met Rome I criteria received 400 mg of rifaximin 3 times daily for 10 days or placebo; rifaximin resulted in greater improvement in global IBS symptoms and a lower bloating score over 10 weeks of follow-up.[1] These previous data suggested that a nonabsorbable antibiotic altered the natural history of IBS symptoms (the first treatment to be shown to alter the natural history of IBS at least over the short term). These results have

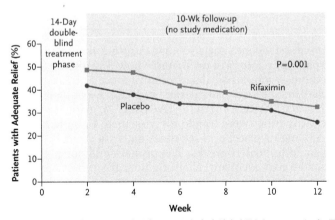

FIGURE 4.—Percentage of Patients with Adequate Relief of Global IBS Symptoms in the TARGET 1 and TARGET 2 Studies Combined. Adequate relief was defined as self-reported relief from symptoms for at least 1 week of every 2-week period. The P value was calculated on the basis of a longitudinal data analysis with the use of a generalized estimating equation model, with fixed effects of treatment, analysis center, and week. Similar figures for the individual TARGET 1 and TARGET 2 trials are shown in the Supplementary Appendix. (Reprinted from Pimentel M, for the TARGET Study Group. Rifaximin therapy for patients with irritable bowel syndrome without constipation. *N Engl J Med.* 2011;364:22-32, Copyright 2011, Massachusetts Medical Society. All rights reserved.)

been confirmed in the TARGET 1 and 2 Phase III trials. Although a higher dose was used and the new study excluded constipation-predominant IBS applying Rome III criteria, similar results were obtained (see Fig 4, with a number needed to treat of approximately 10). However, many questions remain. How durable is the effect (as the figure indicates, the effect wears off, and clinical experience suggests all patients relapse within several months). Strategies to maintain response and the effect of retreatment are also uncertain (some respond to retreatment, others do not). We do not know whether breath testing to identify possible small bowel bacterial overgrowth predicts response (it may not). Furthermore, we do not know how this drug works and why only a minority of patients respond to it. Therefore, a conservative approach to the use of off-label rifaximin for IBS seems appropriate until more data emerge.

N. J. Talley, MD, PhD

Reference

1. Pimentel M, Park S, Mirocha J, Kane SV, Kong Y. The effect of a nonabsorbed oral antibiotic (rifaximin) on the symptoms of the irritable bowel syndrome: a randomized trial. *Ann Intern Med.* 2006;145:557-563.

Physical Activity Improves Symptoms in Irritable Bowel Syndrome: A Randomized Controlled Trial
Johannesson E, Simrén M, Strid H, et al (Univ of Gothenburg, Sweden)
Am J Gastroenterol 106:915-922, 2011

Objectives.—Physical activity has been shown to be effective in the treatment of conditions, such as fibromyalgia and depression. Although these conditions are associated with irritable bowel syndrome (IBS), no study has assessed the effect of physical activity on gastrointestinal (GI) symptoms in IBS. The aim was to study the effect of physical activity on symptoms in IBS.

Methods.—We randomized 102 patients to a physical activity group and a control group. Patients of the physical activity group were instructed by a physiotherapist to increase their physical activity, and those of the control group were instructed to maintain their lifestyle. The primary end point was to assess the change in the IBS Severity Scoring System (IBS-SSS).

Results.—A total of 38 (73.7 % women, median age 38.5 (19—65) years) patients in the control group and 37 (75.7 % women, median age 36 (18—65) years) patients in the physical activity group completed the study. There was a significant difference in the improvement in the IBS-SSS score between the physical activity group and the control group (−51 (−130 and 49) vs. −5 (−101 and 118), $P = 0.003$). The proportion of patients with increased IBS symptom severity during the study was significantly larger in the control group than in the physical activity group.

Conclusions.—Increased physical activity improves GI symptoms in IBS. Physically active patients with IBS will face less symptom deterioration compared with physically inactive patients. Physical activity should be used as a primary treatment modality in IBS.

▶ The initial management of irritable bowel syndrome (IBS) typically includes dietary manipulation (classically with the slow introduction of increased fiber or a fiber supplement), reassurance, and stress reduction. However, many patients fail this approach and require medical therapy, although most drugs prescribed target individual symptoms rather than altering the natural history of the disorder. Uncontrolled data indicate that patients who attend a formal IBS class do better than control subjects; in these classes, instructions regarding stress reduction and diet are provided, and patients may be asked to increase their physical activity.[1] This is the first randomized controlled trial to test the efficacy of physical activity in IBS. The results are interesting because increased physical activity did appear to improve gastrointestinal symptoms, rather than simply improving sense of well-being (which exercise is known to do in many settings). Further work is necessary to confirm that physical activity is efficacious in IBS, but on the basis of the available evidence, clinicians should consider counseling their patients to increase their activity and providing encouragement and assistance for those who can do so.

N. J. Talley, MD, PhD

Reference

1. Saito YA, Prather CM, Van Dyke CT, Fett S, Zinsmeister AR, Locke GR 3rd. Effects of multidisciplinary education on outcomes in patients with irritable bowel syndrome. *Clin Gastroenterol Hepatol.* 2004;2:576-584.

Constipation

Vitamin D and Pelvic Floor Disorders in Women: Results From the National Health and Nutrition Examination Survey
Badalian SS, Rosenbaum PF (SUNY Upstate Med Univ, Syracuse, NY)
Obstet Gynecol 115:795-803, 2010

Objective.—To estimate the prevalence of vitamin D deficiency in women with pelvic floor disorders and to evaluate possible associations between vitamin D levels and pelvic floor disorders.

Methods.—Using 2005–2006 National Health and Nutrition Examination Survey data, we performed a cross-sectional analysis of nonpregnant women older than 20 years of age with data on both pelvic floor disorders and vitamin D measurements (n = 1,881). Vitamin D levels lower than 30 ng/mL were considered insufficient. The prevalence of demographic factors, pelvic floor disorders, and vitamin D levels were determined, accounting for the multi-stage sampling design; odds ratios (OR) and 95% confidence intervals (CI) were calculated to evaluate associations between vitamin D levels and pelvic floor disorders with control for known risk factors.

Results.—One or more pelvic floor disorders were reported by 23% of women. Mean vitamin D levels were significantly lower for women reporting at least one pelvic floor disorder and for those with urinary incontinence, irrespective of age. In adjusted logistic regression models, we observed significantly decreased risks of one or more pelvic floor disorders with increasing vitamin D levels in all women aged 20 or older (OR, 0.94; 95% CI, 0.88—0.99) and in the subset of women 50 years and older (OR, 0.92; 95% CI, 0.85—0.99). Additionally, the likelihood of urinary incontinence was significantly reduced in women 50 and older with vitamin D levels 30 ng/mL or higher (OR, 0.55; 95% CI, 0.34—0.91).

Conclusion.—Higher vitamin D levels are associated with a decreased risk of pelvic floor disorders in women.

▶ Pelvic floor disorders have been associated with osteoporosis. Vitamin D has been associated with severe osteoporosis but also muscle weakness. The study used data from the NHANES survey of Americans to show that lower vitamin D levels might predict pelvic floor disorders, especially pelvic organ prolapse and urinary and fecal incontinence. It appeared that lower levels of vitamin stores were associated with risk of pelvic floor disorders at all ages in adult women. Women older than 50 who had vitamin D levels higher than 30 had significantly fewer pelvic floor disorders than those with low levels. These symptoms were primarily urinary. The proposed mechanisms are related to the role of vitamin D in detrusor muscle function. Although one could conclude that vitamin D supplementation may be helpful, the possibility of a confounding explanation is possible. For example, vitamin D levels might be associated with sun exposure as a result of outdoor exercise; however, vitamin D deficiency can also occur in those exposed to sunlight. Nonetheless, this study will prompt more studies to understand the link between vitamin D stores and pelvic floor disorders and indeed other functional complaints.

J. A. Murray, MD

Methane on Breath Testing Is Associated with Constipation: A Systematic Review and Meta-analysis

Kunkel D, Basseri RJ, Makhani MD, et al (Cedars-Sinai Med Ctr, Los Angeles, CA; et al)
Dig Dis Sci 56:1612-1618, 2011

Background.—A growing body of literature suggests an association between methane and constipation. Studies also link degree of methane production to severity of constipation and have shown constipation is improved following antibiotics.

Aims.—We aim to conduct a systematic review and meta-analysis to examine the cumulative evidence regarding the association between methane and constipation.

Methods.—A literature search was performed using MEDLINE and Embase to identify studies where the presence (or absence) of methane was assessed in constipated subjects. Search terms included "methane," "breath test," constipation," "motility," "transit," "irritable bowel syndrome" and/or "IBS." Pooled odds ratios were generated using a random effects model. In a separate analysis, studies that measured intestinal transit in methane and nonmethane subjects were systematically reviewed. Results Nine studies met inclusion criteria for the metaanalysis. Among these, 1,277 subjects were examined by breath testing ($N = 319$ methane producers and $N = 958$ methane non-producers). Pooling all studies, a significant association was found between methane on breath test and constipation (OR = 3.51, CI = 2.00–6.16). Among adults only, methane was significantly associated with constipation (OR = 3.47, CI = 1.84–6.54). Similar results were seen when only examining subjects with IBS (OR = 3.60, CI = 1.61–8.06). The systematic review identified eight additional papers which all demonstrated an association between methane and delayed transit.

Conclusions.—We demonstrate that methane present on breath testing is significantly associated with constipation in both IBS and functional constipation. These results suggest there may be merit in using breath testing in constipation. Moreover, methane may be used to identify candidates for antibiotic treatment of constipation.

▶ There is accumulating evidence that methane production in the gut, which arises from the intestinal flora, is linked to constipation. Approximately 15% of the population produces methane, and the acquisition of methane-producing bacteria appears to occur just after birth and persists for life. Animal model work supports the view that methane is linked to constipation, and this systematic review of the literature provides further support that, in humans, methane gas production is an important mechanism. This opens up the concept of use of antibiotics in a subset of patients with constipation who are methane producers, although this hypothesis needs to be rigorously tested in randomized, controlled trials. Whether rifaximin, a nonabsorbable antibiotic, will have any benefit in this setting is unclear, but the link between methane gas and constipation appears to be a conceptual advance of which gastroenterologists should at least be aware.

N. J. Talley, MD, PhD

The prevalence of chronic constipation and faecal incontinence among men and women with symptoms of overactive bladder
Coyne KS, Cash B, Kopp Z, et al (United BioSource Corporation, Bethesda, MD; Univ of Health Science, Bethesda, MD; Pfizer, Inc, NY; et al)
BJU Int 107:254-261, 2011

Objective.—To estimate the prevalence and overlap of overactive bladder (OAB), chronic constipation (CC) and faecal incontinence (FI) among a general population sample of adults in the USA.

Patients and Methods.—A cross-sectional internet-based survey of randomly selected panel members who were ≥40 years of age was conducted. Participants reported how often they experienced symptoms of OAB, CC and FI using Likert scales and modified Rome III criteria. Analyses were conducted to examine the overall prevalence of OAB, CC and FI in men and women separately and to characterize the extent of overlap between these conditions in participants with OAB vs those without OAB, and those participants with continent vs incontinent OAB.

Results.—The response rate for the survey was 62.2% and the final sample (N= 2000) included 927 men and 1073 women. The overall prevalence of OAB [defined as a response of ≥ 'sometimes' to urinary urgency (i.e. 'sometimes' or more often) or 'yes' to urinary urgency incontinence (UUI)] was 26.1% in men and 41.2% in women. The overall prevalence of CC was significantly lower in men than in women (15.3 vs 26.3%), but both men and women with OAB were significantly more likely to report CC (22.3 and 35.9% vs 5.7 and 6.7%, respectively, $P < 0.0001$). The overall prevalence of FI reported 'rarely' or more was 16.7% of men and 21.9% of women. Men and women with OAB were significantly more likely to report FI than those without OAB. FI was also more common in participants with incontinent OAB than in those with continent OAB. Logistic regressions controlling for demographic factors and comorbid conditions suggest that OAB status is a very strong predictor of CC, FI and overlapping CC and FI (odds ratios, range 3.55-7.96).

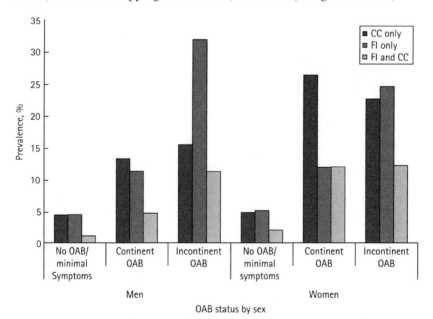

FIGURE 1.—Chronic constipation (CC) and faecal incontinence (FI) by overactive bladder (OAB) status. (Reprinted from Coyne KS, Cash B, Kopp Z, et al. The prevalence of chronic constipation and faecal incontinence among men and women with symptoms of overactive bladder. *BJU Int.* 2011;107:254-261, with permission from BJU International.)

Conclusions.—Chronic constipation, FI and overlapping CC and faecal incontinence occur more frequently in patients with OAB and should be considered when evaluating and treating patients with OAB. These findings suggest a shared pathophysiology among these conditions. Additional study is needed to determine if successful treatment of one or more of these conditions is accompanied by commensurate improvement in symptoms referable to the other organ system (Fig 1).

▶ The relationship between urinary symptoms and functional gastrointestinal disorders is poorly understood. In this population-based study from the United States, urinary urgency was applied as a surrogate measure of overactive bladder (although this is not necessarily the only explanation). Regardless, those experiencing urinary urgency were also more likely to report constipation and fecal incontinence (Fig 1). The frequent coexistence of functional urinary and gastrointestinal symptoms suggests the possibility of a common etiology, perhaps related to smooth muscle dysfunction. A systemic inflammatory response might theoretically drive such multiorgan dysfunction, and in a subset with irritable bowel syndrome (IBS), elevated cytokine levels have been observed. However, it is unclear how many of the subjects in this study also had IBS. However, mechanical compression in the setting of severe constipation might account for bladder dysfunction and explain a portion of the observations in this study. Fecal incontinence was loosely defined in the study and was rare (around 1%) using a stricter more clinically applicable cutoff, so these data should be considered with caution.

N. J. Talley, MD, PhD

Survivors of Childhood Cancer Have Increased Risk of Gastrointestinal Complications Later in Life

Goldsby R, Chen Y, Raber S, et al (UCSF Benioff Children's Hosp; Univ of Alberta, Edmonton, Canada; et al)
Gastroenterology 140:1464-1471, 2011

Background & Aims.—Children who receive cancer therapy experience numerous acute gastrointestinal (GI) toxicities. However, the long-term GI consequences have not been extensively studied. We evaluated the incidence of long-term GI outcomes and identified treatment-related risk factors.

Methods.—Upper GI, hepatic, and lower GI adverse outcomes were assessed in cases from participants in the Childhood Cancer Survivor Study, a study of 14,358 survivors of childhood cancer who were diagnosed between 1970 and 1986; data were compared with those from randomly selected siblings. The median age at cancer diagnosis was 6.8 years (range, 0−21.0 years), and the median age at outcome assessment was 23.2 years (5.6−48.9 years) for survivors and 26.6 years (1.85−6.2 years) for siblings. Rates of self-reported late GI complications (occurred 5 or more years after cancer diagnosis) were determined and associated with patient characteristics and cancer treatments, adjusting for age, sex, and race.

Results.—Compared with siblings, survivors had increased risk of late-onset complications of the upper GI tract (rate ratio [RR], 1.8; 95% confidence interval [CI], 1.6—2.0), liver (RR, 2.1; 95% CI, 1.8—2.5), and lower GI tract (RR, 1.9; 95% CI, 1.7—2.2). The RRs for requiring colostomy/ ileostomy, liver biopsy, or developing cirrhosis were 5.6 (95% CI, 2.4—13.1), 24.1 (95% CI, 7.5—77.8), and 8.9 (95% CI, 2.04—0.0), respectively. Older age at diagnosis, intensified therapy, abdominal radiation, and abdominal surgery increased the risk of certain GI complications.

Conclusions.—Individuals who received therapy for cancer during childhood have an increased risk of developing GI complications later in life (Fig 1).

▶ This is a fascinating study that suggests certain functional gastrointestinal (GI) disorders in addition to organic disease may develop up to 20 or more

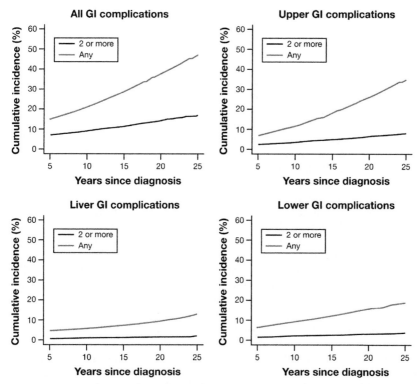

FIGURE 1.—Cumulative incidence of GI conditions (any, red; 2 or more, black) among 5-year survivors. For interpretation of the references to color in this figure legend, the reader is referred to web version of this article. (Reprinted from Goldsby R, Chen Y, Raber S, et al. Survivors of childhood cancer have increased risk of gastrointestinal complications later in life. *Gastroenterology.* 2011;140:1464-1471, Copyright 2011, with permission from the AGA Institute.)

years after treatment for childhood cancer (Fig 1). In particular, dyspepsia, constipation, and diarrhea were associated with surviving childhood cancer. The comparison with sibling controls was reasonable, although how representative they are of the general population is unclear. It is well recognized that cancer therapy induces significant and unpleasant GI toxicity, including mucositis, nausea and vomiting, esophagitis, and enteritis. The present study raises the hypothesis that acute inflammation (or possibly severe symptoms alone) from chemoradiation can "wind up" the enteric or central nervous system (or both), and after a long latent period, unexplained GI symptoms may develop. Bias is possible in this study (how many cancer survivors had recent symptoms because of cancer recurrence is, for example, uncertain), but overall the research suggests more vigilance by clinicians who follow such patients in adult practice.

N. J. Talley, MD, PhD

Constipation and Colonic Transit Times in Children With Morbid Obesity
vd Baan-Slootweg OH, Liem O, Bekkali N, et al (Emma's Children's Hosp/
AMC, Amsterdam, the Netherlands; et al)
J Pediatr Gastroenterol Nutr 52:442-445, 2011

Objectives.—The aim of the study was to determine the frequency of functional constipation according to the Rome III criteria in children with morbid obesity and to evaluate by measuring colonic transit times (CTTs) whether decreased colonic motility is present in these children.

Patients and Methods.—Ninety-one children with morbid obesity ages 8 to 18 years, entering a prospective, randomized controlled study evaluating the effect of an outpatient versus inpatient treatment program of obesity, participated. All of the children filled out a standardized questionnaire regarding their bowel habits, and CTTs were measured using radioopaque markers. Food diaries were also recorded to evaluate their diet.

Results.—A total of 19 children (21%) had functional constipation according to the Rome III criteria, whereas 1 child had functional nonretentive fecal incontinence. Total CTT exceeded 62 hours in only 10.5% of the children with constipation, and among them, 2 had a total CTT of >100 hours. In the nonconstipated group 8.3% had a delayed CTT. Furthermore, no difference was found between the diet of children with or without constipation, specifically not with respect to fiber and fat intake.

Conclusions.—Our study confirms a high frequency of functional constipation in children with obesity, using the Rome III criteria. However, abnormal colonic motility, as measured by CTT, was delayed in only a minority of patients. No relation was found between constipation in these children and fiber or fat intake (Table 1).

▶ Traditionally, it has been assumed that patients with obesity are more likely to suffer from chronic constipation, presumably related to inactivity and slow

TABLE 1.—Total and Segmental CTTs

Transit Time, h	Children with Constipation (n = 19)	Children without Constipation (n = 72)
Total colon		
Median	26.4	26.4
25th–75th percentiles	14.4–52.8	12.0–40.2
Delayed >62 h, %	10.5	8.3
Ascending colon		
Median	4.8	2.4
25th–75th percentiles	0–12.0	2.4–9.6
Delayed >18 h, %	5.3	5.6
Descending colon		
Median	2.4	2.4
25th–75th percentiles	0–7.2	0–9.0
Delayed >20 h, %	15.8	9.7
Rectosigmoid		
Median	16.8	14.4
25th–75th percentiles	4.8–38	4.8–25.8
Delayed >34 h, %	26.3	17.7

Mann-Whitney U test was used. $P < 0.05$ was deemed significant.
CTT = colonic transit time.

colonic transit. In the present study, total colonic transit time was measured by a simple but accurate radio-opaque marker method. Overall, the prevalence of symptomatic constipation was 21% in children with morbid obesity based on the Rome III criteria. However, children with obesity and constipation were no more likely to have slow colonic transit than obese children without constipation (Table 1). Diet also failed to explain constipation in this cohort of children, so what is the underlying explanation? It seems likely that pelvic floor dysfunction would be an important cause in a subset, although anorectal manometry and balloon expulsion testing was not conducted in the present study. Notably there was greater holdup of the radio-opaque markers in the pelvis in the constipation subgroup (Table 1), although this is not an accurate test for pelvic floor dysfunction, and the differences were not reported to be significant (possibly a type II error because of the small sample size). On another note, there is no convincing evidence from adult population-based studies that obesity is linked to chronic constipation; indeed, well-conducted epidemiological research suggests that young adults with obesity are significantly more likely to suffer from diarrhea for unexplained reasons.[1]

N. J. Talley, MD, PhD

Reference

1. Talley NJ, Howell S, Poulton R. Obesity and chronic gastrointestinal tract symptoms in young adults: a birth cohort study. *Am J Gastroenterol.* 2004;99:1807-1814.

Miscellaneous

Esomeprazole With Clopidogrel Reduces Peptic Ulcer Recurrence, Compared With Clopidogrel alone, in Patients With Atherosclerosis

Hsu P-I, Lai K-H, Liu C-P (Chia-Nan Univ of Pharmacy and Science, Tainan, Taiwan; Kaohsiung Veterans General Hosp and Natl Yang-Ming Univ, Taiwan)
Gastroenterology 140:791-798, 2011

Background & Aims.—We performed a prospective, randomized, controlled study to compare the combination of esomeprazole and clopidogrel vs clopidogrel alone in preventing recurrent peptic ulcers in patients with atherosclerosis and a history of peptic ulcers. We also investigated the effects of esomeprazole on the antiplatelet action of clopidogrel.

Methods.—From January 2008 to January 2010, long-term clopidogrel users with histories of peptic ulcers who did not have peptic ulcers at an initial endoscopy examination were assigned randomly to receive the combination of esomeprazole (20 mg/day, before breakfast) and clopidogrel (75 mg/day, at bedtime), or clopidogrel alone for 6 months. A follow-up endoscopy examination was performed at the end of the sixth month and whenever severe symptoms occurred. Platelet aggregation tests were performed on days 1 and 28 for 42 consecutive patients who participated in the pharmacodynamic study.

Results.—The cumulative incidence of recurrent peptic ulcer during the 6-month period was 1.2% among patients given the combination of esomeprazole and clopidogrel (n = 83) and 11.0% among patients given clopidogrel alone (n = 82) (difference, 9.8%; 95% confidence interval, 2.6%–17.0%; $P = .009$). In the group given the combination therapy, there were no differences in the percentages of aggregated platelets on days 1 and 28 (31.0% ± 20.5% vs 30.1% ± 16.5%).

Conclusions.—Among patients with atherosclerosis and a history of peptic ulcers, the combination of esomeprazole and clopidogrel reduced recurrence of peptic ulcers, compared with clopidogrel alone. Esomeprazole does not influence the action of clopidogrel on platelet aggregation (Fig 1).

▶ Clipodogrel may be slightly more effective than aspirin in the prevention of overall ischemic events, but what are the upper gastrointestinal (GI) risks, and how are these best prevented in clinical practice? Clopidogrel can induce upper GI bleeding, and this study suggests that 11% of patients with a peptic ulcer disease history may develop recurrent peptic ulceration from long-term use of clopidogrel. Prevention of peptic ulceration may be problematic because of concerns about an interaction between clopidogrel and proton pump inhibitors (omeprazole is both a substrate and an inhibitor of CYP2C19 and in vitro has been shown to decrease clopidogrel's inhibitory effect on platelets, leading to a potential loss of benefit of clopidogrel). In the current trial, ulcer disease was largely prevented by coadministration of a proton pump inhibitor (esomeprazole), and this was safe with no increase in ischemic events in the combination

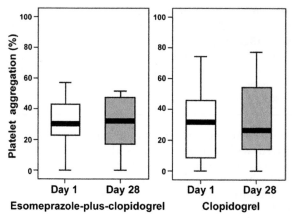

FIGURE 1.—Mean ADP-induced platelet aggregation on days 1 and 28. In the esomeprazole-plus-clopidogrel group, there were no differences between the PPAs on day 1 and day 28 (31.0% vs 30.1%; $P = .851$). In the clopidogrel group, the PPAs on days 1 and 28 also were similar (32.8% vs 35.0%; 95% confidence interval, -13.2 to 8.7; $P = .675$). In addition, there were no differences in the mean PPA between the 2 groups of patients on either day 1 or day 28. (Reprinted from Hsu P-I, Lai K-H, Liu C-P. Esomeprazole with clopidogrel reduces peptic ulcer recurrence, compared with clopidogrel alone, in patients with atherosclerosis. *Gastroenterology.* 2011;140:791-798, Copyright 2011, with permission from the AGA Institute.)

arm (although here the study was underpowered). Notably in this study, the patients were instructed to take esomeprazole before breakfast and clopidogrel at bedtime based on their half-lives, and no interaction was detected (Fig 1). A 14- to 16-hour separation may help minimize any theoretical interaction, although the jury is out whether this potential interaction is clinically relevant anyway, despite the current Food and Drug Administration warning. For example, a major trial failed to show any increase in cardiovascular events in the clopidogrel-omeprazole arm.[1] However, it seems reasonable not to prescribe a PPI to patients on clopidogrel who do not have any major indication for therapy, but in those at high risk of ulcer complications, PPI therapy should still be considered. Nonetheless, avoidance of omeprazole (and the isomer esomeprazole) and separating the dosing would be sensible based on current knowledge.

N. J. Talley, MD, PhD

Reference

1. Bhatt DL, Cryer BL, Contant CF, et al. Clopidogrel with or without omeprazole in coronary artery disease. *N Engl J Med.* 2010;363:1909-1917.

Prevention of peptic ulcers with esomeprazole in patients at risk of ulcer development treated with low-dose acetylsalicylic acid: A randomised, controlled trial (OBERON)

Scheiman JM, Devereaux PJ, Herlitz J, et al (Univ of Michigan Med Ctr, Ann Arbor; McMaster Univ, Hamilton, Ontario, Canada; Sahlgrenska Univ Hosp, Gothenburg, Sweden; et al)
Heart 97:797-802, 2011

Objective.—To determine whether once-daily esomeprazole 40 mg or 20 mg compared with placebo reduces the incidence of peptic ulcers over 26 weeks of treatment in patients taking low-dose acetylsalicylic acid (ASA) and who are at risk for ulcer development.

Design.—Multinational, randomised, blinded, parallelgroup, placebo-controlled trial.

Setting.—Cardiology, primary care and gastroenterology centres (n=240).

Patients.—Helicobacter pylori-negative patients taking daily low-dose ASA (75–325 mg), who fulfilled one or more of the following criteria: age ≥18 years with history of uncomplicated peptic ulcer; age ≥60 years with either stable coronary artery disease, upper gastrointestinal symptoms and five or more gastric/duodenal erosions, or low-dose ASA treatment initiated within 1 month of randomisation; or age ≥65 years. All patients were ulcer-free at study entry.

Interventions.—Once-daily, blinded treatment with esomeprazole 40 mg, 20 mg or placebo for 26 weeks.

Main Outcome Measures.—The primary end point was the occurrence of endoscopy-confirmed peptic ulcer over 26 weeks.

Results.—A total of 2426 patients (52% men; mean age 68 years) were randomised. After 26 weeks, esomeprazole 40 mg and 20 mg significantly reduced the cumulative proportion of patients developing peptic ulcers; 1.5% of esomeprazole 40 mg and 1.1% of esomeprazole 20 mg recipients, compared with 7.4% of placebo recipients, developed peptic ulcers (both p<0.0001 vs placebo). Esomeprazole was generally well tolerated.

Conclusions.—Acid-suppressive treatment with once-daily esomeprazole 40 mg or 20 mg reduces the occurrence of peptic ulcers in patients at risk for ulcer development who are taking low-dose ASA (Fig 2).

▶ Low-dose aspirin is known to reduce cardiovascular risk, but there is a price: increased gastrointestinal (GI) toxicity—in particular, peptic ulcer disease and upper GI bleeding. Enteric coating or buffering aspirin probably provides no additional protection. Concomitant *Helicobacter pylori* infection, advanced age, and a past history of peptic ulcer increase the risk of ulcer disease on aspirin, which is often silent in the elderly until bleeding occurs. In the present study, patients at increased risk of ulceration but who were serologically *H pylori* negative were randomized to the proton pump inhibitor (PPI) esomeprazole 40 mg and 20 mg once daily or placebo over 6 months. They observed that PPI reduced the incidence of endoscopy-confirmed peptic ulcer disease versus placebo, but a higher dose added no benefit (Fig 2). These observations confirm other trial

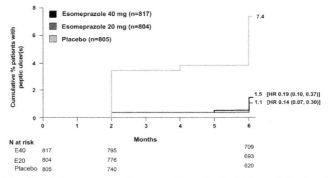

FIGURE 2.—Cumulative percentage of patients with peptic ulcer(s) by week 26 (intention-to-treat population, Kaplane—Meier curve). (Reprinted from Scheiman JM, Devereaux PJ, Herlitz J, et al. Prevention of peptic ulcers with esomeprazole in patients at risk of ulcer development treated with low-dose acetylsalicylic acid: a randomised, controlled trial (OBERON). *Heart.* 2011;97:797-802 Copyright 2011, with permission from the BMJ Publishing Group Ltd.)

data,[1] and presumably the findings translate into lower ulcer complications on PPI as well, although the study was not powered to detect such uncommon events. The PPI produced similar protection in those taking higher doses (up to 325 mg) and lower doses (75—100 mg) of aspirin. About 20% of patients who were truly *H pylori* infected were accidentally included in the study (because they had false-negative *H pylori* serology results), but PPI was equally protective in *H pylori*-positive and -negative cases. These results suggest that in patients at high risk of ulcer disease requiring low dose aspirin for cardiovascular protection, coprescribing a PPI is reasonable to consider and is supported by expert opinion.[2]

N. J. Talley, MD, PhD

References

1. Yeomans N, Lanas A, Labenz J, et al. Efficacy of esomeprazole (20 mg once daily) for reducing the risk of gastroduodenal ulcers associated with continuous use of low-dose aspirin. *Am J Gastroenterol.* 2008;103:2465-2473.
2. Abraham NS, Hlatky MA, Antman EM, et al. ACCF/ACG/AHA 2010 expert consensus document on the concomitant use of proton pump inhibitors and thienopyridines: a focused update of the ACCF/ACG/AHA 2008 expert consensus document on reducing the gastrointestinal risks of antiplatelet therapy and NSAID use. *Am J Gastroenterol.* 2010;105:2533-2549.

Gluten Causes Gastrointestinal Symptoms in Subjects Without Celiac Disease: A Double-Blind Randomized Placebo-Controlled Trial

Biesiekierski JR, Newnham ED, Irving PM, et al (Monash Univ Dept of Medicine and Gastroenterology, Box Hill, Victoria, Australia; et al)
Am J Gastroenterol 106:508-514, 2011

Objectives.—Despite increased prescription of a gluten-free diet for gastrointestinal symptoms in individuals who do not have celiac disease, there is minimal evidence that suggests that gluten is a trigger. The aims of this study were to determine whether gluten ingestion can induce symptoms in non-celiac individuals and to examine the mechanism.

Methods.—A double-blind, randomized, placebo-controlled rechallenge trial was undertaken in patients with irritable bowel syndrome in whom celiac disease was excluded and who were symptomatically controlled on a gluten-free diet. Participants received either gluten or placebo in the form of two bread slices plus one muffin per day with a gluten-free diet for up to 6 weeks. Symptoms were evaluated using a visual analog scale and markers of intestinal inflammation, injury, and immune activation were monitored.

Results.—A total of 34 patients (aged 29–59 years, 4 men) completed the study as per protocol. Overall, 56 % had human leukocyte antigen (HLA)-DQ2 and/or HLA-DQ8. Adherence to diet and supplements was very high. Of 19 patients (68%) in the gluten group, 13 reported that symptoms were not adequately controlled compared with 6 of 15 (40%) on placebo ($P = 0.0001$; generalized estimating equation). On a visual analog scale, patients were significantly worse with gluten within 1 week for overall symptoms ($P = 0.047$), pain ($P = 0.016$), bloating ($P = 0.031$), satisfaction with stool consistency ($P = 0.024$), and tiredness ($P = 0.001$). Anti-gliadin antibodies were not induced. There were no significant changes in fecal lactoferrin, levels of celiac antibodies, highly sensitive C-reactive protein, or intestinal permeability. There were no differences in any end point in individuals with or without DQ2/DQ8.

Conclusions.—" Non-celiac gluten intolerance " may exist, but no clues to the mechanism were elucidated.

▶ Dietary manipulation appears to be of growing importance in the management of irritable bowel syndrome (IBS). There is limited evidence that fiber supplements (especially psyllium) can provide a benefit, although focusing on those with constipation and going slow is key to reducing bloating and noncompliance. More recent data suggest that removal of certain poorly absorbed short-chain carbohydrates (a low fermentable oligosaccharides, disaccharides, monosaccharides and polyols diet) also appears to be useful based on evidence from Australia.[1] A second novel approach to dietary management in IBS is application of a gluten-free diet. Celiac disease is the great imitator in gastroenterology; patients with unrecognized celiac disease can present with classic IBS-like symptoms that appear to respond to gluten withdrawal. In this landmark Australian study, the authors assessed in a double-bind randomized trial the efficacy of a gluten-free diet in IBS where celiac disease was excluded (although half of them were HLA-DQ2 or DQ8 positive, indicating a potential genetic risk for celiac disease). They assessed treatment over only 6 weeks but observed that not only did gastrointestinal symptoms decrease on a gluten-free diet, but also fatigue improved. Other uncontrolled data suggest that 6 months of gluten withdrawal might be beneficial.[2] The findings support the concept that a subset of patients with IBS have gluten sensitivity that may in part explain their IBS symptoms, although the duration of needed dietary intervention and the durability of the response are unknown. Trialing a gluten-free diet now represents a reasonable strategy for patients with resistant IBS symptoms. The problem with a gluten-free diet is that it is restrictive, and compliance can be difficult. However, this is a safe strategy that accumulating evidence now supports; a translation into practice does not seem unreasonable in selected cases.

N. J. Talley, MD, PhD

References

1. Ong DK, Mitchell SB, Barrett JS, et al. Manipulation of dietary short chain carbohydrates alters the pattern of gas production and genesis of symptoms in irritable bowel syndrome. *J Gastroenterol Hepatol.* 2010;25:1366-1373.
2. Wahnschaffe U, Ullrich R, Riecken EO, Schulzke JD. Celiac disease-like abnormalities in a subgroup of patients with irritable bowel syndrome. *Gastroenterology.* 2001;121:1329-1338.

Epidemiology of Peptic Ulcer Disease: Endoscopic Results of the Systematic Investigation of Gastrointestinal Disease in China
Li Z, Zou D, Ma X, et al (Second Military Med Univ, Shanghai, China; et al)
Am J Gastroenterol 105:2570-2577, 2010

Objectives.—Complications of peptic ulcer disease (PUD) are common in China. Population-based estimates of the prevalence of PUD are needed to quantify and characterize the population at risk of these complications.

Methods.—As part of a large epidemiological study, 3,600 randomly selected residents of Shanghai (aged 18—80 years) were asked to undergo endoscopy and to provide blood samples for *Helicobacter pylori* serology. All participants also completed a general information questionnaire and Chinese versions of the reflux disease questionnaire (RDQ) and Rome II questionnaire. Associations between PUD and other factors were analyzed using a multiple logistic regression model.

Results.—In total, 3,153 individuals (87.6%) completed the survey. All underwent blood tests, and 1,030 patients (32.7%) agreed to undergo endoscopy. Results from 1,022 patients were suitable for analysis. In all, 176 participants (17.2%) had PUD (62 with gastric ulcer; 136 with duodenal ulcer). The prevalence of *H. pylori* infection was 73.3% in the total population and 92.6% among those with PUD. *H. pylori* infection was associated with the presence of PUD (odds ratio (OR), 6.77; 95% confidence interval (CI), 2.85—16.10). The majority (72.2%) of individuals with PUD had none of the upper gastrointestinal symptoms assessed by the RDQ. PUD was not significantly associated with symptom-defined gastroesophageal reflux disease (GERD) (OR, 0.80; 95% CI, 0.32—2.03), reflux esophagitis (OR, 1.46; 95% CI, 0.76—2.79) or dyspepsia (OR, 1.69; 95% CI, 0.94—3.04).

Conclusions.—The prevalence of endoscopically confirmed PUD in this Shanghai population (17.2%) is substantially higher than in Western

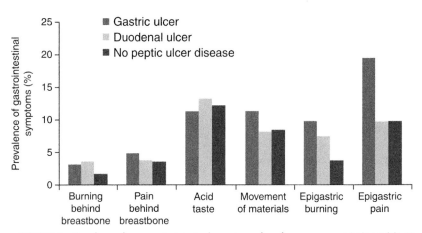

FIGURE 1.—Prevalence of upper gastrointestinal symptoms of any frequency or severity in participants with gastric ulcer, duodenal ulcer, or no peptic ulcer disease. (Reprinted from Li Z, Zou D, Ma X, et al. Epidemiology of peptic ulcer disease: endoscopic results of the systematic investigation of gastrointestinal disease in China. *Am J Gastroenterol.* 2010;105:2570-2577, Copyright 2010, with permission from Macmillan Publishers Ltd: American Journal of Gastroenterology.)

populations (4.1%). The majority of individuals with PUD were asymptomatic (Fig 1).

▶ This is a nice population-based study from China showing a remarkably high prevalence of *Helicobacter pylori* in this part of the world. The health implications of this infection are great, and further work to evaluate the long-term benefits (and risks) of population-based screening and eradication of *H pylori* are needed. Notably, peptic ulcer disease is more prevalent in China (17%) than in the West (4% to 6%) based on this work, but another important observation was how poorly symptoms identify those with a peptic ulcer in China (Fig 1); others have made similar observations in the West.[1] Ulcer disease cannot be diagnosed without endoscopy and may unfairly be blamed for symptoms in clinical practice. Esophagitis at endoscopy was more common in individuals with a gastroduodenal ulcer (10%) than in those without a peptic ulcer (6%), but no significant association was seen; gastroesophageal reflux disease is less common in China, probably because atrophic gastritis with lower gastric acid production is so much more common (presumably secondary to the high background rate of *H pylori* infection). There were some limitations of this study (only about one-third agreed to the endoscopy arm, and aspirin or nonsteroidal anti-inflammatory drug use was not assessed), but the study presents a good snapshot of the burden of upper gastrointestinal disease in China in the early 21st century.

N. J. Talley, MD, PhD

Reference

1. Aro P, Storskrubb T, Ronkainen J, et al. Peptic ulcer disease in a general adult population: the Kalixanda study: a random population-based study. *Am J Epidemiol.* 2006;163:1025-1034.

Small Bowel Homing T Cells Are Associated With Symptoms and Delayed Gastric Emptying in Functional Dyspepsia

Liebregts T, Adam B, Bredack C, et al (Univ Hosp Schleswig-Holstein, Kiel, Germany; Hanson Inst, Adelaide, South Australia, Australia; et al)
Am J Gastroenterol 106:1089-1098, 2011

Objectives.—Immune activation may have an important pathogenic role in the irritable bowel syndrome (IBS). While little is known about immunologic function in functional dyspepsia (FD), we have observed an association between cytokine secretion by peripheral blood mononuclear cells (PBMCs) and symptoms in IBS. Upper gastrointestinal inflammatory diseases are characterized by enhanced small bowel homing α4-, β7-integrin, chemokine receptor 9 (CCR9) positive T lymphocytes. We hypothesized that increased cytokine release and elevated circulating small bowel homing T cells are linked to the severity of symptoms in patients with FD. Thus, we aimed to (i) compare cytokine release in FD and healthy controls (HCs), (ii) quantify "gut homing" T cells in FD compared with HC and patients with IBS, and (iii) correlate the findings to symptom severity and gastric emptying.

Methods.—PBMC from 45 (*Helicobacter pylori negative*) patients with FD (Rome II) and 35 matched HC were isolated by density gradient centrifugation and cultured for 24 h. Cytokine production (tumor necrosis factor (TNF)-α, interleukin (IL)-1 β, IL-6, IL-10) was measured by enzyme-linked immunosorbent assay. CD4+ α4β7 + CCR9+ T cells were quantified by flow cytometry in FD, HC and 23 patients with IBS. Gastric emptying was measured by scintigraphy. Symptom severity was assessed utilizing the standardized Gastrointestinal Symptom Score.

Results.—FD patients had significantly higher TNF-α (107.2 ± 42.8 vs. 58.7 ± 7.4 pg/ml), IL-1β (204.8 ± 71.5 vs. 80.2 ± 17.4 pg/ml), and IL-10 (218 ± 63.3 vs. 110.9 ± 18.5 pg/ml) levels compared with HC, and enhanced gut homing lymphocytes compared with HC or IBS. Cytokine release and CD4 + α4β7 + CCR9 + lymphocytes were correlated with the symptom intensity of pain, cramps, nausea, and vomiting. Delayed gastric emptying was significantly associated ($r=0.78$, $P=0.021$) with CD4 + α4β7 + CCR9 + lymphocytes and IL-1β, TNF-α, and IL-10 secretion.

Conclusions.—Cellular immune activation with increased small bowel homing T cells may be key factors in the clinical manifestations of *H. pylori*-negative FD.

▶ Functional dyspepsia, characterized by epigastric pain, postprandial fullness, or early satiety, affects about 10% of the US population, but the cause remains unknown. Mechanisms thought to be relevant include altered gastric emptying (usually slow in about a quarter of cases) and gastric hypersensitivity or failure of fundic relaxation (also affecting a subset), but treatments remain suboptimal. This novel study suggests a new mechanism may be key—namely, immune activation that occurs in a subset of patients with functional dyspepsia. This is in line with other data that strongly suggest immune activation occurs in a subset of patients with irritable bowel syndrome.[1] Furthermore, a distinct population of small bowel T cells were linked to symptoms in this patient population, as was delayed gastric emptying. It is unclear whether this infiltration of T cells is a direct cause of symptoms or an epiphenomenon, and further work is needed. The observations are, however, consistent with other novel work showing that excess eosinophils, but not mast cells, occur in the duodenum in a subset of patients with functional dyspepsia.[2] All of these abnormalities may be secondary to increased intestinal permeability and exposure to food or bacterial antigens in functional dyspepsia, which turns on the immune response and could explain gastroduodenal motor and sensory dysfunction through abnormal reflex responses. The importance of these observations are that anti-inflammatory therapy may be useful in at least a subset of patients with functional dyspepsia, although further work is necessary to characterize the mechanisms so that logical interventions can be devised.

N. J. Talley, MD, PhD

References

1. Liebregts T, Adam B, Bredack C, et al. Immune activation in patients with irritable bowel syndrome. *Gastroenterology.* 2007;132:913-920.
2. Walker MM, Salehian SS, Murray CE, et al. Implications of eosinophilia in the normal duodenal biopsy - an association with allergy and functional dyspepsia. *Aliment Pharmacol Ther.* 2010;31:1229-1236.

Non-Ulcer Dyspepsia

Risk factors for impaired health-related quality of life in functional dyspepsia

Van Oudenhove L, Vandenberghe J, Vos R, et al (Univ of Leuven, Belgium)
Aliment Pharmacol Ther 33:261-274, 2011

Background.—The influence of patient characteristics on HRQoL in functional dyspepsia is poorly understood.

Aim.—To determine the contribution of gastric sensorimotor function, psychosocial factors & 'somatization' to HRQoL in functional dyspepsia.

Methods.—In 259 tertiary care functional dyspepsia patients, we studied gastric sensorimotor function with barostat. We measured psychosocial factors and 'somatization' using self-report questionnaires. HRQoL was assessed using the SF-36 physical and mental composite scores (PCS, MCS). Bivariate associations between gastric sensorimotor function, psychosocial factors and 'somatization' on the one hand and PCS and MCS on the other were estimated. Variables significantly associated with PCS or MCS in bivariate analysis were entered into hierarchical multiple linear regression models.

Results.—Mean PCS was 40.1 ± 9.5; mean MCS was 45.1 ± 10.8. 'Somatization' ($P < 0.0001$) and chronic fatigue ($P = 0.002$) were significantly associated with impaired PCS ($R^2 = 0.52$, $P < 0.0001$). The effects of abuse history and depression were 'mediated' by 'somatization'. Trait anxiety ($P = 0.02$), alexithymia ($P = 0.06$), depression ($P = 0.06$), positive affect ($P < 0.0001$), negative affect ($P = 0.002$) and generalised anxiety disorder ($P = 0.01$) were significantly associated with impaired MCS ($R^2 = 0.67$, $P < 0.0001$).

Conclusions.—'Somatization' is the most important risk factor for impaired physical HRQoL in functional dyspepsia; it 'mediates' the effect of abuse history and depression. Mental HRQoL is mainly explained by psychosocial factors (Fig 3).

▶ Functional dyspepsia (FD) classically presents as early satiety, postprandial fullness, or epigastric pain; a subset of patients (up to 40%) have failure of gastric relaxation (impaired accommodation), while a third have gastric hypersensitivity that can be assessed by the gastric barostat. This novel research suggests that somatization is a key mediator of impaired quality of life in FD, and other risk factors such as depression and abuse in the past may act through

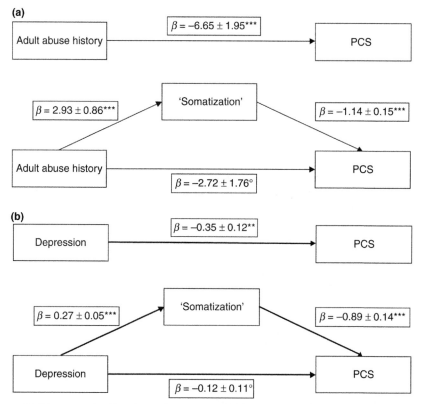

FIGURE 3.—(a) The effect of overall adult abuse history on SF-36 physical composite score is fully 'mediated' by 'somatization'. ***$P < 0.001$; °$P = 0.13$. Sobel test for significance of indirect effect: $Z = -3.11$, $P = 0.002$. (b) The effect of depression on SF-36 physical composite score is fully 'mediated' by 'somatization'. ***$P < 0.001$; **$P < 0.005$; °$P = 0.28$. Sobel test for significance of indirect effect: $Z = -4.12$, $P < 0.0001$. PCS, physical composite score. (Reprinted from Van Oudenhove L, Vandenberghe J, Vos R, et al. Risk factors for impaired health-related quality of life in functional dyspepsia. *Aliment Pharmacol Ther.* 2011;33:261-274, with permission from Blackwell Publishing Ltd.)

this pathway (Fig 3). Notably, somatization was identified by simply counting somatic symptoms that appeared to be unexplained, and, as conceptualized, it is not necessarily a true psychiatric syndrome; indeed, there is exciting speculation that cytokine elevations might account for extraintestinal symptoms in FD and irritable bowel syndrome and explain the apparent link to somatization in these conditions.[1] This study, on the other hand, suggests the effect of abuse and depression may lead to alterations in central nervous system function (eg, reduce normal down-regulation of pain control pathways), leading to increased expression of extraintestinal complaints and impairing quality of life. A novel aspect of this work was the inclusion of measurements of gastric sensitivity and accommodation measured by the barostat. While gastric accommodation was not important in quality-of-life impairment in FD, gastric discomfort was possibly of relevance when considered with somatization, although the results were far from convincing. Perhaps increased gastric sensitivity to balloon distention represents a signal indicating a general tendency for patients with FD to feel sensations others would not process centrally. A causal link between FD and psychological factors, however, is not established, but more research here may help clinicians create better management plans for these patients in practice.

N. J. Talley, MD, PhD

Reference

1. Liebregts T, Adam B, Bredack C, et al. Immune activation in patients with irritable bowel syndrome. *Gastroenterology*. 2007;132:913-920.

Randomised clinical trial: identification of responders to short-term treatment with esomeprazole for dyspepsia in primary care - a randomised, placebo-controlled study

Meineche-Schmidt V, Christensen E, Bytzer P (Univ of Copenhagen, Denmark)
Aliment Pharmacol Ther 33:41-49, 2011

Background.—Response to proton pump inhibitor (PPI) treatment in dyspepsia is unpredictable.

Aim.—To identify symptoms associated with response to esomeprazole in order to target patients for empirical treatment.

Methods.—Eight hundred and five uninvestigated, primary care patients with upper GI symptoms that were considered to be acid-related were randomised to 2 weeks' treatment with esomeprazole 40 mg or placebo. The study population was divided into a model sample ($N = 484$) and a validation sample ($N = 321$). We developed a therapeutic index to predict PPI response from the model sample and tested this in the validation sample.

Results.—Response to PPI was found in 68% of patients (44% in placebo arm). Bothersome heartburn and early satiety were associated with increased likelihood of PPI response, whereas dull abdominal pain,

TABLE 4.—Pocket Chart for Easy Direct Calculation of Therapeutic Index to Predict Response to PPI

Presence of Symptom	Yes	No	Points
Bothersome heartburn	+19	+9	
Early satiety	+12	0	
Dull pain quality	−14	0	
Pain relieved by bowel movement	−13	0	
Nausea in women	−9	0	
Sum of points =			
Therapeutic Index (TI) = Sum of points multiplied by 0.1 =			

Interpretation: TI > 2: excellent response to esomeprazole; TI 1–2: good response to esomeprazole; TI 0–1: fair response to esomeprazole; TI < 0: no or little response to esomeprazole.

pain relieved by bowel movements and nausea in women were associated with a decreased likelihood of PPI response. Patients in the validation sample could be classified as having a 'very high' (*n* = 55), 'high' (*n* = 123), 'medium' (*n* = 78) or 'low' (*n* = 65) probability of PPI response. The therapeutic gains over placebo were 55%, 31%, 20% and 22%, respectively.

Conclusions.—In patients with uninvestigated dyspepsia, PPI responders can be reliably identified by a simple pocket chart using symptoms and patient characteristics (ClinicalTrials.gov NCT00318968) (Table 4).

▶ Dyspepsia in primary and secondary care is typically managed by prescription of a proton pump inhibitor trial. It is well recognized that many patients, especially those with nonulcer dyspepsia, have a suboptimal response or will have no response to acid suppression therapy, which adds unnecessary costs. Previous research has suggested that those with heartburn and dyspepsia are more likely to respond to acid suppression, but a subset of those with predominant epigastric pain will also respond. However, an optimal method of picking out those with dyspepsia who are likely and unlikely to respond to a proton pump inhibitor has been elusive. The present trial suggests that a simple set of questions can be scored and will help identify who to treat with a proton pump inhibitor and when to consider alternatives (Table 4). Strengths of the current study include its large sample size, rigorous randomization and blinding methodology, and use of a development and validation sample (note that developing a predictive set of items from a data set such as this is prone to bias in a positive direction, often not confirmed in validation testing). A weakness of the study remains the inclusion of only patients thought to have an acid-related symptom pattern (and the inclusion of those with predominant heartburn who we already know have an excellent chance of response); the validity of the items across all comers with dyspepsia remains to be established.

N. J. Talley, MD, PhD

Longitudinal and Cross-Sectional Factors Associated With Long-Term Clinical Course in Functional Dyspepsia: A 5-Year Follow-Up Study

Kindt S, Van Oudenhove L, Mispelon L, et al (Univ of Leuven, Belgium)
Am J Gastroenterol 106:340-348, 2011

Objectives.—Functional dyspepsia (FD) is a heterogeneous disorder with different pathophysiological mechanisms underlying the symptom pattern, but little is known about its clinical course. The aims of this study were to study the long-term evolution of symptoms in a clinical FD population and to identify factors associated with outcome.

Methods.—FD patients who previously underwent gastric function testing and filled out a dyspepsia symptom score (DSS) were contacted. At follow-up, patients indicated whether symptoms had worsened, remained unchanged, improved, or disappeared. Anxiety and depression, DSS, chronic fatigue symptoms, irritable bowel syndrome (IBS) comorbidity, and FD-specific quality of life (QoL) were assessed using mailed questionnaires. Bivariate associations between different patient characteristics and DSS and QoL at follow-up were tested; multiple linear regression was used to identify factors associated with the outcomes, both longitudinally and cross-sectionally.

Results.—Data were obtained from 253 patients (84.9% of the eligible and consenting population ($n=298$) and 53.2% of the original population ($n=476$)). The mean duration of follow-up was 68 ± 2 months. Disappeared, improved, unchanged, and worsened symptoms were reported by 17.4, 38.3, 30.8, and 13.4% of the patients, respectively. Correlations between dyspepsia symptoms at initial visit and follow-up were small to moderate in magnitude. DSS at initial visit and trait anxiety were longitudinally associated with DSS at follow-up, with a trend found for weight loss; depression, chronic fatigue, and IBS at follow-up were cross-sectionally associated with DSS. Trait anxiety, weight loss, and DSS at initial visit were independently associated with QoL at follow-up; depression as well as DSS and chronic fatigue at follow-up were cross-sectionally associated.

Conclusions.—About half of FD patients reported disappeared or improved symptoms after a mean follow-up of 5 years. Although stability of symptom levels is low to moderate, DSS at initial visit, trait anxiety, and initial weight loss are more strongly associated with outcome than gastric sensorimotor function (Fig 2).

▶ Functional dyspepsia (FD) is a common but often under-recognized syndrome characterized by meal-induced symptoms (typically fullness or inability to finish a normal sized meal, or epigastric pain or burning). Patients with chronic unexplained dyspepsia are often mislabeled as having gastroesophageal reflux disease (if epigastric pain or burning predominates) or irritable bowel syndrome (IBS) (if fullness - often miscalled bloating - predominates). FD, like IBS or gastroparesis, can occur after an episode of infectious gastroenteritis, although the majority recall no precipitating infection. The prognosis has

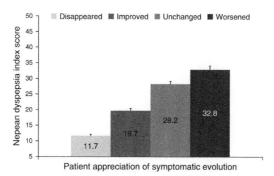

FIGURE 2.—Association between patient appreciation of symptomatic evolution and quality of life at follow-up. All pairwise differences are significant after Tukey correction for multiple comparisons; all P values are <0.0001, except for the comparison between the "unchanged" and "worsened" group, $P = 0.03$. (Reprinted from Kindt S, Van Oudenhove L, Mispelon L, et al. Longitudinal and cross-sectional factors associated with long-term clinical course in functional dyspepsia: a 5-year follow-up study. *Am J Gastroenterol.* 2011;106:340-348, Copyright 2011, with permission from Macmillan Publishers Ltd: American Journal of Gastroenterology.)

remained somewhat unclear, so this large prospective well characterized cohort study with a mean duration just over 5 years in tertiary care is of interest. Notably, in this study around 50% of the patients with FD improved (Fig 2). However, deranged gastric physiology did not predict the prognosis, suggesting these abnormalities (eg, slow gastric emptying), while a biomarker of the disorder, do not identify irreversible damage and link poorly if at all with symptoms. On the other hand, the presence of trait anxiety (or anxiety proneness) did predict continuation of symptoms and may reflect a way clinicians can indirectly assess the likely activity of the disorder. Other studies have observed a large subset with symptoms of FD that can transform into IBS and related functional GI disorders,[1] but this was not measured in this study. The good news from this research is that patients with FD can be reassured that they have a good chance of experiencing spontaneous symptom resolution; predictors of this beneficial response are beginning to emerge. Reassurance and explanation remain mainstays of management of FD in 2012.

N. J. Talley, MD, PhD

Reference

1. Halder SL, Locke GR 3rd, Schleck CD, Zinsmeister AR, Melton LJ 3rd, Talley NJ. Natural history of functional gastrointestinal disorders: a 12-year longitudinal population-based study. *Gastroenterology.* 2007;133:799-807.

3 Pancreaticobiliary Disease

ERCP

Large Balloon Dilation vs. Mechanical Lithotripsy for the Management of Large Bile Duct Stones: A Prospective Randomized Study
Stefanidis G, Viazis N, Pleskow D, et al (Athens Naval Hosp, Greece; Evangelismos Hosp, Athens, Greece; Beth Israel Deaconness Med Ctr, Boston, MA; et al)
Am J Gastroenterol 106:278-285, 2011

Objectives.—The removal of large bile duct stones (>12 mm) after endoscopic sphincterotomy (EST) remains a challenging issue in therapeutic endoscopy. The aim of this prospective, randomized, controlled trial was to compare the effectiveness and complications of EST followed by large balloon dilation (LBD) with that of EST followed by mechanical lithotripsy (ML) for the management of large bile duct stones.

Methods.—A total of 90 patients with large bile duct stones (12−20 mm) were randomized to EST followed by LBD ($n = 45$) or EST followed by ML ($n = 45$). Success rate was determined with a final cholangiogram, whereas type and rate of post-procedure complications were assessed prospectively.

Results.—Complete bile duct stone removal was accomplished in 97.7% of patients subjected to EST−LBD as compared with 91.1% of those subjected to EST−ML ($P = 0.36$). Post-procedure complications were observed in two (4.4%) patients subjected to EST−LBD and in nine (20%) patients subjected to EST−ML (P0.049). Rates of pancreatitis were similar between the two groups (one case in each), as was post-endoscopic retrograde cholangio pancreatography (ERCP) hemorrhage (one case in each group). None of the patients subjected to EST−LBD developed cholangitis, while this was seen in six patients subjected to EST−ML (0.0 vs. 13.3%, $P = 0.026$). One patient subjected to EST−ML developed perforation, which was successfully managed conservatively. None of our patients with complications died.

Conclusions.—EST followed by LBD is equally effective as EST followed by ML for the removal of large bile duct stones, although it is associated with fewer complications.

▶ This is an interesting randomized study comparing efficacy and complications of biliary sphincterotomy followed by mechanical lithotripsy (ML) versus large balloon dilation (LBD) in patients who had bile duct stones that were between 12 and 20 mm in size that could not be removed with an extraction balloon. Ninety patients qualified for inclusion in the study, and there were no differences in patient characteristics between the 2 groups. The success rate of stone removal was high (> 90%), and there was no difference in efficacy between the 2 techniques irrespective of stone size. The balloon size was determined by taking into account the estimated stone diameter and was never larger than the maximal diameter of the duct. The dilatation time of 10 to 12 seconds is much shorter than previous studies and was a deliberate decision based on the theoretical risk of causing pancreatitis with prolonged dilatation; to date there is no published evidence surrounding this decision.

Surprisingly, there was a high rate of cholangitis in the ML group (13%, $P = .026$) with no cases reported in the LBD group. The reasons for this, as discussed by the authors, were common bile duct trauma and sphincterotomy-related edema or inadequacy; an additional mechanism could be intrahepatic duct obstruction secondary to stone fragments. Most of these patients had a plastic stent placed at time of initial endoscopic retrograde cholangiopancreatography (ERCP) for suspected retained stones. Other risks, such as pancreatitis and bleeding, were similar between groups, and approximately 25% of both groups had a stent placed and second ERCP to complete stone extraction.

For the study to demonstrate a difference between the 2 techniques with a power of 80%, more than double the number of patients who participated would have needed to be enrolled; therefore, a type II error may well account for this nonsuperiority result. It took 4 years to enroll 90 patients, so further recruitment was felt to be impractical, and safety concerns because of an increase in procedure-related cholangitis in the ML group led to a decision to terminate the study early.

No information regarding procedure time was included, and one has to question the adequacy of proximal duct clearance and technique of stent placement to accrue such a high rate of cholangitis with ML. Regardless, this study does confirm the efficacy and safety of balloon dilatation to facilitate large stone removal, and for the first time has demonstrated that short dilating times are sufficient to permit adequate stone clearance.

S. M. Philcox, FRACP, MBBS (Hons), BMedSc

Pancreatic stents for prophylaxis against post-ERCP pancreatitis: a meta-analysis and systematic review

Choudhary A, Bechtold ML, Arif M, et al (Univ of Missouri School of Medicine, Columbia; et al)

Gastrointest Endosc 73:275-282, 2011

Background.—Acute pancreatitis is a common complication of ERCP. Several randomized, controlled trials (RCTs) have evaluated the use of pancreatic stents in the prevention of post-ERCP pancreatitis with varying results.

Objective.—We conducted a meta-analysis and systematic review to assess the role of prophylactic pancreatic stents for prevention of post-ERCP pancreatitis.

Design.—MEDLINE, Cochrane Central Register of Controlled Trials and Database of Systematic Reviews, PubMed, and recent abstracts from major conference proceedings were searched. RCTs and retrospective or prospective, nonrandomized studies comparing prophylactic stent with placebo or no stent for post-ERCP pancreatitis were included for the meta-analysis and systematic review. Standard forms were used to extract data by 2 independent reviewers. The effect of stents (for RCTs) was analyzed by calculating pooled estimates of post-ERCP pancreatitis, hyperamylasemia, and grade of pancreatitis. Separate analyses were performed for each outcome by using the odds ratio (OR) or weighted mean difference. Random- or fixed-effects models were used. Publication bias was assessed by funnel plots. Heterogeneity among studies was assessed by calculating I^2 measure of inconsistency.

Setting.—Systematic review and meta-analysis of patients undergoing pancreatic stent placement for prophylaxis against post-ERCP pancreatitis.

Patients.—Adult patients undergoing ERCP.

Interventions.—Pancreatic stent placement for the prevention of post-ERCP pancreatitis.

Main Outcome Measurements.—Post-ERCP pancreatitis, hyperamylasemia, and complications after pancreatic stent placement.

Results.—Eight RCTs (656 subjects) and 10 nonrandomized studies met the inclusion criteria (4904 subjects). Meta-analysis of the RCTs showed that prophylactic pancreatic stents decreased the odds of post-ERCP pancreatitis (odds ratio, 0.22; 95% CI, 0.12-0.38; $P < .01$). The absolute risk difference was 13.3% (95% CI, 8.8%-17.8%). The number needed to treat was 8 (95% CI, 6-11). Stents also decreased the level of hyperamylasemia (WMD, -309.22; 95% CI, -350.95 to -267.49; $P \leq .01$). Similar findings were also noted from the nonrandomized studies.

Limitations.—Small sample size of some trials, different types of stents used, inclusion of low-risk patients in some studies, and lack of adequate study of long-term complications of pancreatic stent placement.

Conclusions.—Pancreatic stent placement decreases the risk of post-ERCP pancreatitis and hyperamylasemia in high-risk patients.

▶ Pancreatitis is a relatively common, potentially avoidable complication of endoscopic retrograde cholangiopancreatography (ERCP) that occurs in approximately 5% to 12% of ERCPs, with higher rates reported in high-risk patients, such as those undergoing pancreatic duct manometry. Meta-analyses and randomized controlled trials (RCTs) of strategies to reduce this risk have found reduced pancreatitis rates with the use of nonsteroidal anti-inflammatory agents and endoscopic techniques, such as the use of wire cannulation, minimization of contrast injection, early needle-knife use, and pancreatic duct stent placement. This meta-analysis revisits stenting of the pancreatic duct and includes 8 RCTs with a total of 656 patients; 3 of these studies were published subsequent to previously published meta-analyses on this subject.[1,2] Ten nonrandomized studies, including 4904 patients, were also systematically reviewed. All the RCTs used short 2- to 5-cm 5-F stents, with 1 study including 7-F stents. The majority of stents were flanged. There was variability in the length of time the stents were kept in place from less than 7 days to 2 weeks and in the indication for ERCP. No publication bias was detected using funnel plot. Results of the meta-analysis are in keeping with those of earlier studies that pancreatic duct stenting does reduce the incidence of post-ERCP pancreatitis (odds ratio, 0.22; 95% confidence interval, 0.12-0.38; $P < .01$) with a number needed to treat of 8 (Fig 3 in the original article). There was also a reduction in post-ERCP amylasemia ($P < .01$) and a significant decrease in the odds of mild to moderate pancreatitis with no reduction in the incidence of severe pancreatitis. The systematic review of nonrandomized studies also showed a reduction in the incidence of pancreatitis with a wide variation in pancreatitis rates in the control group from 6% to 66% that decreased to 0% to 20% with stenting; these studies included high-risk patients, and a statistically significant reduction was seen in only half the studies. This study confirms the utility of pancreatic duct stenting in reducing the risk of ERCP-related pancreatitis. At least in the studies included in this meta-analysis, 5-F short (< 3 cm), flanged stents were the preferred choice, although subgroup analysis did not show any significant differences with respect to length or presence of flanges. A recent retrospective study[3] has suggested longer, 4-F stents may be superior to shorter stents, so the jury is still out on the precise characteristics of the stents. Patient selection remains the Holy Grail to minimize the risk of causing pancreatitis in patients who don't actually need stenting, so further study is clearly required.

S. M. Philcox, FRACP, MBBS (Hons), BMedSc

References

1. Singh P, Das A, Isenberg G, et al. Does prophylactic pancreatic stent placement reduce the risk of post-ERCP acute pancreatitis? A meta-analysis of controlled trials. *Gastrointest Endosc.* 2004;60:544-550.
2. Andriulli A, Forlano R, Napolitano G, et al. Pancreatic duct stents in the prophylaxis of pancreatic damage after endoscopic retrograde cholangiopancreatography: a systematic analysis of benefits and associated risks. *Digestion.* 2007;75:156-163.

3. Iqbal S, Shah S, Dhar V, Stavropoulos SN, Stevens PD. Is there any difference in outcomes between long pigtail and short flanged prophylactic pancreatic duct stents? *Dig Dis Sci.* 2011;56:260-265.

Endoscopic Biliary Sphincterotomy is Not Required for Transpapillary SEMS Placement for Biliary Obstruction

Banerjee N, Hilden K, Baron TH, et al (Univ of Utah School of Medicine, Salt Lake City; Mayo Clinic, Rochester, MN)
Dig Dis Sci 56:591-595, 2011

Background.—Endoscopic retrograde cholangiopancreatography with biliary self-expanding metal stent placement is the preferred method of providing biliary drainage for pancreaticobiliary malignancies. Some endoscopists routinely perform biliary sphincterotomy to facilitate biliary stent placement and potentially minimize pancreatitis with transpapillary self-expanding metal stent placement.

Aims.—Our hypothesis was that biliary sphincterotomy has no effect on the success rate of transpapillary self-expanding metal stent placement and increases procedure-related complications.

Methods.—In a retrospective analysis, outcomes of two groups were compared: (1) self-expanding metal stent placement without biliary sphincterotomy, (2) self-expanding metal stent placement with biliary sphincterotomy during the same procedure. Complications and stent patency rates were evaluated.

Results.—There were 104 subjects included in the study. Post-sphincterotomy bleeding ($p = 0.001$) was associated with biliary sphincterotomy performed immediately prior to self-expanding metal stent placement. Importantly, self-expanding metal stent placement without biliary sphincterotomy was always technically successful and self-expanding metal stent placement without biliary sphincterotomy was not associated with pancreatitis.

Conclusions.—Patients who undergo biliary sphincterotomy during transpapillary self-expanding metal stent placement experience more immediate complications than those who do not. Biliary sphincterotomy was not associated with longer stent patency. Self-expanding metal stent placement without a biliary sphincterotomy was not associated with pancreatitis regardless of the type of self-expanding metal stent used (covered or uncovered). Of the patients without a biliary sphincterotomy, 100% had successful stent placement, further arguing against its use in this setting.

▶ Placement of self-expanding metal stents (SEMS) for malignant obstruction of the bile duct is commonly performed. Endoscopic sphincterotomy (ES) is concurrently performed by some proceduralists with the justification that it may reduce the risk of pancreatitis by minimizing pancreatic duct orifice occlusion by the stent. In addition, there is some thought that it may improve stent function by permitting maximal stent dilatation at the level of the distal common bile duct

(CBD). This is a retrospective cohort study comparing complication rates associated with transpapillary biliary SEMS placement between patients who did or did not undergo ES immediately prior to stent placement. Patients receiving fully internalized biliary SEMS were excluded, as were those patients who had previously undergone pancreaticoduodenectomy or ES.

A total of 104 patients were identified on review of a procedural database from a single US center over a 10-year period. Twenty-seven patients (26%) had ES performed prior to SEMS placement, and 77 patients (74%) did not. Malignancy was diagnosed by a positive imaging modality study or consistent cytology on CBD brushings or endoscopic ultrasound-guided fine-needle aspiration (EUS-FNA). Stents used in this study included the uncovered biliary Wallflex Stent, the uncovered or partially covered biliary Wallstent, the Alimaxx-B biliary stent, and the Wilson-Cook Zilver Stent. A variety of tumors accounted for the biliary obstruction, including pancreatic adenocarcinoma, cholangiocarcinoma, and metastatic cancer; however, the study also included 8 patients with refractory benign biliary strictures. Fifty-seven percent of the cohort had distal CBD strictures and 19% had strictures in the mid-CBD; the remainder were more proximal, with one patient with malignant gastric outlet obstruction stented prophylactically. Two-thirds of the stents placed were uncovered.

Table 3 in the original article outlines the results; the only statistically significant difference between the groups was that bleeding was more common in the patients who underwent ES (18.5%). There was a trend toward having delayed complications in the no-ES group; however, this did not reach statistical significance.

This study demonstrates there is no advantage to performing ES when placing a SEMS for malignant biliary obstruction, and suggests that the immediate complication of ES-related bleeding is significantly higher. The post-ES bleeding rate of 18% is very high in this cohort compared with the 1.34% found in a recent review of 21 studies involving 16,855 patients between 1987 and 2003.[1] Clearly, the low patient numbers in this study predispose to type II errors, but this rate is concerning, particularly as patients with a coagulopathy were excluded from the study. The authors' explanation that this may be caused by pressure on the sphincterotomy site by the stent is incomplete; one would have to infer the pressure exerted by the stent was either inappropriately extending the sphincterotomy and rupturing adjacent blood vessels or may have caused ischemia to the surrounding tissue with subsequent necrosis followed by bleeding.

Seventeen patients in the cohort underwent repeat ERCP, 65% of whom were in the non-ES group. The most common indication was for known or suspected stent obstruction, and no particular relationship was identified to explain the increased incidence in the non-ES group. The authors mention briefly that there was no difference in patency rates between covered and uncovered SEMS used in the study, which is the same finding reported in a recent much larger multicenter randomized controlled trial.[2]

In conclusion, it is clear that ES should definitely not be performed prior to SEMS placement for malignant biliary obstruction.

S. M. Philcox, FRACP, MBBS (Hons), BMedSc

References

1. Andriulli A, Loperfido S, Napolitano G, et al. Incidence rates of post-ERCP complications: a systematic survey of prospective studies. *Am J Gastroenterol.* 2007;102: 1781-1788.
2. Kullman E, Frozanpor F, Söderlund C, et al. Covered versus uncovered self-expandable nitinol stents in the palliative treatment of malignant distal biliary obstruction: results from a randomized, multicenter study. *Gastrointest Endosc.* 2010;72:915-923.

Chronic Pancreatitis

Type of *CFTR* Mutation Determines Risk of Pancreatitis in Patients With Cystic Fibrosis

Ooi CY, Dorfman R, Cipolli M, et al (The Hosp for Sick Children, Toronto, Ontario, Canada; Azienda Ospedaliera Universitaria Integrata di Verona, Italy; et al)

Gastroenterology 140:153-161, 2011

Background & Aims.—Different mutations in the cystic fibrosis gene (CFTR) are associated with different functional status of the exocrine pancreas. We investigated whether CFTR genotypes determine the risk of pancreatitis in patients with cystic fibrosis (CF).

Methods.—Patients with pancreatic-sufficient CF were identified from 2 CF population-based databases (N = 277; 62 with pancreatitis and 215 without pancreatitis); patients' genotypes and clinical characteristics were analyzed. The loss of pancreatic function associated with each CFTR genotype was determined based on the pancreatic insufficiency prevalence (PIP) score.

Results.—Patients with pancreatitis were more likely to have genotypes associated with mild (70%) than moderate-severe (30%) PIP scores ($P = .004$). The cumulative proportion of patients who developed pancreatitis through to the age of 50 years was significantly greater for genotypes associated with mild (50%) than moderate-severe (27%) PIP scores ($P = .006$). The genotype associated with mild PIP scores had a hazard ratio of 2.4 for pancreatitis (95% confidence interval, 1.3—4.5; $P = .006$). Patients with pancreatitis were diagnosed with CF at an older median age than those without pancreatitis (14.9 years [interquartile range, 9.5—27.7] vs 9.3 years [interquartile range, 1.5—21.4]; $P = .003$) and had lower mean levels of sweat chloride than patients without pancreatitis (74.5 ± 26.2 mmol/L vs 82.8 ± 25.2 mmol/L; $P = .03$).

Conclusions.—Specific CFTR genotypes are significantly associated with pancreatitis. Patients with genotypes associated with mild phenotypic effects have a greater risk of developing pancreatitis than patients with genotypes associated with moderate-severe phenotypes. This observation provides further insight into the complex pathogenesis of pancreatitis (Fig 1).

▶ Chronic pancreatitis (CP) is a progressive inflammatory condition that causes structural damage to the pancreas and clinically is manifest by abdominal pain

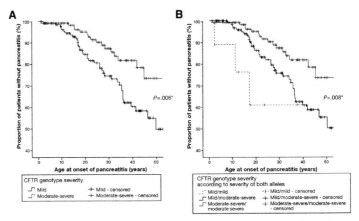

FIGURE 1.—Survival curves comparing time to pancreatitis in patients grouped according to severity of *CFTR* genotype. (*A*) Kaplan—Meier estimate of the proportion of patients with PS-CF who have not developed pancreatitis through to the age of 50 years for mild and severe *CFTR* genotype groups. (*B*) Kaplan—Meier estimate of the proportion of patients with PS-CF who have not developed pancreatitis through to the age of 50 years stratified according to the severity of both *CFTR* alleles. The survival tables (below each curve) indicate the number of patients/"survivors" at risk for pancreatitis at 0, 10, 20, 30, 40, and 50 years, respectively. (Reprinted from Ooi CY, Dorfman R, Cipolli M, et al. Type of *CFTR* mutation determines risk of pancreatitis in patients with cystic fibrosis. *Gastroenterology.* 2011;140:153-161, Copyright 2011, with permission from the AGA Institute.)

and pancreatic insufficiency. While the most common cause in adults is alcohol, as many as one-third of adult patients have idiopathic CP (ICP), and in the pediatric population, hereditary causes such as autosomal recessive cystic fibrosis (CF) account for most cases. CF results from mutations in the CF transmembrane conductance regulator (*CFTR*) gene, and some adults with certain mutations in this gene (eg, p.R75Q) may develop pancreatitis alone with no other clinical manifestations of CF. In addition, mutations in the serine protease 1 gene (*PRSS1*) on chromosome 7q35 are associated with autosomal dominant hereditary pancreatitis, and mutations in the serine protease inhibitor Kazal type 1 gene (*SPINK1*), in particular, the high-risk N34S and P55S haplotypes, have been associated with CP; *SPINK1* is a potent trypsin inhibitor activated by acute inflammation.

This study investigated the role of *CFTR* and *SPINK1* variants in ICP by genotyping the *CFTR* gene and exon 3 of the *SPINK1* gene in 2 independent populations with ICP and compared the results with controls. In addition, the authors looked at both calcium and bicarbonate conductance in *CFTR* p.R75Q polarized cell lines to find a physiological reason for its association with pancreatitis.

Fig 1 summarizes the patient and control groups. Twenty-nine of the 80 patients (36%) were found to be positive for a *SPINK1* exon 3 variant with a median onset of pancreatitis at age 13 as compared with age 34 in those 51 patients who were *SPINK1* negative (*P* < .001). When compared with the control populations, there was an overall odds ratio (OR) of 18 to develop pancreatitis in those with *SPINK1* variants, particularly N34S. Those 7 patients who carried 2 *SPINK1* mutations had an OR of 106 to develop pancreatitis compared with controls.

Multiple *CFTR* variants were identified and grouped according to their reported association with either severe or mild CF; those variants with no reported association were labeled as other. Both severe and mild CF variants were more common in the ICP patient group compared with controls; however, the other group was not. More than two-thirds of patients with a *SPINK1* mutation also had *CFTR* mutations, compared with 23% of controls. In those patients with ICP but without *SPINK1* mutations, *CFTR* mutations were also more common compared with controls (27.5% vs 14.5%). The 2 most common *CFTR* mutations found in this study were F508del and p.R75Q. Patients with both *SPINK1* and either of these 2 mutations had a markedly elevated risk of pancreatitis with an OR of 84.4, mostly associated with the F508del mutation. The combination of *SPINK1* and p.R75Q mutations was of particular interest, as this *CFTR* variant is not associated with typical CF phenotype and still demonstrated an OR of 25 with increased risk of pancreatitis.

For the second part of the study, HEK293 cell lines were used to express both wild-type *CFTR* and the p.R75Q mutant gene. Currents in a chloride solution did not demonstrate any significant difference in conductance; however, there was a 4-fold decrease in current with the p.R75Q mutant compared with wild type in a bicarbonate solution. This supports the hypothesis that this particular mutant expresses its phenotype by impaired bicarbonate conductance.

In conclusion, this study is of particular interest, as it takes the previously recognized association of transheterozygous *CFTR* and *SPINK1* variants markedly increasing the risk of pancreatitis in patients without clinical evidence of CF and goes on to definitively show that there are specific *CFTR* and *SPINK1* mutations that significantly increase this risk and in combination increase this risk further. In addition, the authors have also demonstrated that the increased risk in the p.R75Q *CFTR* variant is specifically associated with impaired bicarbonate conductance but not chloride conductance, thereby offering an explanation as to why the classic CF phenotype is absent.

S. M. Philcox, FRACP, MBBS (Hons), BMedSc

Outcome of Patients With Type 1 or 2 Autoimmune Pancreatitis
Maire F, Le Baleur Y, Rebours V, et al (Diderot-Paris VII Univ, Clichy, France; et al)
Am J Gastroenterol 106:151-156, 2011

Objectives.—Autoimmune pancreatitis (AIP) is better described than before, but there is still no international consensus for definition, diagnosis, and treatment. Our aims were to analyze the short- and long-term outcome of patients with focus on pancreatic endocrine and exocrine functions, to search for predictive factors of relapse and pancreatic insufficiency, and to compare patients with type 1 and type 2 AIP.

Methods.—All consecutive patients followed up for AIP in our center between 1999 and 2008 were included. Two groups were defined: (a) patients with type 1 AIP meeting HISORt (Histology, Imaging, Serology, Other organ involvement, and Response to steroids) criteria; (b) patients with definitive/probable type 2 AIP including those with histologically confirmed idiopathic duct-centric pancreatitis (definitive) or suggestive imaging, normal serum IgG4, and response to steroids (probable). AIP-related events and pancreatic exocrine/endocrine insufficiency were looked for during follow-up. Predictive factors of relapse and pancreatic insufficiency were analyzed.

Results.—A total of 44 patients (22 males), median age 37.5 (19–73) years, were included: 28 patients (64%) with type 1 AIP and 16 patients (36%) with type 2 AIP. First-line treatment consisted of steroids or pancreatic resection in 59 and 27% of the patients, respectively. Median follow-up was 41 (5–130) months. Steroids were effective in all treated patients. Relapse was observed in 12 patients (27%), after a median delay of 6 months (1–70). Four patients received azathioprine because of steroid resistance/dependence. High serum IgG4 level, pain at time of diagnosis, and other organ involvement were associated with relapse (P<0.05). At the end point, pancreatic atrophy was observed in 35% of patients. Exocrine and endocrine insufficiencies were present in 34 and 39% of the patients, respectively. At univariate analysis, no factor was associated with exocrine insufficiency, although female gender (P=0.04), increasing age (P=0.006), and type 1 AIP (P=0.001) were associated with the occurrence of diabetes. Steroid/azathioprine treatment did not prevent pancreatic insufficiency. Type 2 AIP was more frequently associated with inflammatory bowel disease than type 1 AIP (31 and 3%, respectively), but relapse rates were similar in both groups.

Conclusions.—Relapse occurs in 27% of AIP patients and is more frequent in patients with high serum IgG4 levels at the time of diagnosis. Pancreatic atrophy and functional insufficiency occur in more than one-third of the patients within 3 years of diagnosis. The outcome of patients with type 2 AIP, a condition often associated with inflammatory bowel disease, is not different from that of patients with type 1 AIP, except for diabetes.

▶ Autoimmune pancreatitis (AIP) is a rare condition that can be mistaken for pancreatic cancer[1] given its similar radiological appearance and clinical presentation, so it is an important differential to consider. This article is a retrospective review of patients in a single center in France who were diagnosed with either type 1 or type 2 AIP over a 9-year period. The aim of the review was to document outcomes regarding pancreatic endocrine and exocrine function, to identify predictors of relapse and pancreatic insufficiency, and to see if there were differences between each type of AIP.

The selection of patients included in the study was based both on the Mayo Histology, Imaging, Serology, Other organ involvement, and Response to steroids (HISORt) criteria[2] for type 1 patients and a reasonable, but not universally accepted, definition of type 2 patients; this is consistent with recently published international consensus guidelines.[3] There were 28 type 1 patients and 16 type 2 patients identified over the 9-year period of the study, demonstrating how uncommon the disease is. Twelve patients were initially thought to have pancreatic cancer (27%) and underwent surgery, with an additional 26 patients commenced on steroids, 4 of whom also required azathioprine. Six patients required no treatment. Twelve patients relapsed, with a median time to relapse of 6 months, and most were treated again with steroids, with a 90% response rate.

There were several differences between the 2 groups that were statistically significant: The patients with type 2 were younger (median age 27 vs 48 years) and were more likely to have inflammatory bowel disease (5 vs 1 patients). Patients with type 1 were more likely to have other organ involvement (5 vs 2 patients) and have an elevated serum immunoglobulin (Ig) G4; this was seen in 12 patients with type 1 (43%) and in none with type 2. Type 1 patients were also more likely to be diabetic (16 patients, ie, 57% vs 1 patient), with an increase from 3 patients at the start to 17 patients by the finish. These data are suggestive of an association between type 1 AIP and the development of diabetes, although other factors, such as pancreatic surgery, age, or steroid use, may also play a role in this finding. Thirty-five percent of patients developed exocrine insufficiency, with no significant difference between the 2 types. Factors predictive of relapse included high serum IgG4 levels (odds ratio 5.5), abdominal pain as a presenting symptom, and other organ involvement.

This study is naturally limited by the retrospective observational design but raises several interesting points. All patients in this study responded to treatment, with 1 in 4 patients relapsing; relapse was associated with elevated serum IgG4 levels. Azathioprine was shown to be effective in avoiding relapse despite steroid cessation, although follow-up was limited to 3 years in these patients. Diabetes, particularly insulin-requiring, commonly developed in patients with type 1 AIP, although this may reflect older age, higher exposure to pancreatic surgery, and steroid use in this group. There were no significant differences between the 2 groups regarding exocrine insufficiency.

There was not enough information provided to assess whether the diagnostic criteria were used in a prospective or retrospective fashion; with 1 in 4 patients in this cohort undergoing unnecessary surgery, it is hoped that future studies will report these data prospectively. Although we were told 35% of the cohort developed pancreatic changes on imaging throughout the study, no initial imaging data were presented. Endoscopic ultrasound was underused, with only 25% of the cohort undergoing this assessment; it appeared that only 1 in 3 patients were identified as having elevated tissue IgG4 at fine-needle aspiration (FNA). No information was provided as to whether this was a core biopsy that has been shown to be superior to FNA. Future studies will hopefully provide guidance as to the prospective utility of the HISORt criteria and whether there is clinical benefit and cost-effectiveness to assess all pancreatic masses with these guidelines in mind.

S. M. Philcox, FRACP, MBBS (Hons), BMedSc

References

1. Song Y, Liu QD, Zhou NX, Zhang WZ, Wang DJ. Diagnosis and management of autoimmune pancreatitis: experience from China. *World J Gastroenterol.* 2008; 14:601-606.
2. Chari ST. Diagnosis of autoimmune pancreatitis using its five cardinal features: introducing the Mayo Clinic's HISORt criteria. *J Gastroenterol.* 2007;42:39-41.
3. Shimosegawa T, Chari ST, Frulloni L, et al. International consensus diagnostic criteria for autoimmune pancreatitis: guidelines of the International Association of Pancreatology. *Pancreas.* 2011;40:352-358.

A 6-month, open-label clinical trial of pancrelipase delayed-release capsules (Creon) in patients with exocrine pancreatic insufficiency due to chronic pancreatitis or pancreatic surgery

Gubergrits N, Malecka-Panas E, Lehman GA, et al (Donetsk Natl Med Univ, Ukraine; Med Univ of Lodz, Poland; Indiana Univ Med Ctr, Indianapolis; et al)
Aliment Pharmacol Ther 33:1152-1161, 2011

Background.—Pancreatic enzyme replacement therapy (PERT) is necessary to prevent severe maldigestion and unwanted weight loss associated with exocrine pancreatic insufficiency (EPI) due to chronic pancreatitis (CP) or pancreatic surgery (PS).

Aim.—To assess the long-term safety and efficacy of pancrelipase (pancreatin) delayed-release capsules (Creon) in this population.

Methods.—This was a 6-month, open-label extension of a 7-day, double-blind, placebo-controlled study enrolling patients ≥18 years old with confirmed EPI due to CP or PS who were previously receiving PERT. Patients received individualised pancrelipase doses as directed by investigators (administered as Creon 24 000-lipase unit capsules).

Results.—Overall, 48 of 51 patients completed the open-label phase; one withdrew due to the unrelated treatment-emergent adverse event (TEAE) of cutaneous burns and two were lost to follow-up. The mean age was 50.9 years, 70.6% of patients were male, 76.5% had CP and 23.5% had undergone PS. The mean ± s.d. pancrelipase dose was 186 960 ± 74 640 lipase units/day. TEAEs were reported by 22 patients (43.1%) overall. Only four patients (7.8%) had TEAEs that were considered treatment related. From double-blind phase baseline to end of the open-label period, subjects achieved a mean ± s.d. body weight increase of 2.7 ± 3.4 kg ($P < 0.0001$) and change in daily stool frequency of −1.0 ± 1.3 ($P < 0.001$). Improvements in abdominal pain, flatulence and stool consistency were observed.

Conclusions.—Pancrelipase was well tolerated over 6 months and resulted in statistically significant weight gain and reduced stool frequency in patients with EPI due to CP or PS previously managed with standard PERT.

▶ Exocrine pancreatic insufficiency leads to malabsorption and is often associated with weight loss and malnutrition. Pancreatic enzyme supplementation has been a well-accepted part of the management of these patients for many years; however, this is the first study to demonstrate meaningful increases in body weight and reduction in stool frequency over 6 months of treatment with an acceptable side-effect profile. The mean weight gain was 2.7 ± 3.4 kg, and there was a significant decrease in daily stool frequency from 2.8 to 1.8. The doses of enzyme replacement were higher than reported previously with a mean daily dosage of 186 960 ± 74 640 units of lipase, although the response was not dose dependent. No change was demonstrated in symptoms, such as abdominal pain, stool consistency or flatulence, clinical global improvement scores, or quality of life measures. Treatment-related adverse events occurred in 7.8% of patients and included mild abdominal pain, flatulence, diarrhea, and weight gain in a patient with a body mass index of 35.

Although healthy skepticism should be applied to any nonrandomized and company-funded research, this study does suggest enzyme supplementation has potential value in those patients with confirmed pancreatic insufficiency caused by chronic pancreatitis or pancreatic surgery, at least in terms of weight gain. The doses used in this study are higher than previously reported, and further study on optimal dosing schedules should be performed.

S. M. Philcox, FRACP, MBBS (Hons), BMedSc

Acute Pancreatitis

A Step-up Approach or Open Necrosectomy for Necrotizing Pancreatitis
van Santvoort HC, for the Dutch Pancreatitis Study Group (Univ Med Ctr, Utrecht, the Netherlands; et al)
N Engl J Med 362:1491-1502, 2010

Background.—Necrotizing pancreatitis with infected necrotic tissue is associated with a high rate of complications and death. Standard treatment is open necrosectomy. The outcome may be improved by a minimally invasive step-up approach.

Methods.—In this multicenter study, we randomly assigned 88 patients with necrotizing pancreatitis and suspected or confirmed infected necrotic tissue to undergo primary open necrosectomy or a step-up approach to treatment. The step-up approach consisted of percutaneous drainage followed, if necessary, by minimally invasive retroperitoneal necrosectomy. The primary end point was a composite of major complications (new-onset multiple-organ failure or multiple systemic complications, perforation of a visceral organ or enterocutaneous fistula, or bleeding) or death.

Results.—The primary end point occurred in 31 of 45 patients (69%) assigned to open necrosectomy and in 17 of 43 patients (40%) assigned to the step-up approach (risk ratio with the step-up approach, 0.57; 95% confidence interval, 0.38 to 0.87; P=0.006). Of the patients assigned to the step-up approach, 35% were treated with percutaneous drainage only. New-onset multiple-organ failure occurred less often in patients assigned to the step-up approach than in those assigned to open necrosectomy (12% vs. 40%, P=0.002). The rate of death did not differ significantly between groups (19% vs. 16%, P=0.70). Patients assigned to the step-up approach had a lower rate of incisional hernias (7% vs. 24%, P=0.03) and new-onset diabetes (16% vs. 38%, P=0.02).

Conclusions.—A minimally invasive step-up approach, as compared with open necrosectomy, reduced the rate of the composite end point of major complications or death among patients with necrotizing pancreatitis and infected necrotic tissue. (Current Controlled Trials number, ISRCTN13975868.)

▶ This is a very elegant randomized multicenter study from the Netherlands, which is known for high-quality multicenter trials in the field of acute pancreatitis. Eighty-eight patients underwent randomization to open necrosectomy or a step-up approach, initially with percutaneous or endoscopic drainage followed by video-assisted retroperitoneal debridement (VARD). Interestingly, 42% of those who underwent the open procedure required additional surgical intervention, and 33% required further percutaneous drainage. Of those who underwent the step-up approach, 35% required only percutaneous or endoscopic drainage without further intervention, with a further 60% undergoing VARD. Thirty-three percent required additional debridement procedures, and 27% required further percutaneous drainage. A significant advantage of the step-up approach was demonstrated with respect to major complications or death with a risk ratio (RR) of 0.57 (95% confidence interval, 0.38-0.87) in favor of the step-up approach, and new-onset organ failure was less common in this group as well with absolute RR of 28, which translates to an number needed to treat of 3.5. Mortality was not statistically different between the 2 groups, with around 1 in 5 to 6 patients passing away despite either intervention.

This study concisely demonstrates why most centers are no longer performing open necrosectomy as first-line debridement of complicated pancreatic necrosis. Whether VARD will be the mainstay compared with even less invasive approaches such as endoscopic necrosectomy remains to be seen; several groups have reported equivalent data with the latter approach, and more data are emerging to support its use primarily.[1,2] However, according to this study, VARD is unequivocally superior to open necrosectomy and should be the treatment of choice in units performing this procedure.

S. M. Philcox, FRACP, MBBS (Hons), BMedSc

References

1. Gardner TB, Coelho-Prabhu N, Gordon SR, et al. Direct endoscopic necrosectomy for the treatment of walled-off pancreatic necrosis: results from a multicenter U.S. series. *Gastrointest Endosc.* 2011;73:718-726.
2. Seifert H, Biermer M, Schmitt W, et al. Transluminal endoscopic necrosectomy after acute pancreatitis: a multicentre study with long-term follow-up (the GEPARD Study). *Gut.* 2009;58:1260-1266.

Direct endoscopic necrosectomy for the treatment of walled-off pancreatic necrosis: results from a multicenter U.S. series
Gardner TB, Coelho-Prabhu N, Gordon SR, et al (Dartmouth-Hitchcock Med Ctr, Lebanon, NH; Mayo Clinic, Rochester, MN; et al)
Gastrointest Endosc 73:718-726, 2011

Background.—Direct endoscopic necrosectomy (DEN) for treatment of walled-off pancreatic necrosis (WOPN) has been performed as an alternative to operative or percutaneous therapy.

Objective.—To report the largest combined experience of DEN performed for WOPN.

Design.—Retrospective chart review.

Setting.—Six U.S. tertiary medical centers.

Patients.—A total of 104 patients with a history of acute pancreatitis and symptomatic WOPN since 2003.

Interventions.—DEN for WOPN.

Main Outcome Measurements.—Resolution or near-resolution of WOPN without the need for surgical or percutaneous intervention and procedural complications.

Results.—Successful resolution was achieved in 95 of 104 patients (91%). Of the patients in whom it failed, 5 died during follow-up before resolution, 2 underwent operative drainage for persistent WOPN, 1 required surgery for massive bleeding on fistula tract dilation, and 1 died periprocedurally. The mean time to resolution from the initial DEN was 4.1 months. The first débridement was performed a mean of 63 days after the initial onset of acute pancreatitis. In 73%, the entry was transgastric with median tract dilation diameter of 18 mm. The median number of procedures was 3 with 2 débridements. Complications occurred in approximately 14% and included 5 retrogastric perforations/pneumoperitoneum, which were managed nonoperatively. Univariate analysis identified a body mass index >32 as a risk factor for failed DEN.

Limitations.—Retrospective, highly specialized centers.

Conclusions.—This large, multicenter series demonstrates that transmural, minimally invasive endoscopic débridement of WOPN performed in the United States is an efficacious and reproducible technique with an acceptable safety profile.

▶ Historically, patients with symptomatic walled-off pancreatic necrosis (WOPN) have been managed surgically. Over the past 15 years, however, there has been a shift toward minimally invasive approaches, including laparoscopic (mainly video-assisted retroperitoneal debridement or VARD), percutaneous, and endoscopic. This study is a US-based multicenter retrospective case series reporting their experience with a minimally invasive endoscopic approach to debridement of necrotic pancreatic tissue following severe pancreatitis.

Successful resolution of WOPN was achieved in 95 of 104 patients (91%), with a mean number of 3.7 procedures over 4.1 months (3.5-4.6). Endoscopic ultrasound was used to guide the procedure in 45% of cases, and recurrence was seen in just 6%. Lesions measuring up to 34 cm in maximal cross-sectional diameter were included, and debridement was performed most often via a transgastric route following balloon-dilation of a fistula tract to an average of 18 mm in diameter. The overall complication rate was 14%, and most of these were managed medically without the need for reintervention or surgery; there were 2 procedure-related, 2 deaths, and 2 patients who required nonendoscopic intervention for uncontrolled bleeding. These results are equivalent or superior to comparable surgical series.

Despite the limitations of noncomparative retrospective data collection, these results are very encouraging and reflect the changing face of the management of these patients. There are no randomized studies comparing endoscopic debridement with other minimally invasive approaches, and the Pancreatitis, Necrosectomy Versus Step-Up Approach (PANTER) trial really only compared percutaneous drainage and VARD with open surgery because only 2 patients underwent endoscopic debridement[1]; it is to be hoped that this type of comparison will be published in the future. Intuitively, the most logical approach would be a step-up approach to management following a multidisciplinary patient review to guide the selection of the most appropriate approach for an individual patient. Which particular minimally invasive technique should be used will inevitably be influenced by the locally available expertise at any particular institution.

S. M. Philcox, FRACP, MBBS (Hons), BMedSc

Reference

1. Besselink MG, van Santvoort HC, Nieuwenhuijs VB, et al. Minimally invasive 'step-up approach' versus maximal necrosectomy in patients with acute necrotising pancreatitis (PANTER trial): design and rationale of a randomised controlled multicenter trial [ISRCTN13975868]. *BMC Surg.* 2006;6:6.

Pancreatic Ductal Complications

External Pancreatic Duct Stent Decreases Pancreatic Fistula Rate After Pancreaticoduodenectomy: Prospective Multicenter Randomized Trial

Pessaux P, Fédération de Recherche en Chirurgie (French) (Université de Strasbourg, France; et al)
Ann Surg 253:879-885, 2011

Objective.—Pancreatic fistula (PF) is a leading cause of morbidity and mortality after pancreaticoduodenectomy (PD). The aim of this multicenter prospective randomized trial was to compare the results of PD with an external drainage stent versus no stent.

Methods.—Between 2006 and 2009, 158 patients who underwent PD were randomized intraoperatively to either receive an external stent inserted across the anastomosis to drain the pancreatic duct (n = 77) or no stent (n = 81). The criteria of inclusion were soft pancreas and a diameter of wirsung <3 mm. The primary study end point was PF rate defined as amylase-rich fluid (amylase concentration >3 times the upper limit of normal serum amylase level) collected from the peripancreatic drains after postoperative day 3. CT scan was routinely done on day 7.

Results.—The 2 groups were comparable concerning demographic data, underlying pathologies, presenting symptoms, presence of comorbid illness, and proportion of patients with preoperative biliary drainage. Mortality, morbidity, and PF rates were 3.8%, 51.8%, and 34.2%, respectively. Stented group had a significantly lower overall PF (26% vs. 42%; $P = 0.034$), morbidity (41.5% vs. 61.7%; $P = 0.01$), and delayed gastric emptying (7.8% vs. 27.2%; $P = 0.001$) rates compared with nonstented group. Radiologic or surgical intervention for PF was required in 9 patients in the stented group and 12 patients in the nonstented group. There were no significant differences in mortality rate (3.7% vs. 3.9%; $P = 0.37$) and in hospital stay (22 days vs. 26 days; $P = 0.11$).

Conclusion.—External drainage of pancreatic duct with a stent reduced. PF and overall morbidity rates after PD in high risk patients (soft pancreatic texture and a nondilated pancreatic duct). This study is registered at http://www.clinicaltrials.gov: Clinical trial ID# NCT01068886.

▶ As the authors point out, pancreatic fistula remains the Achilles heel of pancreaticoduodenectomy (PD). Over the past 30 years, extensive efforts and discussions have focused on this exact topic. Single-institution series have offered all manner of intraoperative and perioperative management in attempts to decrease the risk of pancreatic anastomotic leak. Techniques have ranged from obliteration of the remnant pancreatic duct by latex injection, to dunking the entire open end of the gland into the bowel, both intended to avoid the creation of an anastomosis to the pancreatic duct entirely. Through all these years, there has not been a definitive answer to what is the best technique for minimizing pancreatic leak and fistula after PD.

Herein the authors have completed a prospective, randomized controlled trial of stenting the pancreatic anastomosis with an externalized stent versus no stenting at all. This is a multicenter study and is well conceived and executed. The external stents were used in "high-risk" cases, defined as a soft pancreatic parenchyma and no ductal dilation. The analysis is sound, and the authors acknowledge the weaknesses of the study, a major one being the lack of control for surgeon experience and anastomotic technique.

The authors find that external stenting in this "high-risk" group reduced pancreatic anastomotic leak and fistula and decreased overall morbidity.

Of course we all like data that support our biases. It has been several years since I have performed much pancreatic surgery, but during the last year of my training and in my first few years in practice, I would perform 15 to 20 PD annually. It was always my practice to bring a small pediatric feeding tube across the anastomosis and externalize the end. I would leave the stent to drain until around postoperative day 5 when I would obtain a contrast study through the external stent and base its management on the results. Anecdotally, I felt like my partners who were not using stents were more frequently at Morbidity and Mortality with leaks and fistulae than I was seeing in my patients, not something easily discussed among competitive pancreatic surgeons. This study would certainly support my bias and anecdotal experience.

C. D. Smith, MD

4 Gastrointestinal Cancers and Benign Polyps

Colon Cancer

Long-term effect of aspirin on colorectal cancer incidence and mortality: 20-year follow-up of five randomised trials
Rothwell PM, Wilson M, Elwin C-E, et al (Univ of Oxford, UK; Karolinska Institutet, Stockholm, Sweden; et al)
Lancet 376:1741-1750, 2010

Background.—High-dose aspirin (≥ 500 mg daily) reduces long-term incidence of colorectal cancer, but adverse effects might limit its potential for long-term prevention. The long-term effectiveness of lower doses (75–300 mg daily) is unknown. We assessed the effects of aspirin on incidence and mortality due to colorectal cancer in relation to dose, duration of treatment, and site of tumour.

Methods.—We followed up four randomised trials of aspirin versus control in primary (Thrombosis Prevention Trial, British Doctors Aspirin Trial) and secondary (Swedish Aspirin Low Dose Trial, UK-TIA Aspirin Trial) prevention of vascular events and one trial of different doses of aspirin (Dutch TIA Aspirin Trial) and established the effect of aspirin on risk of colorectal cancer over 20 years during and after the trials by analysis of pooled individual patient data.

Results.—In the four trials of aspirin versus control (mean duration of scheduled treatment 6·0 years), 391 (2·8%) of 14033 patients had colorectal cancer during a median follow-up of 18·3 years. Allocation to aspirin reduced the 20-year risk of colon cancer (incidence hazard ratio [HR] 0·76, 0·60–0·96, p=0·02; mortality HR 0·65, 0·48–0·88, p=0·005), but not rectal cancer (0·90, 0·63–1·30, p=0·58; 0·80, 0·50–1·28, p=0·35). Where subsite data were available, aspirin reduced risk of cancer of the proximal colon (0·45, 0·28–0·74, p=0·001; 0·34, 0·18–0·66, p=0·001), but not the distal colon (1·10, 0·73–1·64, p=0·66; 1·21, 0·66–2·24, p=0·54; for incidence difference p=0·04, for mortality difference p=0·01). However, benefit increased with scheduled duration of treatment, such that allocation to aspirin of 5 years or longer reduced risk of proximal colon cancer by about 70% (0·35, 0·20—0·63; 0·24, 0·11—0·52; both p<0·0001) and also reduced risk of rectal cancer (0·58, 0·36—0·92, p=0·02; 0·47, 0·26—0·87, p=0·01). There was no increase in benefit at doses of aspirin greater than 75 mg daily, with an absolute reduction of 1·76% (0·61—2·91; p=0·001) in 20-year risk of any fatal colorectal cancer after 5-years scheduled treatment with 75—300 mg daily. However, risk of fatal colorectal cancer was higher on 30 mg versus 283 mg daily on long-term follow-up of the Dutch TIA trial (odds ratio 2·02, 0·70—6·05, p=0·15).

Interpretation.—Aspirin taken for several years at doses of at least 75 mg daily reduced long-term incidence and mortality due to colorectal cancer. Benefit was greatest for cancers of the proximal colon, which are not otherwise prevented effectively by screening with sigmoidoscopy or colonoscopy (Table 3).

▶ For decades, aspirin has been recognized as potential chemoprevention for colorectal cancer (CRC). In many respects it is an ideal agent because it is widely available, simple to administer (once-daily dosing), and inexpensive. Multiple lines of epidemiologic, cohort, and retrospective evidence support the concept that aspirin and related inhibitors of cyclo-oxygenase II reduce the rate and mortality of CRC. Because development of CRC is relatively uncommon and takes many years, trials in this field have used adenoma

TABLE 3.—Effect of Aspirin (75—1200 mg) Versus Control on Long-Term Risk of Colorectal Cancer

| | | All Patients | | Scheduled Treatment Duration ≥5 Years | | |
	Events	Hazard Ratio (95% CI)	P	Events	Hazard Ratio (95% CI)	P
All cancers	397	0·76 (0·63-0·94)	0·01	316	0·68 (0·54-0·87)	0·002
Proximal colon	69	0·45 (0·28-0·74)	0·001	61	0·35 (0·20-0·63)	<0·0001
Distal colon	100	1·10 (0·73-1·64)	0·66	75	1·14 (0·69-1·86)	0·61
Colon (site unspecified)	109	0·74 (0·51-1·07)	0·11	93	0·81 (0·52-1·25)	0·34
All colon	278	0·76 (0·60-0·96)	0·02	229	0·75 (0·58-0·97)	0·03
Rectum	119	0·90 (0·63-1·30)	0·58	87	0·58 (0·36-0·92)	0·02
Fatal cancers	240	0·66 (0·52-0·86)	0·002	193	0·57 (0·42-0·78)	<0·0001
Proximal colon	41	0·34 (0·18-0·66)	0·001	37	0·24 (0·11-0·52)	<0·0001
Distal colon	44	1·21 (0·66-2·24)	0·54	30	1·24 (0·58-2·65)	0·58
Colon (site unspecified)	89	0·61 (0·40-0·94)	0·02	75	0·71 (0·44-1·17)	0·18
All colon	174	0·65 (0·48-0·88)	0·005	142	0·63 (0·45—0·87)	0·006
Rectum	70	0·80 (0·50—1·28)	0·35	54	0·47 (0·26-0·87)	0·01

Numbers differ slightly from those quoted for case-fatality in the main text because of inclusion of data from SALT. Stratified by site of tumour and by scheduled duration of treatment allocated in the initial randomised trial in a pooled analysis (Cox regression, stratified by trial) of the Thrombosis Prevention Trial, the Swedish Aspirin Low Dose Trial (SALT), the UK-TIA Aspirin Trial, and the British Doctors Aspirin Trial. The p values are taken from a Cox model stratified by study and the analysis of patients with longer scheduled trial treatments includes all events from the time of random assignment. The p values therefore differ slightly from those obtained from the log-rank test in analyses from different timepoints in figure 2. Two colorectal cancers at different sites are included in four patients in whom it was not possible to establish which cancer was responsible for death.

recurrence rates after colonoscopic polypectomy as a surrogate for cancer prevention. These studies have consistently demonstrated a reduction in recurrence of approximately 20%.

Multiple trials with placebo control in prevention of vascular disease have enrolled large numbers of patients on a variety of doses of aspirin. Long-term follow-up of 2 such studies showed a reduction in CRC risk, but the dose of aspirin was high (500 mg/d or higher). Bleeding complications associated with this dose of aspirin could negate the protective effect and limit the potential for chemoprevention. For example, the bleeding risk associated with daily aspirin use (including hemorrhagic stroke) makes the recommendation for daily acetylsalicylic acid prophylaxis against myocardial infarction, a much more common lethal condition than CRC, a controversial recommendation in average-risk subjects. Thus, although the complication rate of daily aspirin is definitely dose-dependent, the effect of dose on risk of CRC is unknown.

Indirect observational studies have suggested that higher doses of aspirin were necessary, and 2 large trials of low-dose alternate-day aspirin failed to show protection against CRC. However, the duration of the follow-up was 10 years, which may be insufficient to demonstrate a protective effect for cancer.

To try to address these deficiencies, these European authors examined the outcomes of 5 randomized trials of daily aspirin of various doses and obtained CRC rates after 20 years of follow-up. This important study made several key points highlighted in Table 3 from the article. Doses as low as 75 mg per day lowered the risk of CRC, which was almost exclusively due to reductions in right-sided colon cancer. The observation that mortality was reduced more than incidence suggests that aspirin might mitigate against the aggressiveness of CRC, perhaps especially proximal cancers that have a distinct pathobiology and are difficult to detect with colonoscopy.

Overall, the relative 70% and absolute 1.5% reduction in CRC mortality has implications for clinical practice. In patients with a secondary indication for antiplatelet treatment, aspirin should be favored over other drugs. Furthermore, reduced CRC mortality must be calculated in the finely balanced analysis of reduced cardiovascular mortality with major bleeding risk; this additional benefit of aspirin could tip the balance in favor of more patients qualifying for treatment. Finally, from an endoscopist's point of view, the importance of right-sided colon cancer prevention cannot be overemphasized. The failure of colonoscopy and polypectomy to reduce proximal colon cancer has been a consistent finding in recent large-scale observational studies. Daily aspirin combined with colonoscopy (possibly with less frequent surveillance intervals) could be synergistic and improve outcomes at reduced cost for CRC screening.

R. K. Pearson, MD

High prevalence of colorectal neoplasm in patients with non-alcoholic steatohepatitis

Wong VW-S, Wong GL-H, Tsang SW-C, et al (The Chinese Univ of Hong Kong, China; Tseung Kwan O Hosp, Hong Kong, China)
Gut 60:829-836, 2011

Objective.—Non-alcoholic fatty liver disease (NAFLD) affects 20—40% of the general adult population. Due to shared risk factors, it is postulated that NAFLD patients have an increased risk of colorectal neoplasm and should be a target group for screening. The aim of this study was to examine the prevalence of colorectal neoplasm in NAFLD patients and the risk of colorectal neoplasm in relation to the severity of NAFLD histology.

Design.—Cross-sectional study.

Setting.—University hospital with case recruitment from the community and clinics.

Patients.—Subjects aged 40—70 years were recruited for colonoscopic screening from two study cohorts: (1) community subjects; and (2) consecutive patients with biopsy proven NAFLD. In the community cohort, hepatic fat was measured by proton-magnetic resonance spectroscopy.

Main Outcome Measures.—Prevalence of colorectal adenomas. Advanced colorectal neoplasm was defined as cancer or adenomas with villous architecture or high grade dysplasia.

Results.—NAFLD patients (N=199) had a higher prevalence of colorectal adenomas (34.7% vs 21.5%; p=0.043) and advanced neoplasms (18.6% vs 5.5%; p=0.002) than healthy controls (N=181). Thirteen of 29 (45%) NAFLD patients with advanced neoplasms had isolated lesions in the right sided colon. Among patients with biopsy proven NAFLD, patients with non-alcoholic steatohepatitis (N=49) had a higher prevalence of adenomas (51.0% vs 25.6%; p=0.005) and advanced neoplasms (34.7% vs 14.0%; p=0.011) than those with simple steatosis (N=86). After adjusting for demographic and metabolic factors, non-alcoholic steatohepatitis remained associated with adenomas (adjusted OR 4.89, 95% CI 2.04 to 11.70) and advanced neoplasms (OR 5.34, 95% CI 1.92 to 14.84). In contrast, the prevalence of adenomas and advanced neoplasms was similar between patients with simple steatosis and control subjects.

Conclusions.—Non-alcoholic steatohepatitis is associated with a high prevalence of colorectal adenomas and advanced neoplasms. The adenomas are found more commonly in the right sided colon. Colorectal cancer screening is strongly indicated in this high risk group (Table 1).

▶ A "strong" family history has been accepted as a useful tool for defining risk for colorectal cancer (CRC) and figures into screening and surveillance guidelines. On one end of the spectrum are the autosomal dominant inherited syndromes, such as hereditary nonpolyposis colon cancer (HNPCC) with their very high risk of CRC, which should be monitored with very early and frequent colonoscopy. Familial colorectal cancer (FCC) is generally defined as a clustering of CRC without features or evidence of HNPCC or other

TABLE 1.—Clinical Characteristics of NAFLD and Control Subjects

Characteristics	Biopsy-Proven NAFLD (N=135)	NAFLD by ^{1}H-MRS (N=64)	Controls (N=181)
Age (SD), years	50.8 (8.5)	50.3 (5.8)	48.5 (5.8)
Male gender, n (%)	74 (54.8)	37 (57.8)	66 (36.5)
Ever smoker, n (%)	10 (7.4)	11 (17.2)	30 (16.6)
Colorectal cancer in first degree relatives, n (%)	8 (5.9)	6 (9.4)	9 (5.0)
BMI (SD), kg/m^2	27.7(4.0)	24.9 (2.8)	22.3 (3.6)
Male	28.3 (3.6)	25.2 (2.5)	22.8 (2.4)
Female	26.9 (4.4)	24.4 (3.2)	22.1 (4.1)
Waist circumference (SD), cm	95.0 (10.0)	88.3 (7.5)	79.4 (8.4)
Male	97.2 (9.6)	90.9 (5.7)	84.0 (7.4)
Female	92.2 (9.8)	84.6 (8.2)	76.8 (7.8)
Fasting glucose (SD), mmol/l	6.3 (2.0)	5.8 (1.8)	5.0 (0.5)
Total cholesterol (SD), mmol/l	5.1 (1.5)	5.6 (1.0)	5.5 (3.1)
HDL cholesterol (SD), mmol/l	1.0 (1.5)	1.4 (0.3)	1.6 (0.4)
LDL cholesterol (SD), mmol/l	2.5 (2.7)	3.4 (0.9)	3.3 (2.0)
Triglycerides (SD), mmol/l	2.1 (1.5)	1.9 (1.3)	1.2 (0.7)
ALT (SD), IU/l	65 (39)	33 (17)	24 (20)
AST (SD), IU/l	45 (27)	22 (8)	21 (6)
Diabetes, n (%)	72 (53.3)	9 (14.3)	4 (2.2)
Hypertension, n (%)	64 (47.4)	15 (23.4)	24 (13.3)
Hepatic triglyceride content (SD), %	–	11.0 (5.7)	1.8 (1.3)
Steatosis grade, 1/2/3	51/54/29	–	–
Lobular inflammation, 0/1/2/3	62/65/6/1	–	–
Ballooning, 0/1/2	44/87/3	–	–
Fibrosis stage, 0/1/2/3/4	51/50/13/11/9	–	–
NAFLD activity score (range)	3 (0–6)	–	–
Non-alcoholic steatohepatitis, n (%)	49 (36.3)	–	–

ALT, alanine aminotransferase; AST, aspartate aminotransferase; BMI, body mass index; HDL, high density lipoprotein. ^{1}H-MRS, proton-magnetic resonance spectroscopy; LDL, low density lipoprotein; NAFLD, non-alcoholic fatty liver disease.

syndromes. Patients in this category are far more common in clinical practice. Substantial literature exists, indicating a relative risk of 4 to 6 in the lifetime risk of developing cancer. However, the adenoma detection rate is based on small retrospective studies.

This study from the Netherlands fills in several gaps. Using standard definitions of a high-risk family based either on age under 50 of a single first-degree relative with CRC or number of first-degree relatives affected, these investigators prospectively recruited subjects from FCC kindreds for a study examining surveillance intervals after polypectomy (3 vs 6 years). This report summarizes the yield of the 456 subjects' (from 317 families) first colonoscopy.

As summarized in Table 1, the detection rate of both adenomas and advanced adenomas justifies the attention paid to these kindreds in guidelines for CRC screening. Using published prevalence data from the literature for the average-risk general population, this study indicates a doubling of the risk of adenomas and advanced lesions in this cohort. This study will go forward to address the question of whether surveillance intervals need to be adjusted in these patients, but this result highlights the importance of an accurate family history in stratifying risk for CRC.

R. K. Pearson, MD

Endoscopic Mucosal Resection Outcomes and Prediction of Submucosal Cancer From Advanced Colonic Mucosal Neoplasia

Moss A, Bourke MJ, Williams SJ, et al (Westmead Hosp, Sydney, New South Wales, Australia; et al)
Gastroenterology 140:1909-1918, 2011

Background & Aims.—Large sessile colonic polyps usually are managed surgically, with significant morbidity and potential mortality. There have been few prospective, intention-to-treat, multicenter studies of endoscopic mucosal resection (EMR). We investigated whether endoscopic criteria can predict invasive disease and direct the optimal treatment strategy.

Methods.—The Australian Colonic Endoscopic (ACE) resection study group conducted a prospective, multicenter, observational study of all patients referred for EMR of sessile colorectal polyps that were 20 mm or greater in size (n = 479, mean age, 68.5 y; mean lesion size, 35.6 mm). We analyzed data on lesion characteristics and procedural, clinical, and histologic outcomes. Multiple logistic regression analysis identified independent predictors of EMR efficacy and recurrence of adenoma, based on findings from follow-up colonoscopy examinations.

Results.—Risk factors for submucosal invasion were as follows: Paris classification 0—IIa+c morphology, nongranular surface, and Kudo pit pattern type V. The most commonly observed lesion (0—IIa granular) had a low rate of submucosal invasion (1.4%). EMR was effective at completely removing the polyp in a single session in 89.2% of patients; risk factors for lack of efficacy included a prior attempt at EMR (odds ratio [OR], 3.8; 95% confidence interval, 1.77—7.94; $P = .001$) and ileocecal valve involvement (OR, 3.4; 95% confidence interval, 1.20—9.52; $P = .021$). Independent predictors of recurrence after effective EMR were lesion size greater than 40 mm (OR, 4.37; 95% confidence interval, 2.43—7.88; $P < .001$) and use of argon plasma coagulation (OR, 3.51; 95% confidence interval, 1.69—7.27; $P = .0017$). There were no deaths from EMR; 83.7% of patients avoided surgery.

Conclusions.—Large sessile colonic polyps can be managed safely and effectively by endoscopy. Endoscopic assessment identifies lesions at increased risk of containing submucosal cancer. The first EMR is an important determinant of patient outcome—a previous attempt is a significant risk factor for lack of efficacy.

▶ Prevention of colorectal cancer (CRC) with colonoscopy screening and endoscopic polypectomy is credited with the decreased rate of CRC in the United States. It is the primary factor for favoring colonoscopy over other modalities as the gold standard for screening. Most polyps are small or pedunculated and can be easily removed with widely available expertise in snare and biopsy techniques. Increasingly, large, flat, and sessile lesions are being recognized, particularly in the right colon. The higher failure rate in detecting these polyps likely accounts for the disappointing rates of missed cancers (especially right sided) after colonoscopy screening. Sessile polyps are associated with higher rates of advanced neoplasia, including invasive cancer. When these lesions are large, recommendations for surgery are often made despite its morbidity and even mortality risks. Endoscopic mucosal resection (EMR) is increasingly used to manage these polyps and is the subject of this well-executed prospective multicenter observational study from Australia reporting on the outcomes and complications from more than 400 polyps greater than 2 cm in size.

The results of this study clearly support the use of EMR with excellent safety and efficacy; overall, 84% of patients avoided surgery. This is clearly high-risk endoscopy with a perforation rate of 1.3% and a 2.9% bleeding rate. Certainly these complications compare favorably to surgical resection. The failure rate was approximately 14% with the majority being attempted but incomplete resections. This rate is artificially high given that any polyp injected but failing to lift was deemed a failure of EMR. During careful standardized follow-up examinations, the recurrence rate was 20%, highlighting the importance of the surveillance colonoscopy within 6 months.

The technique employed is standard EMR with all polyps undergoing a submucosal injection of a saline/dye solution to "lift" the lesion and provide a cushion or safety zone for snare resection. The endoscopists in this multi-center trial favored a sequential inject and resect technique or piecemeal resection rather than en bloc resection. For larger lesions, en bloc resection is associated with lower rates of residual adenoma at follow-up but also higher rates of perforation. To reduce the residual polyp rate, these authors used small snares to remove a collar of normal mucosa surrounding the neoplasm, which may explain the excellent outcomes reported with this technique.

The observation that previous failed attempt at resection reduces the success rate substantially highlights the importance of training in this technique. When done properly in endoscopy referral centers, colonic EMR is safe and effective for large, flat, and sessile lesions. The majority will be cured, and patients can avoid surgical resection.

R. K. Pearson, MD

Inflammatory Markers Are Associated With Risk of Colorectal Cancer and Chemopreventive Response to Anti-Inflammatory Drugs

Chan AT, Ogino S, Giovannucci EL, et al (Massachusetts General Hosp and Harvard Med School, Boston; Brigham and Women's Hosp and Harvard Med School, Boston)
Gastroenterology 140:799-808, 2011

Background & Aims.—Aspirin and nonsteroidal anti-inflammatory drugs (NSAIDs) lower the risk of colorectal cancer (CRC). We investigated whether plasma inflammatory markers were associated with risk of CRC and if use of anti-inflammatory drugs was differentially associated with risk of CRC according to levels of inflammatory markers.

Methods.—We measured levels of high-sensitivity C-reactive protein (CRP), interleukin (IL)-6, and the soluble tumor necrosis factor receptor 2 (sTNFR-2) in blood samples from 32,826 women, collected from

1989 to 1990. Through 2004, we documented 280 cases of incident CRC; each case was matched for age to 2 randomly selected participants without cancer (controls). Information on anti-inflammatory drug (aspirin and NSAIDs) use was collected biennially.

Results.—Compared with women in the lowest quartile of plasma levels of sTNFR-2, women in the highest quartile had an increased risk of CRC (multivariate relative risk [RR], 1.67; 95% confidence interval [CI], 1.05−2.68; *P* for trend = .03). Among women with high baseline levels of sTNFR-2, those who initiated aspirin/NSAID use after blood collection had significant reductions in subsequent risk of CRC (multivariate RR, 0.39; 95% CI, 0.18−0.86). In contrast, among women with low baseline levels of sTNFR-2, initiation of aspirin/NSAID use was not associated with significant risk reduction (multivariate RR, 0.86; 95% CI, 0.41−1.79). Plasma levels of CRP and IL-6 were not significantly associated with CRC risk.

Conclusions.—Plasma levels of sTNFR-2, but not CRP or IL-6, are associated with an increased risk of CRC. Anti-inflammatory drugs appear to reduce risk of CRC among women with high, but not low, baseline levels of sTNFR-2. Certain subsets of the population, defined by inflammatory markers, may obtain different benefits from anti-inflammatory drugs (Tables 3 and 4).

▶ It is widely accepted that aspirin and nonsteroidal antiinflammatory drug (NSAID) use reduces the risk of colorectal cancer (CRC) and precursor adenoma. There is also considerable evidence in experimental models and clinical studies that chronic inflammation increases the risk of cancer, including the well-accepted cancer risk associated with inflammatory bowel disease. Any role for chronic inflammation in sporadic CRC is undefined; but certainly serological markers for chronic inflammation, such as C-reactive protein (CRP), have been associated with several diseases, including obesity, diabetes, and vascular disease. Previous attempts to relate these markers of inflammation to CRC have been equivocal.

This study exploited the Nurses' Health Study that began in 1976 when more than 100 000 US female nurses answered questions at baseline and every 2 years thereafter about their health, lifestyle, medications, including aspirin and NSAIDS, and diagnoses. In 1989, blood samples were collected from 32 826 of the participants, and these subjects make up the cohort used in this interesting study. After blood collection, 286 incident CRCs were identified through 2004 and matched 2:1 with controls. Stored blood samples were then assayed for 3 markers of chronic inflammation.

As Table 3 demonstrates, levels of soluble tumor necrosis factor receptor 2 (sTNFR-2), but not CRP or interleukin-6, correlate with the risk of CRC. To ensure that undiagnosed CRC itself was not responsible for the high marker level, CRCs diagnosed within 2 years of the sample draw were excluded, and the relative risk of CRC remained unchanged. Controlling for other conditions associated with chronic inflammation (eg, diabetes, obesity) did not change the results. In a previous study, aspirin and NSAID use in the same cohort was shown to be associated with a lower risk of CRC. In an interesting analysis,

TABLE 3.—RR of Colorectal Cancer According to Plasma Inflammatory Markers

Analyte	Quartiles				P_{trend}[a]
	1	2	3	4	
CRP					
Median (*mg/L*)	0.39	0.95	2.13	5.37	
No. of cases/controls	77/133	68/138	75/142	60/142	
Age-adjusted RR (95% CI)[b]	1.00 (referent)	0.85 (0.57–1.27)	0.91 (0.61–1.35)	0.73 (0.48–1.10)	.13
Multivariate-adjusted RR (95% CI)[c]	1.00 (referent)	0.79 (0.51–1.21)	0.89 (0.57–1.39)	0.65 (0.40–1.05)	.17
IL-6					
Median (*pg/mL*)	0.65	1.02	1.45	3.04	
No. of cases/controls	63/138	70/138	71/138	75/139	
Age-adjusted RR (95% CI)[b]	1.00 (referent)	1.11 (0.73–1.68)	1.13 (0.74–1.70)	1.17 (0.78–1.78)	.52
Multivariate-adjusted RR (95% CI)[c]	1.00 (referent)	1.13 (0.73–1.74)	1.11 (0.72–1.72)	1.18 (0.75–1.85)	.55
sTNFR-2					
Median (*pg/mL*)	1900	2345	2743	3463	
No. of cases/controls	54/138	63/139	80/139	80/139	
Age-adjusted RR (95% CI)[b]	1.00 (referent)	1.18 (0.76–1.82)	1.50 (0.98–2.30)	1.51 (0.98–2.33)	.04
Multivariate-adjusted RR (95% CI)[c]	1.00 (referent)	1.22 (0.78–1.92)	1.53 (0.98–2.40)	1.67 (1.05–2.68)	.03

NOTE. Quartiles of plasma inflammatory markers are based on the distribution in the controls. For CRP, women were categorized according to cut points of never-users or ever-users of postmenopausal hormones. For CRP, the median values in the table represent never-users of postmenopausal hormones. The corresponding values for ever-users of postmenopausal hormones were 0.68 mg/L for quartile 1, 1.62 mg/L for quartile 2, 3.15 mg/L for quartile 3, and 6.71 mg/L for quartile 4. One case and 2 controls had insufficient plasma for IL-6 measurements. Three cases had insufficient plasma for sTNFR-2 measurements.

[a]Tests for linear trend were conducted using the median values for each quartile of analyte.

[b]Age-adjusted models including adjustment for age at blood draw, date of blood draw.

[c]Multivariate models were adjusted for age at blood draw, date of blood draw, body mass index (quintiles), physical activity (quintiles of metabolic equivalent task score hours per week), current or past smoking (yes or no), menopause status, current postmenopausal hormone use (yes or no), prior lower gastrointestinal endoscopy (yes or no), colorectal cancer in parent or sibling (yes or no), regular use of multivitamins (yes or no), regular use of aspirin or NSAIDs (≥2 tablets/week), energy-adjusted intake (including supplements) of calcium and folate (quintiles), servings of beef, pork, or lamb as a main dish (0–3 times/month, 1 time/week, 2–4 times/week, 5+ times/week), and alcohol consumption (0, 0.1–4.9, 5.0–14.9, or + 15 g/day).

TABLE 4.—RR of Colorectal Cancer According to Initiation of Regular Aspirin or NSAID Use After Blood Draw, Stratified by sTNFR-2 Level

Characteristic	Nonuser after blood draw	Regular user after blood draw
All sTNF-R2 levels		
No. of cases/controls	109/177	34/84
Age-adjusted RR (95% CI)[a]	1.00	0.65 (0.41−1.04)
Multivariable-adjusted RR (95% CI)[b]	1.00	0.67 (0.41−1.09)
sTNFR-2 level greater than or equal to the median (2636 pg/mL)		
No. of cases/controls	59/83	15/43
Age-adjusted RR (95% CI)[a]	1.00	0.49 (0.25−0.97)
Multivariable-adjusted RR (95% CI)[b]	1.00	0.39 (0.18−0.86)
sTNFR-2 level less than the median (2636 pg/mL)		
No. of cases/controls	48/94	19/41
Age-adjusted RR (95% CI)[a]	1.00	0.91 (0.48−0.74)
Multivariable-adjusted RR (95% CI)[b]	1.00	0.86(0.41−1.79)

NOTE. This analysis was restricted to the 404 participants who denied regular use of aspirin (≥2 standard 325-mg tablets/week) or NSAIDs (≥2 tablets/week) on the most recent questionnaire before blood draw. Nonusers after blood draw denied regular use of aspirin on any questionnaire after blood draw but before diagnosis. Regular users after blood draw reported regular use after the most recent questionnaire after blood draw but before diagnosis.
[a]Age-adjusted models including adjustment for matching factors (age at blood draw, date of blood draw).
[b]Multivariate RRs and 95% CIs were adjusted for the same factors as the multivariate model in Table 3 with the exception of regular use ofaspirin/NSAIDs.

the investigators examined the risk of CRC according to levels of sTNFR-2 among 286 women who were not using these agents at the time of the blood draw. Table 4 shows a protective effect of initiating aspirin or NSAIDs in women with inflammatory markers above the median but not in those below.

The authors go to great lengths in detailing the limitations of this case-control study, including the obvious restriction to women. However, this provocative study demonstrated an association with an inflammatory marker and CRC and supports a role for chronic inflammation in the pathogenesis of CRC. Furthermore, it suggests the possibility of using a biomarker for inflammation to predict who might benefit from prophylaxis against CRC with aspirin or NSAIDS. Given the risks associated with its use, this would be a welcome addition to the clinician advising patients about chemoprevention with aspirin.

R. K. Pearson, MD

Pancolonic chromoendoscopy with indigo carmine versus standard colonoscopy for detection of neoplastic lesions: a randomised two-centre trial
Pohl J, Schneider A, Vogell H, et al (Dr. Horst-Schmidt-Klinik, Wiesbaden, Germany; Stadtkrankenhaus Korbach, Germany; et al)
Gut 60:485-490, 2011

Objective.—Colonoscopy is the accepted gold standard for detecting colorectal adenomas, but the miss rate, especially for small and flat lesions, remains unacceptably high. The aim of this study was to determine whether enhanced mucosal contrast using pancolonic chromoendoscopy (PCC) allows higher rates of adenoma detection.

Methods.—In a prospective, randomised two-centre trial, PCC (with 0.4% indigo carmine spraying during continuous extubation) was compared with standard colonoscopy (control group) in consecutive patients attending for routine colonoscopy. The histopathology of the lesions detected was confirmed by evaluating the endoscopic resection or biopsy specimens.

Results.—A total of 1008 patients were included (496 in the PCC group, 512 in the control group). The patients' demographic characteristics and indications for colonoscopy were similar in the two groups. The proportion of patients with at least one adenoma was significantly higher in the PCC group (46.2%) than in the control group (36.3%; p=0.002). Chromoendoscopy increased the overall detection rate for adenomas (0.95 vs 0.66 per patient), flat adenomas (0.56 vs 0.28 per patient) and serrated lesions (1.19 vs 0.49 per patient) (p<0.001). There was a non-significant trend towards increased detection of advanced adenomas (103 vs 81; p=0.067). Mean extubation times were slightly but significantly longer in the PCC group in comparison with the control group (11.6 ± 3.36 min vs 10.1 ± 2.03 min; p<0.001).

Conclusions.—Pancolonic chromoendoscopy markedly enhances adenoma detection rates in an average-risk population and is practicable enough for routine application (Table 2).

▶ As a gold standard for screening for colorectal cancer, colonoscopy has to detect and resect adenomatous polyps to prevent cancer. Unfortunately, the miss rate for polyps with standard colonoscopy remains unacceptably high at 10% to 25%. This has been especially true for the right colon, where difficult sessile or flat lesions predominate and likely account for the failure of colonoscopy to protect against colon cancer in this site.

Technically, especially for flat lesions, low contrast between normal mucosa and adenomatous mucosa probably contributes substantially to the difficulty in recognizing these polyps with standard white light endoscopy. Strategies directed at increasing the mucosal contrast would increase adenoma detection

TABLE 2.—Pathological Features of the Evaluated Lesions

Histopathology	PCC	Control Group	P Value
Adenoma, n (ml/p, min—max)	470 (0.95, 0—10)	338 (0.66, 0—9)	<0.001
Flat adenoma, n (ml/p, min—max)	280 (0.56, 0—5)	144 (0.28, 0—5)	<0.001
Advanced neoplasia, n (ml/p, min—max)	103 (0.21, 0—4)	81 (0.16, 0—5)	0.067
Carcinoma (n)	12	12	
Serrated lesion, n (ml/p, min—max)	592 (1.19, 0—12)	253 (0.49, 0—9)	<0.001
Others (n)	1	3	
Total, n (ml/p, min—max)	1075 (2.17, 0—14)	606 (1.18, 0—10)	<0.001

Differences in numbers of lesions (ml/p) were compared using Mann-Whitney U test. Definition of advanced neoplasia: adenoma ≥1 cm, adenoma with high-grade intraepithelial neoplasia, carcinoma.
PCC, pancolonic chromoendoscopy; mL/p: mean lesions per patient ± SD.

and improve the capacity for colonoscopy to reduce colon cancer rates; however, these techniques have been criticized for average-risk screening because of the increased time associated with these methods and the increased reported polyps detected are often small lesions of uncertain clinical significance.

Chromoendoscopy is a technique of enhancing mucosal contrast with the use of dye spraying by making fine surface details visible by highlighting with accumulating dye in the grooves and crypt openings in the normal and aberrant mucosa. In this multicenter prospective randomized trial from Germany, pancolonic chromoendoscopy (PCC) with indigo carmine was compared with standard colonoscopy. Both arms used high-definition endoscopes. The spray technique involved the insertion of a dye-spraying catheter in the instrument's working channel (it is small enough that suction is still functional), and 0.4% indigo carmine was applied in low-volume continuous fashion during withdrawal from the cecum to diffusely cover the mucosa while avoiding excess dye accumulation.

As Table 2 from the article shows, the PCC increased adenoma detection rate substantially in this large study of 1200 screening and diagnostic/surveillance examinations. The absolute number of adenomas, as well as the number of patients in whom polyps were found, was increased. As previously noted, the increased polyps detected were primarily small and flat; a modest trend (non-statistically significant) toward increased detection of advanced neoplasia is nevertheless promising. Although the procedural time was increased, it was on average by less than 2 minutes.

As described with all-quality metrics in colonoscopy screening, the effect of PCC on detection rates were operator dependent; 4 of 5 endoscopists had increased detection rates. Another "limitation" of the study was that only 50% of the subjects were for average-risk screening, possibly increasing the overall yield of lesions.

In summary, PCC confers a significant advantage in polyp detection rate compared with standard colonoscopy. The authors confidently state that although a learning curve is involved, the technique used in this study is easy to use. This strengthens the argument for incorporating dye enhancement in colonoscopy screening programs. In many centers it is already used in high-risk populations.

R. K. Pearson, MD

Analysis of Administrative Data Finds Endoscopist Quality Measures Associated With Postcolonoscopy Colorectal Cancer

Baxter NN, Sutradhar R, Forbes SS, et al (Univ of Toronto, Ontario, Canada)
Gastroenterology 140:65-72, 2011

Background & Aims.—Most quality indicators for colonoscopy measure processes; little is known about their relationship to patient outcomes. We investigated whether characteristics of endoscopists, determined from administrative data, are associated with development of postcolonoscopy colorectal cancer (PCCRC).

Methods.—We identified individuals diagnosed with colorectal cancer in Ontario from 2000 to 2005 using the Ontario Cancer Registry. We determined performance of colonoscopy using Ontario Health Insurance Plan data. Patients who had complete colonoscopies 7 to 36 months before diagnosis were defined as having a PCCRC. Patients who had complete colonoscopies within 6 months of diagnosis had detected cancers. We determined if endoscopist factors (volume, polypectomy and completion rate, specialization, and setting) were associated with PCCRC using logistic regression, controlling for potential covariates.

Results.—In the study, 14,064 patients had a colonoscopy examination within 36 months of diagnosis; 584 (6.8%) with distal and 676 (12.4%) with proximal tumors had PCCRC. The endoscopist's specialty (nongastroenterologist/nongeneral surgeon) and setting (nonhospital-based colonoscopy) were associated with PCCRC. Those who underwent colonoscopy by an endoscopist with a high completion rate were less likely to have a PCCRC (distal: odds ratio [OR], 0.73; 95% confidence interval [CI], 0.54–0.97; $P = .03$; proximal: OR, 0.72; 95% CI, 0.53–0.97; $P = .002$). Patients with proximal cancers undergoing colonoscopy by endoscopists who performed polypectomies at high rates had a lower risk of PCCRC (OR, 0.61; 95% CI, 0.42–0.89; $P < .0001$). Endoscopist volume was not associated with PCCRC.

Conclusions.—Endoscopist characteristics derived from administrative data are associated with development of PCCRC and have potential use as quality indicators.

▶ Colonoscopy remains the most common procedure recommended for screening and prevention of colorectal cancer. There is good evidence to support this position, and there are many advocates of it. However, there is also considerable evidence that the quality of colonoscopy varies and that this variation has a considerable impact on the ultimate outcome, detection, and prevention of colorectal cancer (CRC). Furthermore, several recent large-scale studies have suggested that colonoscopy may be particularly ineffective in prevention of right-sided colon cancer. Whether this primarily represents flaws in colonoscopy screening or in the biological behavior of right-sided colon cancers is hotly debated. Because of the expense and inherent risks associated with colonoscopy screening programs, there has been a call for the development of meaningful performance metrics to assess the quality. The ultimate quality measure would be missed or prevented CRC; however, for the individual endoscopist, these events are too rare to be useful; surrogate endpoints are clearly needed if organizations and payers are to measure quality.

These investigators from Toronto, Canada, have previously exploited a large provincial (Ontario) database for the diagnosis of incident CRC and the single-payer system in Canada to identify missed CRC or "postcolonoscopy CRC" (PCCRC). Linking the billing and diagnostic provincial database, they attempted to measure the characteristics of the performing endoscopist and the rate of missed cancers and used the traditional definition of CRC being diagnosed 7 to 36 months after undergoing a complete colonoscopy.

This was an administrative database study and one of the largest outcomes-based studies of its kind. Although other studies measuring missed cancers have identified scores of patients, this database study had more than 1000; interestingly, the rate was one of the highest at 9%. Similar to virtually all other studies, right-sided cancers were missed at a higher rate than left-sided lesions.

Importantly for gastroenterologists, type of training had a significant impact on the outcome, with gastroenterologists and surgeons having lower rates of PCCRC than nonspecialists. Not surprisingly, completion rate and polypectomy rate were also significantly associated with better outcomes. However, procedure volumes by individual endoscopist did not correlate with PCCRC rate in this study. This might suggest that once trained "correctly," the volume performed is less critical in skill maintenance. However, there must certainly be a minimum number of procedures required.

The authors acknowledge the limitations of this type of administrative database approach. However, the scale of this population-based study, with its strong statistical results, indicates that the approach can yield insights into meaningful quality measurements for colonoscopy. Whether application of any of these measures would truly reduce the number of PCCRC in a population remains to be demonstrated. For example, applying a "polypectomy rate" as opposed to adenoma detection rate as a quality measure could lead to a "gaming" of the system and the removal of trivial lesions to improve the measurement but not the cancer rate. Further studies of this type are necessary to determine the best way to measure and educate endoscopists and ultimately further reduce the risk of CRC.

R. K. Pearson, MD

Pancreaticobiliary Cancer

FOLFIRINOX versus Gemcitabine for Metastatic Pancreatic Cancer
Conroy T, for the Groupe Tumeurs Digestives of Unicancer and the PRODIGE Intergroup (Nancy Univ and Centre Alexis Vautrin, France; et al)
N Engl J Med 364:1817-1825, 2011

Background.—Data are lacking on the efficacy and safety of a combination chemotherapy regimen consisting of oxaliplatin, irinotecan, fluorouracil, and leucovorin (FOLFIRINOX) as compared with gemcitabine as first-line therapy in patients with metastatic pancreatic cancer.

Methods.—We randomly assigned 342 patients with an Eastern Cooperative Oncology Group performance status score of 0 or 1 (on a scale of 0 to 5, with higher scores indicating a greater severity of illness) to receive FOLFIRINOX (oxaliplatin, 85 mg per square meter of body-surface area; irinotecan, 180 mg per square meter; leucovorin, 400 mg per square meter; and fluorouracil, 400 mg per square meter given as a bolus followed by 2400 mg per square meter given as a 46-hour continuous infusion, every

2 weeks) or gemcitabine at a dose of 1000 mg per square meter weekly for 7 of 8 weeks and then weekly for 3 of 4 weeks. Six months of chemotherapy were recommended in both groups in patients who had a response. The primary end point was overall survival.

Results.—The median overall survival was 11.1 months in the FOLFIR-INOX group as compared with 6.8 months in the gemcitabine group (hazard ratio for death, 0.57; 95% confidence interval [CI], 0.45 to 0.73; P<0.001). Median progression-free survival was 6.4 months in the FOLFIRINOX group and 3.3 months in the gemcitabine group (hazard ratio for disease progression, 0.47; 95% CI, 0.37 to 0.59; P<0.001). The objective response rate was 31.6% in the FOLFIRINOX group versus 9.4% in the gemcitabine group (P<0.001). More adverse events were noted in the FOLFIRINOX group; 5.4% of patients in this group had febrile neutropenia. At 6 months, 31% of the patients in the FOLFIR-INOX group had a definitive degradation of the quality of life versus 66% in the gemcitabine group (hazard ratio, 0.47; 95% CI, 0.30 to 0.70; P<0.001).

Conclusions.—As compared with gemcitabine, FOLFIRINOX was associated with a survival advantage and had increased toxicity. FOLFIR-INOX is an option for the treatment of patients with metastatic pancreatic cancer and good performance status. (Funded by the French government and others; ClinicalTrials.gov number, NCT00112658.)

▶ Pancreatic cancer is the fourth leading cause of cancer death in the United States with a 5-year survival rate of 6%. Only the minority of patients (approximately 15%) are eligible for surgical resection, the only realistic chance for cure. For the majority of patients presenting with metastatic disease, the prognosis is particularly grim, with average survival under 6 months. Thus, any advances in the outcome for pancreatic cancer will require improved chemotherapy regimens. Standard of care is single-agent gemcitabine after the pivotal study in 1997 showed its superior survival advantage of 6 weeks (5.6 vs 4.4 months) over bolus infusion fluorouracil. Multiple clinical trials combining gemcitabine with cytotoxic and targeted agents (eg, epidermal growth factor receptor overexpression) have not successfully extended survival in advanced pancreatic cancer. For example, combining irinotecan, oxaliplatin, and fluorouracil/leucovorin had shown synergistic effects in preclinical studies and Phase I clinical trials, suggesting the benefits of this drug combination (FOLFIRINOX). In this Phase III, multicenter trial, patients with measurable metastatic pancreatic cancer (the majority with liver metastases) were randomized to standard gemcitabine versus FOLFIR-INOX. Importantly, the inclusion criteria specified high performance status (Eastern Cooperative Oncology performance status 0 or 1); patients had to be able to function normally with daily living and only limited by strenuous activity.

The improvement in survival and progression-free survival as shown in Fig 1 in the original article is the largest improvement obtained in clinical trials of pancreatic cancer in the modern chemotherapeutic age. FOLFIRINOX is an aggressive multidrug regimen and, as expected, toxicity was high even in these patients with excellent performance status. However, when assessed by quality of life measurement, patients in the FOLFIRINOX arm maintained their scores longer because of the delay in pancreatic cancer progression. For this subgroup of patients, this regimen will become the standard of care for advanced pancreatic cancer. How this regimen will fit into management of patients in the adjuvant setting after surgical resection and for locally advanced, nonmetastatic disease will be the subject of future studies.

R. K. Pearson, MD

Everolimus for Advanced Pancreatic Neuroendocrine Tumors

Yao JC, for the RAD001 in Advanced Neuroendocrine Tumors, Third Trial (RADIANT-3) Study Group (Univ of Texas M D Anderson Cancer Ctr, Houston; et al)
N Engl J Med 364:514-523, 2011

Background.—Everolimus, an oral inhibitor of mammalian target of rapamycin (mTOR), has shown antitumor activity in patients with advanced pancreatic neuroendocrine tumors, in two phase 2 studies. We evaluated the agent in a prospective, randomized, phase 3 study.

Methods.—We randomly assigned 410 patients who had advanced, low–grade or intermediate-grade pancreatic neuroendocrine tumors with radio-logic progression within the previous 12 months to receive everolimus, at a dose of 10 mg once daily (207 patients), or placebo (203 patients), both in conjunction with best supportive care. The primary end point was progression-free survival in an intention-to-treat analysis. In the case of patients in whom radiologic progression occurred during the study, the treat-ment assignments could be revealed, and patients who had been randomly assigned to placebo were offered open-label everolimus.

Results.—The median progression-free survival was 11.0 months with everolimus as compared with 4.6 months with placebo (hazard ratio for disease progression or death from any cause with everolimus, 0.35; 95% confidence interval [CI], 0.27 to 0.45; P<0.001), representing a 65% reduc-tion in the estimated risk of progression or death. Estimates of the propor-tion of patients who were alive and progression-free at 18 months were 34% (95% CI, 26 to 43) with everolimus as compared with 9% (95% CI, 4 to 16) with placebo. Drug-related adverse events were mostly grade 1 or 2 and included stomatitis (in 64% of patients in the everolimus group vs. 17% in the placebo group), rash (49% vs. 10%), diarrhea (34% vs. 10%), fatigue (31% vs. 14%), and infections (23% vs. 6%), which were primarily upper respiratory. Grade 3 or 4 events that were more frequent with everolimus than with placebo included anemia (6% vs. 0%) and hyper-glycemia (5% vs. 2%). The median exposure to everolimus was longer than exposure to placebo by a factor of 2.3 (38 weeks vs. 16 weeks).

Conclusions.—Everolimus, as compared with placebo, significantly pro-longed progression-free survival among patients with progressive advanced pancreatic neuroendocrine tumors and was associated with a low rate of severe adverse events. (Funded by Novartis Oncology; RADIANT-3 ClinicalTrials.gov number, NCT00510068.)

▶ Although there is no question that the prognosis of pancreatic neuroendocrine tumors (PNETs) is much better than for ductal adenocarcinoma,[1] 65% of patients present with late-stage disease and succumb to it, with a median survival of 24 months. Effective chemotherapy is lacking; the only approved medication is streptozocin, and its value in treatment continues to be debated by oncologists. The lack of effective therapy is highlighted by the placebo arm in this randomized trial.

Everolimus is an oral agent in the family of immunosuppressives and antiproliferative agents that act by inhibiting mammalian target of rapamycin (mTOR), a protein kinase that stimulates cell growth, proliferation, and angiogenesis. Its immunosuppressive properties have been exploited in preventing rejection in solid organ transplantation. In vitro, it was observed that PNETs have constitutively activated mTOR through autocrine activation of various growth factors. PNET tumor cell line growth is significantly slowed by mTOR inhibition in vitro. Promising results in Phase II clinical trials led to this worldwide, multicenter placebo-controlled trial of Everolimus in advanced PNET.

As Fig 1 from the original article demonstrates, this was another example of a successful translation of an in vitro observation to a clinical treatment. Patients in the treatment arm had a clinically and statistically significantly longer progression-free survival; indeed, approximately one third of patients were responders at 18 months. As shown in panel C from the study, this benefit included all subgroups of patients, including those with previous exposure to chemotherapy. As expected for this family of agents, toxicity was acceptable and indeed quite low for a cancer trial. Grade 3 or 4 toxicity occurred in only 2% of patients in the treatment arm.

The observation that another oral agent inhibitor of tyrosine kinases (Sunitinib)[1] also improves outcomes gives real optimism for patients with advanced PNET. Future clinical trials will focus on the benefit of combining these agents.

R. K. Pearson, MD

Reference

1. Raymond E, Dahan L, Raoul JL, et al. Sunitinib malate for the treatment of pancreatic neuroendocrine tumors. *N Engl J Med*. 2011;364:501-513.

Magnetic Resonance Imaging Surveillance Detects Early-Stage Pancreatic Cancer in Carriers of a *p16-Leiden* Mutation
Vasen HFA, Wasser M, Van Mil A, et al (Leiden Univ Med Ctr, the Netherlands; et al)
Gastroenterology 140:850-856, 2011

Background & Aims.—Surveillance of high-risk groups for pancreatic cancer might increase early detection and treatment outcomes. Individuals with germline mutations in *p16-Leiden* have a lifetime risk of 15% to 20% of developing pancreatic cancer. We assessed the feasibility of detecting pancreatic cancer at an early stage and investigated the outcomes of patients with neoplastic lesions.

Methods.—Individuals with germline mutations in *p16-Leiden* (N = 79; 31 male; mean age, 56 years; range, 39–72 years) were offered annual surveillance by magnetic resonance imaging (MRI) and magnetic resonance cholangiopancreatography (MRCP). Those found to have neoplastic lesions were offered options for surgery or intensive follow-up. Individuals found to have possible neoplastic lesions were examined again by MRI/MRCP within 2 to 4 months.

Results.—After a median follow-up period of 4 years (range, 0–10 years), pancreatic cancer was diagnosed in 7 patients (9%). The mean age at diagnosis was 59 years (range, 49–72 years). Three of the tumors were present at the first examination, and 4 were detected after a negative result in the initial examination. All 7 patients had a resectable lesion; 5 underwent surgery, 3 had an R0 resection, and 2 had lymph node metastases. Possible precursor lesions (ie, duct ectasias, based on MRCP) were found in 9 individuals (11%).

Conclusions.—MRI/MRCP detects small, solid pancreatic tumors and small duct ectasias. Although surveillance increases the rate of resectability, carriers of a *p16-Leiden* mutation develop agressive tumors (Fig 2).

▶ Pancreatic cancer (PC) has a poor prognosis with a 5-year survival of 5% or less. Curative surgical resection is the only hope for long-term survival, but only 15% to 20% of patients are candidates for surgery because of advanced disease when symptoms are present. Screening for pancreatic cancer for average-risk populations has not been deemed feasible because of the lack of a biomarker.

Approximately 5% to 10% of PC cases are associated with an inherited predisposition. Syndromes associated with an increased risk of PC include

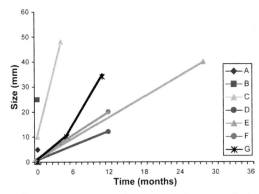

FIGURE 2.—Size of pancreatic tumors at subsequent surveillance examinations. (Reprinted from Vasen HFA, Wasser M, Van Mil A, et al. Magnetic resonance imaging surveillance detects early-stage pancreatic cancer in carriers of a p16-*Leiden* mutation. *Gastroenterology.* 2011;140:850-856, Copyright 2011, with permission from the AGA Institute.)

Peutz-Jeghers syndrome, familial atypical multiple mole melanoma (FAMMM), *BRCA2* carriers (hereditary breast cancer), and Lynch syndrome (HNPCC). FAMMM is associated with germline mutations in the gene known as p16; a specific mutation in kindreds from the Netherlands (p16-Leiden) confers a lifetime risk of PC of 15% to 20% by age 75. Patients can be identified with genetic testing, and these mutation carriers are an ideal population for studies on surveillance for PC.

This exciting study enrolled 79 patients (ages 45-70 years) with documented p16-Leiden germline mutations in a prospective surveillance study using annual MRI/MRCP imaging. After only 4 years of study, 7 cancers were identified. The 7 patients identified with PC all had resectable disease, and 3 had favorable surgical outcomes with clear margins, small tumors, and no lymph node metastases. It is sobering to acknowledge that even when detected in a completely asymptomatic state by screening, PC often is advanced beyond curative resection. The aggressiveness of PC is demonstrated by the fact that 3 of 5 tumors observed in serial examinations increased in size by 1 cm or more in 6 months (Fig 2).

The study also identified duct ectasias or cystic lesions in 11% of patients, most presumably representing intraductal papillary mucinous neoplasia (IPMN) of the branch duct variety. The relationship between PC and duct ectasia is unclear, and operating prophylactically on these lesions is difficult. This is highlighted by the observation in this high-risk kindred that 7 of 9 patients with these small cysts have been followed for more than 5 years without any evidence of progression.

This is by far the most effective surveillance study ever published for PC owing to the high rate of PC in these subjects (nearly 10%). MRI/MRCP is generally well tolerated, avoids ionizing radiation, and is noninvasive. This is a promising advance for the relatively uncommon patients in these high-risk groups. It remains unproven whether this or any other surveillance program will improve the prognosis of this terrible disease.

R. K. Pearson, MD

Feasibility and Yield of Screening in Relatives From Familial Pancreatic Cancer Families

Ludwig E, Olson SH, Bayuga S, et al (Memorial Sloan-Kettering Cancer Ctr, NY)
Am J Gastroenterol 106:946-954, 2011

Objectives.—Pancreatic adenocarcinoma is a lethal disease. Over 80% of patients are found to have metastatic disease at the time of diagnosis. Strategies to improve disease-specific outcome include identification and early detection of precursor lesions or early cancers in high-risk groups. In this study, we investigate whether screening at-risk relatives of familial pancreatic cancer (FPC) patients is safe and has significant yield.

Methods.—We enrolled 309 asymptomatic at-risk relatives into our Familial Pancreatic Tumor Registry (FPTR) and offered them screening with magnetic resonance cholangiopancreaticogram (MRCP) followed by endoscopic ultrasound (EUS) with fine needle aspiration if indicated. Relatives with findings were referred for surgical evaluation.

Results.—As of 1 August 2009, 109 relatives had completed at least one cycle of screening. Abnormal radiographic findings were present on initial screening in 18/109 patients (16.5%), 15 of whom underwent EUS. A significant abnormality was confirmed in 9 of 15 patients, 6 of whom ultimately had surgery for an overall diagnostic yield of 8.3% (9/109). Yield was greatest in relatives >65 years old (35%, 6/17) when compared with relatives 55—65 years (3%, 1/31) and relatives <55 years (3%, 2/61).

Conclusions.—Screening at-risk relatives from FPC families has a significant diagnostic yield, particularly in relatives >65 years of age, confirming prior studies. MRCP as initial screening modality is safe and effective.

▶ Pancreatic cancer (PC) is a devastating illness with a very poor prognosis. Established risk factors for the disease include advancing age, smoking, obesity, and a family history of pancreatic cancer. A positive family history is present in approximately 10% of patients with PC. None of these risk factors has an absolute risk high enough to warrant screening for the disease. Furthermore, there is no serologic test of sufficient accuracy to enrich a population for more expensive or invasive imaging tests, such as CT, MRI, or endoscopic ultrasound scan.

Familial PC is defined by multiple first-degree relatives (generally, 2 or more, or 1 under the age of 50) with PC and no known cancer syndrome. Because of their high absolute risk of PC, these kindreds have been studied in multiple centers in trials of screening. In this study from Memorial Sloan Kettering, 109 kindred members underwent screening initially with magnetic resonance cholangiopancreaticogram (MRCP), and if abnormal ductal changes were identified, endoscopic ultrasound scan (EUS) was performed. Patients with any suspicious lesions determined by cytology or carcinoembryonic antigen levels in aspirated cysts were seen in consultation by surgeons.

While the title of the article and conclusion suggest that the yield in these families is high, skeptics would counter with several cautions. First, only 1 invasive cancer was identified, and 5 other patients underwent resection for premalignant lesions, primarily dysplastic intraductal papillary mucinous neoplasia (IPMN) of the branch duct variety. These are quite common in the general population, and their management and risk are controversial subjects. Whether IPMN represents a higher risk for patients with a family history of PC remains to be established. Second, the false-positive rate for the MRCP screening was approximately 50%. Finally, all of the patients with significant findings on MRCP and EUS were identified on the initial screening round of testing. The role of surveillance in these kindreds remains completely unknown.

While it is tempting to offer screening for patients fearful of this disease because of a family history, this article should inspire caution. PC screening should not be undertaken outside of centers engaged in prospective, clinical trials.

R. K. Pearson, MD

Sunitinib Malate for the Treatment of Pancreatic Neuroendocrine Tumors

Raymond E, Dahan L, Raoul J-L, et al (Hôpital Beaujon, Clichy, France; Hôpital Timone, Marseille, France; Univ of Rennes, France; et al)
N Engl J Med 364:501-513, 2011

Background.—The multitargeted tyrosine kinase inhibitor sunitinib has shown activity against pancreatic neuroendocrine tumors in preclinical models and phase 1 and 2 trials.

Methods.—We conducted a multinational, randomized, double-blind, placebo-controlled phase 3 trial of sunitinib in patients with advanced, well-differentiated pancreatic neuroendocrine tumors. All patients had Response Evaluation Criteria in Solid Tumors-defined disease progression documented within 12 months before baseline. A total of 171 patients were randomly assigned (in a 1:1 ratio) to receive best supportive care with either sunitinib at a dose of 37.5 mg per day or placebo. The primary end point was progression-free survival; secondary end points included the objective response rate, overall survival, and safety.

Results.—The study was discontinued early, after the independent data and safety monitoring committee observed more serious adverse events and deaths in the placebo group as well as a difference in progression-free survival favoring sunitinib. Median progression-free survival was 11.4 months in the sunitinib group as compared with 5.5 months in the placebo group (hazard ratio for progression or death, 0.42; 95% confidence interval [CI], 0.26 to 0.66; $P<0.001$). A Cox proportional-hazards analysis of progression-free survival according to baseline characteristics favored sunitinib in all subgroups studied. The objective response rate was 9.3% in the sunitinib group versus 0% in the placebo group. At the data cutoff point, 9 deaths were reported in the sunitinib group (10%) versus 21 deaths in the placebo group (25%) (hazard ratio for death, 0.41; 95% CI, 0.19 to 0.89; $P=0.02$). The most frequent adverse events in the sunitinib group were diarrhea, nausea, vomiting, asthenia, and fatigue.

Conclusions.—Continuous daily administration of sunitinib at a dose of 37.5 mg improved progression-free survival, overall survival, and the objective response rate as compared with placebo among patients with advanced pancreatic neuroendocrine tumors. (Funded by Pfizer; ClinicalTrials.gov number, NCT00428597.)

▶ Pancreatic neuroendocrine tumors account for between 1% and 2% of all pancreatic cancer but have a much better prognosis than ductal adenocarcinoma. The relatively indolent progress of the disease means more patients are found in a resectable stage at diagnosis (about 35%), and local therapy (resection or percutaneous ablation techniques) directed at liver metastases may have some palliative benefit. However, for the 65% of patients found to have metastatic disease, the average survival is approximately 24 months. Somatostatin analogues are useful in the minority of patients with symptoms related to hormone secretion (eg, Zollinger-Ellison syndrome) and may slow the rate of tumor growth in a subset of patients. Systemic chemotherapy in the form of streptozocin with or without doxorubicin is the only agent approved for the treatment of advanced pancreatic neuroendocrine tumors, but the magnitude of its benefit is debated. At many centers treating these cancers, chemotherapy is reserved for a last resort after a period of observation to establish the aggressiveness of the unresectable pancreatic neuroendocrine tumor and exhaustion of attempts to control liver metastases with ablation.

In vitro studies had established a number of growth factor receptors important in the growth promotion of pancreatic neuroendocrine tumors, including platelet-derived growth factor and stem-cell factor receptor (c-kit). Further, these studies identified vascular endothelial growth factor as a crucial regulator of angiogenesis, a biological event critical in tumor growth. Sunitinib is a small molecule inhibitor of multiple kinases and had been shown to have activity against pancreatic neuroendocrine tumors in several experimental systems and looked promising in phase I and II clinical trials.

In this report of a phase III multicenter placebo-controlled study from the United States, sunitinib lived up to its promise; the study was halted early during an interim analysis because of the superior outcome in patients receiving active agent versus placebo as demonstrated in Fig 1 in the original article. Furthermore, the drug was well tolerated.

The gap between these observations and proven clinical benefit is a broad one, and the oncological literature is well populated with failed phase III studies of agents with well characterized in vitro activity against tumor growth and possible effectiveness in early clinical trials. Thus, it is particularly gratifying when reports like this one appear that confirm the benefits of investigationally directed, rational translational research. This and an accompanying report of another biologically targeted growth inhibitor (everolimus) gives oncologists new treatment options for most patients with pancreatic neuroendocrine tumors that are not cured with surgical resection.

R. K. Pearson, MD

Miscellaneous

High cancer risk and increased mortality in patients with Peutz–Jeghers syndrome

van Lier MGF, Westerman AM, Wagner A, et al (Univ Med Ctr, Rotterdam, The Netherlands; et al)
Gut 60:141-147, 2011

Background.—Peutz–Jeghers syndrome (PJS) is associated with an increased cancer risk. As the determination of optimal surveillance strategies is hampered by wide ranges in cancer risk estimates and lack of data on cancer-related mortality, we assessed cancer risks and mortality in a large cohort of patients with PJS.

Methods.—Dutch PJS patients were included in this cohort study. Patients were followed prospectively between January 1995 and July 2009, and clinical data from the period before 1995 were collected retrospectively. Data were obtained by interview and chart review. Cumulative cancer risks were calculated by Kaplan—Meier analysis and relative cancer and mortality risks by Poisson regression analysis.

Results.—We included 133 PJS patients (48% males) from 54 families, contributing 5004 person-years of follow-up. 49 cancers were diagnosed in 42 patients (32%), including 25 gastrointestinal (GI) cancers. The median age at first cancer diagnosis was 45 years. The cumulative cancer risk was 20% at age 40 (GI cancer 12%), increasing to 76% at age 70 (GI cancer 51%). Cumulative cancer risks were higher for females than for males (p=0.005). The relative cancer risk was higher in PJS patients than in the general population (HR 8.96; 95% CI 6.46 to 12.42), and higher among female (HR 20.40; 95% CI 13.43 to 30.99) than among male patients (HR 4.76; 95% CI 2.82 to 8.04). 42 patients had died at a median age of 45 years, including 28 cancer-related deaths (67%). Mortality was increased in our cohort compared to the general population (HR 3.50; 95% CI 2.57 to 4.75).

Conclusions.—PJS patients carry high cancer risks, leading to increased mortality. The malignancies occur particularly in the GI tract and develop at young age. These results justify surveillance in order to detect malignancies in an early phase to improve outcome (Fig 1, Table 6).

▶ Peutz-Jeghers syndrome (PJS) is an uncommon autosomal dominant disorder well known to gastroenterologists because of its recognizable phenotype characterized by gastrointestinal (GI) hamartomatous polyposis syndrome

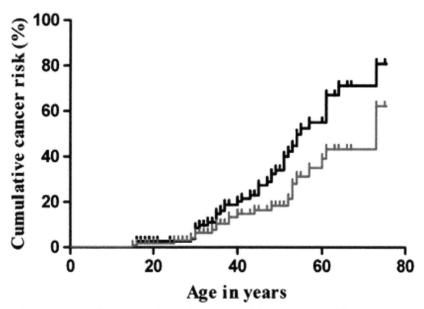

FIGURE 1.—Cumulative cancer risks according to age. Black line: Cumulative risk for any cancer. Grey line: Cumulative risk for gastrointestinal (GI) cancer. (Reprinted from van Lier MGF, Westerman AM, Wagner A, et al. High cancer risk and increased mortality in patients with Peutz—Jeghers syndrome. *Gut.* 2011;60:141-147.)

TABLE 6.—Surveillance Recommendations for Patients with Peutz—Jeghers Syndrome

Examination*	Starting Age	Interval
History, physical examination (including palpation testis) and haemoglobin analysis	10 years	1 year (paediatrician)
Video-capsule endoscopy and/or MRI enteroclysis[†]	10 years	2—3 years
Gastroduodenoscopy	20 years	2—5 years (depending on findings)
Colonoscopy	25—30 years	2—5 years (depending on findings)
MRI and endoscopic ultrasonography pancreas	30 years	1 year, only in a prospective ongoing trial[60]
Breast exam and breast MRI	25 years	1 year
Mammography and breast MRI	30 years	1 year[‡]
Pelvic exam, PAP-smear, transvaginal ultrasonography and CA-125	25—30 years	1 year

In addition, we recommend intra-operative enteroscopy with polyp removal in every indicated laparotomy, to avoid re-laparotomies. If surgery is indicated a laparoscopic approach is preferred when possible.

Editor's Note: Please refer to original journal article for full references.

*Earlier and/or more frequently in symptomatic patients/if clinically indicated.

[†]If video-capsule endoscopy shows polyps it is recommended to perform an MRI enteroclysis to determine the exact localisation and size if the polyps are > 1 cm in diameter are an indication for double-balloon enteroscopy with polypectomy.

[‡]Mammography and MRI alternately performed every 6 months.

coupled with mucocutaneous pigmentation. In at least 90% of subjects with PJS, germline mutations in the serine threonine kinase 11 gene can be identified so that the diagnosis can be established unequivocally in the vast majority. It has long been recognized that the cancer rate in PJS subjects is elevated, but because the syndrome is rare, the estimation of risks has varied significantly depending on the type of population or cohort analyzed; many are quite small. Thus, definitive evidence in support of cancer screening and surveillance have been lacking, as well as mortality rate in this syndrome.

This study from the Netherlands analyzed the cancer and mortality rates in a relatively large cohort of PJS families followed at 2 academic centers over 15 years. While the cumulative cancer rate was lower than some reports, it remains a staggering absolute risk of 76% by age 70 years with approximately half of the cancers being related to the GI tract as shown in Fig 1. The most common non-GI cancers included breast, cervical, and ovarian; the higher rate in women overall makes the relative cancer risk to the general population approach 20-fold.

This study is also the first to demonstrate excess mortality in this syndrome. These observations justify the development of specific surveillance recommendations for these patients outlined in Table 6. Based on the young age of onset of cancer, the guidelines for colorectal cancer screening begin by age 30 years, similar to other inherited cancer syndromes. Small bowel intussusception because of the development of large hamartomatous polyps in this region contributed to 19% of the deaths in the cohort. The authors recommend small bowel screening with either capsule or MR enterography with endoscopic or surgical resection for large hamartomas to prevent this complication.

R. K. Pearson, MD

5 Inflammatory Bowel Disease

Crohn's Disease

Azathioprine versus mesalazine for prevention of postoperative clinical recurrence in patients with Crohn's disease with endoscopic recurrence: efficacy and safety results of a randomised, double-blind, double-dummy, multicentre trial

Reinisch W, on behalf of the International AZT-2 Study Group (Universitätsklinik für Innere Medizin III, Vienna, Austria; et al)
Gut 59:752-759, 2010

Objective.—The aim of the study was to compare azathioprine versus mesalazine tablets for the prevention of clinical recurrence in patients with postoperative Crohn's disease (CD) with moderate or severe endoscopic recurrence.

Methods.—This was a 1 year, double-blind, double-dummy, randomised study which took place in 21 gastroenterology centres in Austria, the Czech Republic, Germany and Israel. The study participants were 78 adults with CD who had undergone resection with ileocolonic anastomosis in the preceding 6–24 months without subsequent clinical recurrence and with a Crohn's disease activity index (CDAI) score <200, but with moderate or severe endoscopic recurrence. The study drugs were azathioprine 2.0–2.5 mg/kg/day or mesalazine 4 g/day over 1 year. The primary end point was therapeutic failure during 1 year, defined as a CDAI score ≥200 and an increase of ≥60 points from baseline, or study drug discontinuation due to lack of efficacy or intolerable adverse drug reaction.

Results.—Treatment failure occurred in 22.0% (9/41) of azathioprine-treated patients and 10.8% (4/37) of mesalazine-treated patients, a difference of 11.1% (95% CI −5.0% to 27.3%, p=0.19). Clinical recurrence was significantly less frequent with azathioprine versus mesalazine (0/41 (0%) vs 4/37 (10.8%), p=0.031), whereas study drug discontinuation due to adverse drug reactions only occurred in azathioprine-treated patients (9/41 (22.0%) vs 0%, p=0.002). The proportion of patients showing ≥1 point reduction in Rutgeerts score between baseline and month 12 was 63.3%

(19/30) and 34.4% (11/32) in the azathioprine and mesalazine groups, respectively (p=0.023).

Conclusions.—In this population of patients with postoperative CD at high risk of clinical recurrence, superiority for azathioprine versus mesalazine could not be demonstrated for therapeutic failure.

▶ The decision on whether to start or resume medical therapy after surgical resection for Crohn's disease (CD) is based on the clinician's prediction of the likelihood of disease recurrence. Immunomodulator or biologic therapy is typically reserved for patients at high risk because of the potential for toxicity. We know that infliximab does reduce endoscopic recurrence after surgery and probably clinical recurrence. Surprisingly, little is known about azathioprine/ 6-mercaptopurine in this setting. Mesalamine (mesalazine) has been previously tested, and while recurrence rates were lower, the effect was small. In this randomized clinical trial, mesalazine is directly compared with azathioprine among adult patients with CD who had undergone resection in the previous 6 to 24 months. Rates of recurrence after surgery vary with time, and this wide variation in time since surgery may have impacted the study results. Patients had to have moderate endoscopic recurrence at study entry, suggesting that overall rates of treatment failure with either therapy should have been higher. However, rates were low, especially in the mesalamine arm. Treatment failure rates were higher in the azathioprine group because of higher rates of adverse reactions leading to medication discontinuation. Among those who could tolerate azathioprine, clinical recurrence was lower and rate of improvement of endoscopy score was higher compared with mesalazine. Unfortunately, the number of patients was too small to determine disease characteristics that led to failure other than therapy. Because the potential of toxicity for azathioprine is high, identifying which patients would benefit from this therapy after surgery is the most important question. Unfortunately, this has yet to be answered.

M. F. Picco, MD, PhD

A Single Dose of Intravenous Zoledronate Prevents Glucocorticoid Therapy-Associated Bone Loss in Acute Flare of Crohn's Disease, a Randomized Controlled Trial
Klaus J, Haenle MM, Schröter C, et al (Univ of Ulm, Germany; et al)
Am J Gastroenterol 106:786-793, 2011

Objectives.—To assess the effectiveness and safety of zoledronate (ZOL) in preventing glucocorticoid therapy-associated bone loss in patients with acute flare of Crohn's disease (CD) in a randomized, double-blind, placebo-controlled trial.

Methods.—Forty CD patients starting a glucocorticoid therapy (60 mg prednisolone per day) for acute flare (CD activity index (CDAI) >220) were randomized to compare the effect of ZOL (4 mg intravenous, $n = 20$) or placebo ($n = 20$) on change in lumbar bone mineral density

(BMD). All patients received calcium citrate (800 mg) and colecalciferol (1,000 IU) daily. Dual energy X-ray absorptiometry (DXA) of the lumbar spine (L1—L4) was performed at baseline and day 90. Follow-up examinations at day 1/7/14/30 and 90 included laboratory tests and adverse event/ serious adverse events reports.

Results.—Thirty-six patients were available for per-protocol analysis. With placebo ($n = 18$), a decrease in BMD was seen (T-score: -0.98 ± 0.8, day 0 and -1.25 ± 0.77, day 90, $P = 0.06$), with ZOL ($n = 18$) BMD increased (-1.15 ± 1.02, day 0 and -0.74 ± 1.09, day 90, $P = 0.03$). The change in BMD under placebo (-0.26 ± 0.21) vs. ZOL ($+0.41 \pm 0.19$) was highly significant ($P = 0.006$). In all, 14 out of 18 patients with ZOL had an increase in BMD ($+0.64 \pm 0.48$), 12 of 18 with placebo a decrease (-0.50 ± 0.39). Changes of clinical findings and laboratory results of inflammation (leukocytes, platelets, and C-reactive protein) were the same in and between groups throughout the study. With ZOL, serum bone degradation marker β-Cross-Laps decreased. Study medication was safe and well tolerated.

Conclusions.—ZOL is effective in preventing glucocorticoid therapy-induced bone loss in patients with acute flare of CD and should be considered whenever a glucocorticoid therapy is started in CD patients.

▶ Bone loss in inflammatory bowel disease (IBD) can be related to the disease itself but more often is directly the result of corticosteroid use. The most dramatic bone loss occurs early in therapy and can be seen at dosages of prednisone as little as 7.5 mg or less daily. Evaluation for bone loss is part of the care of patients with IBD. Active treatment of osteoporosis leads to lower risk of subsequent fracture among patients with IBD. Given that bone loss is so pervasive among patients with IBD taking corticosteroids, should we not focus our efforts on preventing bone loss among our patients? Simple calcium and vitamin D supplementation, although commonly recommended, may fall short, whereas bisphosphonates (the most effective therapy) are usually started after the damage has been done by corticosteroids. Oral bisphosphonates are difficult for patients to take, but once-weekly and once-monthly formulations have enhanced compliance. In this important study, the authors showed that a single dose of zolindronate, at the time when corticosteroids are introduced for the treatment of active Crohn's disease, prevented bone loss in a randomized trial. Unfortunately, follow-up was only 90 days. Although the patient groups were well matched, the sample size was small so that other non-IBD patient-specific factors may have affected the results. However, the effect of zolindronate was dramatic. Zolindronate was given intravenously where compliance was ensured and appeared to be safe. Further studies are needed with larger patient numbers and with the more commonly prescribed oral bisphosphonates. These oral forms may have issues of compliance. We need more data on long-term outcomes, including whether the effects of these agents are sustained and whether there is any risk of long-term adverse outcomes in our IBD population.

M. F. Picco, MD, PhD

Infliximab Therapy Inhibits Inflammation-Induced Angiogenesis in the Mucosa of Patients with Crohn's Disease

Rutella S, Fiorino G, Vetrano S, et al (Catholic Univ Med School, Rome, Italy; Istituto Clinico Humanitas, Milan, Italy)
Am J Gastroenterol 106:762-770, 2011

Objectives.—Inflammation-driven angiogenesis contributes to the pathogenesis of inflammatory bowel disease (IBD). In line with this, the efficacy of inhibitors of angiogenesis has been demonstrated in experimental models of colitis. Currently, the ability of infliximab, an anti-tumor necrosis factor-α (TNF-α) agent that is highly beneficial in patients with IBD, to affect mucosal angiogenesis in patients with Crohn's disease (CD) and ulcerative colitis (UC) is unknown.

Methods.—Patients with active CD ($n = 14$) were treated with infliximab for 1 year, and peripheral blood and intestinal mucosa samples were collected before and after treatment. Mucosal angiogenesis was evaluated by CD31 and Ki-67 staining in endoscopic biopsies at baseline (week 0) and at week 54. The release of vascular endothelial growth factor-A (VEGF-A) by cultured mucosal extracts was measured by enzyme-linked immunosorbent assay (ELISA), before and after administration of infliximab, as well as in cultures of human intestinal fibroblasts (HIFs) stimulated with TNF-α in the presence or absence of infliximab. Migration of human intestinal microvascular endothelial cells (HIMECs) was investigated by migration assays.

Results.—Microvessel density was significantly higher in the mucosa from patients with CD compared with tissue from healthy control individuals. Of the 14 patients, 8 (57%) showed a clinical remission in response to infliximab, which was associated with a significant reduction of microvascular density. Morphometric vessel analysis further confirmed the significant reduction of the area of vascular section after administration of infliximab. Furthermore, the expression levels of the proliferation marker Ki-67 in endothelial cells were significantly reduced after treatment. The mucosal concentration of VEGF-A was also significantly decreased, whereas *in vitro* exposure of HIF to infliximab virtually abolished TNF-α-induced VEGF-A production. These phenomena did not occur in patients who showed no clinical response to infliximab.

Conclusions.—Administration of infliximab downregulates mucosal angiogenesis in patients with CD and restrains production of VEGF-A by mucosal fibroblasts. It is proposed that this ameliorates inflammation-driven angiogenesis in the gut mucosa and contributes to the therapeutic efficacy of blockade of TNF-α.

▶ Why is angiogenesis important in Crohn's disease (CD)? The formation of new blood vessels is integral to chronic inflammatory processes like CD. It also is necessary for the development of malignancy. Previous human studies have concentrated on the effect of tumor necrosis alpha inhibition on immune cells in CD. In this interesting study, the authors show through various methods that inhibition of angiogenesis occurs among patients who were treated and responded to infliximab. The strength of the study is that the results were confirmed by each of the different established methods that measure angiogenesis, including immunostaining, enzyme-linked immunosorbent assay (ELISA), and cell-culture and migration assays. The novel finding here is that the authors established inhibition of angiogenesis in human subjects with CD who received infliximab. The long-term implications are not clear, but this does suggest an important mechanism for controlling inflammation and a potential target for future therapies. Although other therapies also inhibit angiogenesis, their action is also part of an overall effect on the immune system. Angiogenesis as a separate mechanism may also have important implications of the development of stricturing CD or malignancy.

M. F. Picco, MD, PhD

Randomised clinical trial: certolizumab pegol for fistulas in Crohn's disease - subgroup results from a placebo-controlled study

Schreiber S, Lawrance IC, Thomsen OØ, et al (Univ Hosp Schleswig-Holstein, Kiel, Germany; Univ of Western Australia, Fremantle, Australia; Univ of Copenhagen, Denmark; et al)
Aliment Pharmacol Ther 33:185-193, 2011

Background.—Treatment options for fistulizing Crohn's disease (CD) are limited.

Aim.—To examine whether fistula closure is maintained at week 26 following treatment with certolizumab pegol.

Methods.—Patients with draining fistulas at baseline from PRECiSE 2 ($n = 108$) received open-label induction with certolizumab pegol 400 mg at weeks 0 (baseline), 2 and 4. Response was defined as ≥100-point decrease from baseline in the Crohn's Disease Activity Index. Nonresponders (50/108) were excluded. At week 6, responders with draining fistulas ($N = 58$) were randomised to certolizumab pegol 400 mg ($n = 28$) or placebo ($n = 30$) every 4 weeks across weeks 8–24. Fistula closure was evaluated throughout the study, with a final assessment at week 26.

Results.—The majority of patients (55/58) had perianal fistula. At week 26, 36% of patients in the certolizumab pegol group had 100% fistula closure compared with 17% of patients receiving placebo ($P = 0.038$). Protocol-defined fistula closure (≥50% closure at two consecutive post-baseline visits ≥3 weeks apart) was not statistically significant ($P = 0.069$) with 54% and 43% of patients treated with certolizumab pegol and placebo achieving this end point, respectively.

Conclusion.—Continuous treatment with certolizumab pegol improves the likelihood of sustained perianal fistula closure compared with placebo.

▶ Infliximab has proven efficacy in the treatment of penetrating (fistulizing) Crohn's disease (CD). Evidence for adalimumab and certolizumab is lacking, but these agents are generally considered equivalent alternatives. The Pegylated

Antibody Fragment Evaluation in Crohn's Disease: Safety and Efficacy (PRECiSE) trial established certiluzimab as an effective treatment for inflammatory (nonstricturing nonpenetrating) CD. In this post hoc analysis of the PRECiSE trial, the authors identified 58 patients with fistula. Unfortunately, the primary outcome of fistula closure was not met, most likely because of the small sample size and an analysis comparing patients who all received open-label certolizumab induction. Because all patients received induction therapy, fistula closure rates were similar before randomization to active drug or placebo in the maintenance phase and remained similar. There was no true placebo arm. Small sample size allowed for only limited comparisons, and nearly all fistulae were perianal. Although a high proportion of perianal fistula is similar to trials with the other agents of this class, having so few internal fistulae does not allow for any conclusions about an important group of patients. Despite these limitations, the results are encouraging. Secondary outcome of complete fistula closure was higher at week 26. Given that this agent is already an accepted treatment for fistulizing CD, it is unlikely that a dedicated placebo-controlled study will ever be done. We will likely be left to reports from case series and clinical experience that, fortunately, support the efficacy of this agent.

M. F. Picco, MD, PhD

Risk Factors Associated With Progression to Intestinal Complications of Crohn's Disease in a Population-Based Cohort
Thia KT, Sandborn WJ, Harmsen WS, et al (Mayo Clinic, Rochester, MN)
Gastroenterology 139:1147-1155, 2010

Background and Aims.—We sought to assess the evolution of Crohn's disease behavior in an American population-based cohort.

Methods.—Medical records of all Olmsted County, Minnesota residents who were diagnosed with Crohn's disease from 1970 to 2004 were evaluated for their initial clinical phenotype, based on the Montreal Classification. The cumulative probabilities of developing structuring and/or penetrating complications were estimated using the Kaplan-Meier method. Proportional hazards regression was used to assess associations between baseline risk factors and changes in behavior.

Results.—Among 306 patients, 56.2% were diagnosed between the ages of 17 and 40 years. Disease extent was ileal in 45.1%, colonic in 32.0%, and ileocolonic in 18.6%. At baseline, 81.4% had nonstricturing nonpenetrating disease, 4.6% had stricturing disease, and 14.0% had penetrating disease. The cumulative risk of developing either complication was 18.6% at 90 days, 22.0% at 1 year, 33.7% at 5 years, and 50.8% at 20 years after diagnosis. Among 249 patients with nonstricturing, nonpenetrating disease at baseline, 66 changed their behavior after the first 90 days from diagnosis. Relative to colonic extent, ileal, ileocolonic, and upper GI extent were significantly associated with changes in behavior, whereas the association with perianal disease was barely significant.

Conclusions.—In a population-based cohort study, 18.6% of patients with Crohn's disease experienced penetrating or stricturing complications within 90 days after diagnosis; 50% experienced intestinal complications 20 years after diagnosis. Factors associated with development of complications were the presence of ileal involvement and perianal disease.

▶ Crohn's disease (CD) is a heterogeneous disease with varied disease locations and behaviors. Patients with the highest risk of developing of penetrating or stricturing complications would benefit most from the early introduction of immunomodulator or biologic therapies. Early intervention with these agents, termed the top-down approach, may modify the natural history of CD. Studies that attempt to predict the course of CD typically come from tertiary centers and are thus prone to referral bias. These patients tend to be sicker and may be more likely to develop complications. They may not be representative of most patients with this disease. In this population-based study from Olmsted County, Minnesota, one gets a better sense of prognosis among all patients with CD in North America. This report confirms the high rate of complications among patients with CD over time. The reported association of complications with ileal and upper disease was confirmed. The presence of perianal disease also seemed to result in higher rates of complications, but the association was of borderline significance possibly because of less severe perianal disease in the community or small sample size. These reported factors associated with disease progression were present in nearly 75% of patients. These sobering findings, in addition to other reports, suggest the need for studies on earlier intervention with aggressive therapies in an attempt to alter the natural history of CD among these high-risk patients.

M. F. Picco, MD, PhD

The Impact of Thiopurines on the Risk of Surgical Recurrence in Patients With Crohn's Disease After First Intestinal Surgery

Papay P, Reinisch W, Ho E, et al (Med Univ of Vienna, Austria)
Am J Gastroenterol 105:1158-1164, 2010

Objectives.—Smoking and a lack of immunosuppressive (IS) therapy are considered risk factors for intestinal surgery in Crohn's disease (CD). Good evidence for the latter is lacking. The objective of this study was to evaluate the impact of thiopurine treatment on surgical recurrence in patients after first intestinal resection for CD and its possible interaction with smoking.

Methods.—Data on 326 patients after first intestinal resection were retrieved retrospectively, and subjects were grouped according to their postoperative exposure to thiopurines. Treatment with either azathioprine (AZA) or 6-mercaptopurine (6-MP) was recorded on 161 patients (49%). Smoking status was assessed by directly contacting the patients.

Results.—Surgical recurrence occurred in 151/326 (46.3%) patients after a median time of 71 (range 3—265) months. Cox regression revealed a significant reduction of re-operation rate in patients treated with AZA/6-MP for ≥ 36 months as compared with patients treated for 3–35 months, for less than 3 months, and to those without postoperative treatment with AZA/6-MP (P=0.004). Cox regression analysis revealed treatment with thiopurines for ≥ 36 months (hazard ratio (HR) 0.41; 95% confidence interval (CI) 0.23–0.76, P=0.004) and smoking (HR 1.6; 95% CI 1.14–2.4, P=0.008) as independent predictors for surgical recurrence. Furthermore, longer duration of disease tended to be protective (HR 0.99; 95% CI 0.99–1.0, P=0.067).

Conclusions.—Long-term maintenance treatment with AZA/6-MP reduces the risk of surgical recurrence in patients with CD. We also identified smoking as a risk factor for surgical recurrence.

▶ The role of thiopurines in reducing rates of first and subsequent surgeries in Crohn's disease is controversial. Differences in types of patients and study design have led to disparate results. In this retrospective cohort study, the authors attempted to determine the role of thiopurines in preventing second surgical recurrence. This design was different in that previous studies had focused on endoscopic and clinical recurrence. In this study, longer therapy with thiopurines did result in lower rates of surgical recurrence. Patients were stratified based on whether they received thiopurines after first surgery, the duration, and whether they were smokers. Surgical recurrence is a concrete outcome, but the decision to reoperate was not standardized given that it was a retrospective study. Similarly, treatment decisions were also not standardized, and clinical outcomes may have been influenced by disease severity in this referral-based population. The authors did use a propensity score analysis that adjusted for baseline characteristics across subgroups. This adjustment for duration of disease and initial surgery after 1996 was necessary because these were confounding variables in that they influenced both the likelihood of thiopurine therapy and rate of surgical recurrence. The benefit of azathioprine was seen only in those treated for at least 36 months despite an anticipated onset of therapeutic effect of 3 to 6 months. It is not clear why no benefit was seen until 36 months. A comparison of disease characteristics based on duration of treatment with azathioprine would have helped address this, although disease behavior at first surgery did not influence surgical recurrence in the Cox model. This article is important in that it adds to the evidence that thiopurines are effective in preventing disease recurrence after surgery. The retrospective nature of this and other studies may limit their conclusions, but it is unlikely that a large randomized study will ever be done. However, future studies will likely include biologic therapies that have been shown to be more effective in inducing clinical remission in Crohn's disease. Comparisons of these agents with thiopurines in surgical recurrence are clearly needed.

M. F. Picco, MD, PhD

5-Aminosalicylates Prevent Relapse of Crohn's Disease After Surgically Induced Remission: Systematic Review and Meta-Analysis

Ford AC, Khan KJ, Talley NJ, et al (Leeds General Infirmary, UK; McMaster Univ, Hamilton, Ontario, Canada; Univ of Newcastle, New South Wales, Australia)
Am J Gastroenterol 106:413-420, 2011

Objectives.—Evidence from randomized controlled trials (RCTs) for the use of 5-aminosalicylic acid (5-ASA) drugs in Crohn's disease (CD) in remission after a surgical resection is conflicting. We conducted a systematic review and meta-analysis of RCTs to examine this issue.

Methods.—MEDLINE, EMBASE, and the Cochrane central register of controlled trials were searched (through April 2010). Eligible trials recruited adults with luminal CD in remission after a surgical resection and compared 5-ASAs with placebo, or no treatment. Dichotomous data were pooled to obtain relative risk (RR) of relapse of disease activity, with a 95% confidence interval (CI). The number needed to treat (NNT) was calculated from the reciprocal of the risk difference.

Results.—The search strategy identified 3,061 citations. Eleven RCTs were eligible for inclusion containing 1,282 patients. The RR of relapse of CD in remission after surgery with 5-ASA vs. placebo or no therapy was 0.86 (95% CI = 0.74—0.99) (NNT13). Sulfasalazine was of no benefit in preventing relapse in 448 patients (RR0.97; 95% CI = 0.72—1.31), but mesalamine was more effective than placebo or no therapy (RR = 0.80; 95% CI0.70—0.92) in 834 patients, with an NNT of 10.

Conclusions.—Mesalamine is of modest benefit in preventing relapse of CD in remission after surgery. Its use should be considered in those in whom immunosuppressive therapy is either not warranted or contraindicated.

▶ Currently, there is little enthusiasm for the use of mesalamine for Crohn's disease. This conclusion is based on many studies that, while in some cases are conflicting, show little benefit. In this meta-analysis, the authors concluded that mesalamine is beneficial in prophylaxis after surgically induced remission. Mesalamine did show a "modest" benefit, but sulfasalazine did not. While the authors do conduct a careful meta-analysis to allow for bias and study heterogeneity, questions still remain as to the appropriate use of mesalamine among patients with a surgically induced remission. The first concern is the heterogeneity of the patients studied. The authors could not adjust for the location of Crohn's disease or type of resection. Furthermore, we have no information regarding disease behavior. Both these factors may influence response to mesalamine. Behavior is particularly important. Patients included had "luminal disease," which does not distinguish disease confined to the lumen from penetrating or fibrostenotic disease. Each of these behaviors has its own postoperative prognosis. These factors, along with other patient-specific factors, such as smoking, may have influenced relapse rates. The authors suggest that treatment of 10 patients would result in prevention of one relapse. This may very well be the best possible treatment effect that can be expected in a group of low-risk patients in whom immunomodulator or biologic therapy would not be considered. As treatment of Crohn's disease has become more aggressive, this represents very few patients. Other patients in whom immunosuppressive therapy is warranted but contraindicated are much less likely to respond to mesalamine. If there is no other choice, this meta-analysis suggests that there may be some benefit despite the high costs of these medications. Postoperative prophylaxis with mesalamine is marginally better than nothing and may be considered in select patients.

M. F. Picco, MD, PhD

Predictors of Infliximab Failure After Azathioprine Withdrawal in Crohn's Disease Treated With Combination Therapy

Oussalah A, Chevaux J-B, Fay R, et al (Univ Hosp of Nancy, Vandoeuvre-lès-Nancy, France; Jeanne d'Arc Hosp, Dommartin-lès-Toul, France; et al)
Am J Gastroenterol 105:1142-1149, 2010

Objectives.—Whether all Crohn's disease (CD) patients should maintain long-term azathioprine treatment in combination with infliximab remains controversial. We analyzed the predictive factors of infliximab failure after azathioprine withdrawal.

Methods.—This was an observational study from a single referral center. All patients with luminal CD in remission who stopped azathioprine after receiving infliximab in combination with azathioprine for at least 6 months were studied. Cumulative probabilities of infliximab failure-free survival were estimated by the Kaplan–Meier method from the date of azathioprine withdrawal to the date of infliximab failure or last known follow-up. Infliximab failure was defined by: (i) disease flare requiring shortening of the dosing interval or increasing the infliximab dose to 10 mg/kg, or switching to adalimumab; (ii) acute or delayed hypersensitivity reactions leading to infliximab discontinuation; or (iii) CD-related surgery.

Results.—At last known follow-up, 35 out of 48 (73%) patients were infliximab failure free. The survival probabilities were 85% ($\pm$5%) at 12 months and 41% ($\pm$18%) at both 24 and 32 months. Cox proportional-hazards regression identified three predictors of infliximab failure: infliximab–azathioprine exposure duration of $\leq$811 days (hazard ratio (HR) = 7.46, P = 0.01), C-reactive protein > 5 mg/l (HR = 4.79, P = 0.008), and platelet count > 298 10^9/l (HR = 4.75, P = 0.02).

Conclusions.—In CD in clinical remission under azathioprine–infliximab combination therapy, azathioprine withdrawal is associated with a high risk of relapse in patients with a duration of combination therapy of < 27 months and/or the presence of biological inflammation.

▶ This article attempts to address the important question of whether among patients taking infliximab and azathioprine, azathioprine can be safely discontinued after at least 6 months of combination therapy. Van Assche et al[1] had previously shown that continuing combination therapy longer than 6 months did not result in added benefit after 2 years compared with infliximab alone. This study aimed to identify predictors of infliximab failure that were not addressed in the previous study. Unfortunately, this study has important limitations. It was a retrospective observational study with a small number of patients. Patients receiving infliximab added to ongoing azathioprine therapy (step-up therapy) were combined with those receiving initial azathioprine and infliximab. These 2 groups may represent fundamentally different patients with different rates of infliximab failure after withdrawal. In univariate analysis, step-up therapy, not surprisingly, was associated with infliximab failure. One might speculate that these patients had worse disease of possibly longer duration, making them more likely to fail, but specific differences between the groups were not provided. Failure to find a difference in multivariate analysis is probably related to small patient numbers. This is an important problem for all of the 15 predictors that they addressed. The finding of high C-reactive protein and platelets being associated with failure makes sense, as these are markers for inflammation. The finding of higher rates of failure for those treated for less than 27 months is difficult to interpret. It may suggest that that there may be patients who require long-term combination therapy. However, further prospective larger series are needed before definitive conclusions can be made.

M. F. Picco, MD, PhD

Reference

1. Van Assche G, Magdelaine-Beuzelin C, D'Haens G, et al. Withdrawal of immuno-suppression in Crohn's disease treated with scheduled infliximab maintenance: a randomized trial. *Gastroenterology.* 2008;134:1861-1868.

Pathogenesis of postoperative recurrence in Crohn's disease
Ahmed T, Rieder F, Fiocchi C, et al (Cleveland Clinic, OH)
Gut 60:553-562, 2011

The majority of patients with Crohn's disease (CD) require surgery during the course of their disease, but such surgery is typically not curative. Although some studies suggest that the disease state is theoretically reset to its earliest phase following surgery, disease phenotype and natural history of CD do not change significantly after surgery, leading to high rates of recurrence. Factors predisposing to this recurrence are not well defined, so there is a need for and a unique opportunity to develop a better understanding of the pathogenesis of recurrent inflammation and associated risk factors after an ileocolic resection. This paper reviews the postoperative disease outcome and evolution based on defining the combination of the patient's microbial flora, environmental exposure history, immune response and genetic make-up.

▶ The pathogenesis of Crohn's disease (CD) is complex and multifactorial. In this article, the authors discuss factors that influence the onset of CD and its recurrence after ileocolonic resection. Understanding factors that lead to the onset of CD and recurrence after surgery open important avenues for preventive therapy. The potential influences of bacterial flora, environmental factors, smoking, immune response, and genetic factors on disease development and postoperative recurrence are discussed. Clinical correlations and mechanisms are presented.

Bacterial flora influence pathogenesis. Diversion of the fecal stream proximal to a surgical anastomosis leads to absence of recurrence, but exposure to fecal material leads to endoscopic reappearance. Antibiotics have also been shown to reduce recurrence postoperatively. The mechanism of this interaction of bacteria with the host remains unknown, but the authors propose that alterations of gut flora, especially as the result of loss of the ileocecal valve, may be responsible.

Environmental factors were also discussed. The hygiene hypothesis was highlighted and suggests that higher rates of inflammatory bowel disease (IBD) in industrialized societies is due to lack of exposure to microbes and lack of development of immune tolerance. Medications such as nonsteroidal anti-inflammatory agents (NSAIDs), and possibly oral contraceptives, have also been linked to disease flares. Studies on the pathogenesis of NSAID-related injury as it relates to IBD are likely to shed light on pathogenesis.

The most important environmental risk factor for CD is smoking. Despite the largest body of knowledge compared with other environmental factors, little is known regarding the mechanism.

Studies regarding immune response have shown that certain cytokines may be elevated not only in active flares but also in periods of clinical remission. Elevations in periods of clinical remission have been shown to be predictive of relapse. This information may lead to identifying patients who would benefit most from aggressive therapy in the postoperative period.

Genetics remains the most important risk factor for IBD and the area of most intensive research. Identification of the association of ileal CD with NOD2/CARD 15 of chromosome 16 was landmark. Subsequently, multiple other genetic associations have been described. As with the other factors, although genetic association is important, genetic predisposition is neither necessary nor sufficient for the development of IBD.

When one looks at the multiple factors associated with IBD, a complex picture emerges that suggests significant disease heterogeneity. In the future, disease phenotype description will move beyond clinical descriptions of age at onset, disease location, and behavior to include genetic and cytokine profiles. The importance of bacterial and environmental influences on these profiles will lead to better understanding of natural history and selection of appropriate therapies to alter prognosis.

M. F. Picco, MD, PhD

Can Laparoscopic Ileocolic Resection be Performed with Comparable Safety to Open Surgery for Regional Enteritis: Data from National Surgical Quality Improvement Program

Kirat HT, Pokala N, Vogel JD, et al (Cleveland Clinic Foundation, OH)
Am Surg 76:1393-1396, 2010

Laparoscopic ileocolic resection is feasible for Crohn's disease but few studies adjust for the various preoperative, intraoperative, and postoperative variables that may confound comparisons with open surgery. The aim of this study is to compare outcomes after laparoscopic (LICR) and open ileocolic resection (OICR) performed for regional enteritis using National Surgical Quality Improvement Program (NSQIP) data. Retrospective evaluation of data prospectively accrued into the NSQIP database for patients undergoing ileocolic resection for Crohn's by LICR and OICR was performed. LICR (n = 104) and OICR (n = 203) groups had similar age ($P = 0.1$), body mass index ($P = 0.9$), smoking history ($P = 0.6$), steroid use ($P = 0.7$), diabetes ($P = 0.3$), serum albumin ($P = 0.07$), and American Society of Anesthesiologists class ($P = 0.13$). LICR group had more female patients ($P = 0.005$). Complications including surgical site infections ($P = 0.5$), wound dehiscence ($P = 1$), pneumonia ($P = 0.1$), deep vein thrombosis ($P = 0.3$), pulmonary embolism ($P = 1$), urinary infection ($P = 0.1$), and return to the operating room ($P = 0.2$) were similar. LICR had shorter length of hospital stay than OICR ($P < 0.001$). In current practice, as observed with the NSQIP data, LICR, performed by experienced surgeons, is comparable in safety to OICR and is associated with a shorter hospital stay.

▶ Laparoscopic ileocolonic resection (LICR) is becoming the preferred approach over open ileocolonic resection for (OICR) for patients requiring surgery for ileocolonic Crohn's disease. Previous studies have suggested that LICR results in shorter hospital stays and lower costs. However, these studies were relatively small, raising the possibility that preoperative factors may have influenced patient selection for LICR and resulted in better outcomes. This retrospective study considers important patient characteristics through use of the American College of Surgeons National Surgical Quality Improvement Program (NSQIP). This large database allows for adjustment for preoperative factors that may influence outcomes or selection for the laparoscopic approach. The factors chosen were reasonable and comparable between the two groups. However, the possibility for selection bias remains. We are provided little information regarding the indication for surgery except that there was no statistical difference between emergent surgery rates between the two groups; however, these rates were numerically higher (6.4 vs 2.9%) in the OICR group. Behavior of Crohn's disease may influence procedure selection, especially for patients with penetrating disease and resulting fistula who may require OICR. Similarly, underlying disease activity may also influence the type of operation. Neither of these factors was assessed in this analysis. Despite these limitations, the results are reassuring and suggest that the laparoscopic approach is comparable to the open approach with shorter length of stay among experienced surgeons. This finding alone will lead to a greater use of the technique. The authors' conclusion that selected patients who require ileocolonic resection should be considered for the laparoscopic approach is appropriate. The proportion of patients who undergo the laparoscopic approach will likely increase with time as experience grows and more surgeons adopt this technique.

M. F. Picco, MD, PhD

Autologous bone marrow-derived mesenchymal stromal cells in the treatment of fistulising Crohn's disease
Ciccocioppo R, Bernardo ME, Sgarella A, et al (Università degli Studi di Pavia, Italy)
Gut 60:788-798, 2011

Objective.—External fistulas represent a disabling manifestation of Crohn's disease with a difficult curability and a high relapse rate despite a large therapeutic armamentarium. Stem cell therapy is a novel and promising approach for treatment of chronic inflammatory conditions. We therefore investigated the feasibility, safety and efficacy of serial intrafistular injections of autologous bone marrow-derived mesenchymal stromal cells (MSCs) in the treatment of fistulising Crohn's disease.

Patients and Methods.—We enrolled 12 consecutive outpatients (eight males, median age 32 years) refractory to or unsuitable for current available therapies. MSCs were isolated from bone marrow and expanded ex vivo to be used for both therapeutic and experimental purposes. Ten patients (two refused) received intrafistular MSC injections (median 4) scheduled every 4 weeks, and were monitored by surgical, MRI and endoscopic evaluation for 12 months afterwards. The feasibility of obtaining at least 50×10^6 MSCs from each patient, the appearance of adverse events, and the efficacy in terms of fistula healing and reduction of both Crohn's disease and perianal disease activity indexes were evaluated. In addition, the percentage of both mucosal and circulating regulatory T cells expressing FoxP3, and the ability of MSCs to influence mucosal T cell apoptosis were investigated.

Results.—MSC expansion was successful in all cases; sustained complete closure (seven cases) or incomplete closure (three cases) of fistula tracks with a parallel reduction of Crohn's disease and perianal disease activity indexes (p<0.01 for both), and rectal mucosal healing were induced by treatment without any adverse effects. The percentage of mucosal and circulating regulatory T cells significantly increased during the treatment and remained stable until the end of follow up (p<0.0001 and p<0.01, respectively). Furthermore, MSCs have been proven to affect mucosal T cell apoptotic rate.

Conclusions.—Locally injected MSCs represent a feasible, safe and beneficial therapy in refractory fistulising Crohn's disease.

▶ Despite advances in the treatment of Crohn's disease (CD), existing therapies often fall short, especially for patients with penetrating (fistulizing) disease. In this article, the authors present the results of a small case series of 10 patients who received a novel therapy: intrafistula injection of autologous bone marrow—derived mesenchymal stem cells (MSCs). Assessment of fistula response was based on clinical criteria and MRI findings. MSCs derived from bone marrow have been shown to have immunomodulatory properties in both in vitro and in vivo experimental models.[1] Among these are interference with dendritic cells that results in a decreased activation of T cells and decreased production of proinflammatory cytokines and suppression of T-cell proliferation. These actions suggest that MSC would be potentially useful in CD. Experience in humans with CD is limited, but the effects were remarkable in this study. However, this conclusion needs to be tempered by the small sample size and limited follow-up. The long-term effects of this therapy are unknown, and the authors' conclusion that MSCs are safe is open to criticism. In vitro experiments have suggested the potential for malignancy of the MSCs although this has yet to be demonstrated in humans. Furthermore, local immune suppression caused by MSCs could increase the risk of malignancy secondary to the chronic inflammation of inflammatory bowel disease. Despite these questions of safety, further investigation in this area is warranted.

M. F. Picco, MD, PhD

Reference

1. Nauta AJ, Fibbe WE. Immunomodulatory properties of mesenchymal stromal cells. *Blood.* 2007;110:3499-3506.

Dysbiosis of the faecal microbiota in patients with Crohn's disease and their unaffected relatives
Joossens M, Huys G, Cnockaert M, et al (Univ Hosp Gasthuisberg, Leuven, Belgium; Ghent Univ, Belgium)
Gut 60:631-637, 2011

Background and Aims.—A general dysbiosis of the intestinal microbiota has been established in patients with Crohn's disease (CD), but a systematic characterisation of this dysbiosis is lacking. Therefore the composition of the predominant faecal microbiota of patients with CD was studied in comparison with the predominant composition in unaffected controls. Whether dysbiosis is present in relatives of patients with CD was also examined.

Methods.—Focusing on families with at least three members affected with CD, faecal samples of 68 patients with CD, 84 of their unaffected relatives and 55 matched controls were subjected to community fingerprinting of the predominant microbiota using denaturing gradient gel electrophoresis (DGGE). To analyse the DGGE profiles, BioNumerics software and non-parametric statistical analyses (SPSS V.17.0) were used. Observed differences in the predominant microbiota were subsequently confirmed and quantified with real-time PCR.

Results.—Five bacterial species characterised dysbiosis in CD, namely a decrease in *Dialister invisus* (p=0.04), an uncharacterised species of *Clostridium cluster* XIVa (p=0.03), *Faecalibacterium prausnitzii* (p<1.3×10^{-5}) and *Bifidobacterium adolescentis* (p=5.4×10^{-6}), and an increase in *Ruminococcus gnavus* (p=2.1×10^{-7}). Unaffected relatives of patients with CD had less *Collinsella aerofaciens* (p=0.004) and a member of the *Escherichia coli–Shigella* group (p=0.01) and more *Ruminococcus torques* (p=0.02) in their predominant microbiota as compared with healthy subjects.

Conclusion.—Unaffected relatives of patients with CD have a different composition of their microbiota compared with healthy controls. This dysbiosis is not characterised by lack of butyrate-producing bacteria as observed in CD but suggests a role for microorganisms with mucin degradation capacity.

▶ Host-bacterial interactions have long been implicated in the pathogenesis of Crohn's disease (CD). Genetic predisposition, especially *NOD2* gene mutations, have been linked to immune system dysfunction in CD in response to luminal bacteria. Antibiotics have shown efficacy in the treatment of Crohn disease, especially in postoperative prophylaxis and perianal disease. In this article, the authors attempt to identify patterns of bacterial flora unique to CD patients and their unaffected relatives. These bacteria may be important to the pathogenesis of CD. In this article, they isolated 5 bacterial species more common in CD than unaffected relatives or controls. The association of these strains is difficult to interpret. Do they predispose an individual to CD? Are they important to pathogenesis of CD, or are they the result of numerous therapies, such as antibiotics or immune suppressant medication, and have nothing to do with disease at all? Ideally, it would be best to test newly diagnosed patients (prior to therapy). Unaffected relatives have a significantly different bacterial flora than controls. The lack of commonality of these bacterial species among unaffected relatives and controls is also open to different interpretations but is important. Finally, the study was too small to determine if certain bacterial profiles fit with specific disease locations or behaviors. This would be particularly important for ileocolonic disease, which has been associated with *NOD2* gene mutations. Despite these limitations, the article is important both for its results and the methods used. The authors apply a sophisticated methodology that will likely be used in the future to address the complex role of bacteria in the pathogenesis of CD.

M. F. Picco, MD, PhD

Ulcerative Colitis

Adalimumab for induction of clinical remission in moderately to severely active ulcerative colitis: results of a randomised controlled trial

Reinisch W, Sandborn WJ, Hommes DW, et al (Med Univ Vienna, Austria; Mayo Clinic, Rochester, MN; Leiden Univ Med Ctr, Netherlands; et al)
Gut 60:780-787, 2011

Objective.—The aim of this study was to assess the efficacy and safety of adalimumab (ADA), a recombinant human monoclonal antibody against tumour necrosis factor α (TNF), for the induction of clinical remission in anti-TNF naïve patients with moderately to severely active ulcerative colitis.

Methods.—This 8-week, multicentre, randomised, double-blind, placebo-controlled study (NCT00385736), conducted at 94 centres in North America and Europe, enrolled ambulatory adult patients with Mayo score of ≥ 6 points and endoscopic subscore of ≥ 2 points despite treatment with corticosteroids and/or immunosuppressants. Under the original study protocol, 186 patients were randomised (1:1) to subcutaneous treatment with ADA160/80 (160 mg at week 0, 80 mg at week 2, 40 mg at weeks 4 and 6) or placebo. Subsequently, at the request of European regulatory authorities, the protocol was amended to include a second induction group (ADA80/40: 80 mg at week 0, 40 mg at weeks 2, 4 and 6). The primary efficacy endpoint was clinical remission (Mayo score ≤ 2 with no individual subscore >1) at week 8, assessed in 390 patients randomised (1:1:1) to ADA160/80, ADA80/40, or placebo. Safety was assessed in all enrolled patients. Patients, study site personnel, investigators, and the sponsor were blinded to treatment assignment.

Results.—At week 8, 18.5% of patients in the ADA160/80 group (p=0.031 vs placebo) and 10.0% in the ADA80/40 group (p=0.833 vs placebo) were in remission, compared with 9.2% in the placebo group. Serious adverse events occurred in 7.6%, 3.8% and 4.0% of patients in the placebo, ADA80/40, and ADA160/80 groups, respectively. There were two malignancies in the placebo group, none in the ADA groups. There were no cases of tuberculosis and no deaths.

Conclusions.—ADA160/80 was safe and effective for induction of clinical remission in patients with moderately to severely active ulcerative colitis failing treatment with corticosteroids and/or immunosuppressants.

Clinical Trial.—NCT00385736.

▶ Here we are presented with the results of the first large, randomized, controlled trial of adalimumab for the treatment of moderate to severe ulcerative colitis (UC). Unfortunately, the results were not impressive and lead to more questions than answers. The patients selected and the general assessments of the study were similar to the Active Ulcerative Colitis Trials (ACT) studies[1] that established infliximab as an effective treatment for ulcerative colitis. Both studies enrolled outpatients with moderate to severe UC despite corticosteroids (ACT) or immunomodulators (current study) and assessed the outcome at week 8. Although it is difficult to compare these studies directly, response rates were similar, but remission rates for infliximab were numerically higher at week 8 (39% and 34% for ACT1 and ACT 2, respectively) compared with adalimumab (19%). Placebo response rates in this adalimumab trial were also high regarding secondary outcomes, including clinical response, although adalimumab at 160 mg/80 mg was superior to placebo for remission. Why was adalimumab not more impressive? The authors speculate that patient-specific factors, such as body weight and C-reactive protein (CRP) levels, may play a role. Patients weighing less than 82 kg had twice the remission rate compared with those more than 82 kg. This is important because adalimumab dosing is not weight based. Weight-based dosing may lead to better efficacy. Similarly, higher CRP levels were associated with a lack of response, leading the authors to speculate that these patients may also have needed a higher dose. Alternatively, patients with low CRP may have had a higher response rate simply because their disease was not that active compared with those with a higher CRP. These assertions are clearly speculative but are important in planning future studies. Ultimately, this study did meet its primary end point, but questions remain regarding the use and position of this medication in the treatment of moderate to severe UC.

M. F. Picco, MD, PhD

Reference

1. Rutgeerts P, Sandborn WJ, Feagan BG, et al. Infliximab for induction and maintenance therapy for ulcerative colitis. *N Engl J Med.* 2005;353:2462-2476.

An Association Between Dietary Arachidonic Acid, Measured in Adipose Tissue, and Ulcerative Colitis

de Silva PSA, Olsen A, Christensen J, et al (Norfolk and Norwich Univ Hosp NHS Trust, UK; Inst of Cancer Epidemiology, Copenhagen, Denmark; et al)
Gastroenterology 139:1912-1917, 2010

Background & Aims.—Dietary arachidonic acid, an n-6 polyunsaturated fatty acid (n-6 PUFA), might be involved in the etiology of ulcerative colitis (UC). We performed a prospective cohort study to determine whether high levels of arachidonic acid in adipose tissue samples (which reflects dietary intake) are associated with UC.

Methods.—We analyzed data collected from 57,053 men and women in the EPIC-Denmark Prospective Cohort Study from 1993 to 1997. Adipose tissue biopsy samples were collected from gluteal regions at the beginning of the study, the cohort was monitored over subsequent years, and participants who developed UC were identified. A subcohort of 2510 randomly selected participants were used as controls. Concentrations of arachidonic acid were measured in adipose tissue samples. In the analysis, arachidonic acid levels were divided into quartiles; relative risks (RR) were calculated and adjusted for smoking, use of aspirin and nonsteroidal anti-inflammatory drugs, and levels of n-3 PUFAs.

Results.—A total of 34 subjects (56% men) developed incident UC at a median age of 58.8 years (range, 50.0—69.0 years). Those in the highest quartile for arachidonic acid concentrations in adipose tissue had an RR for UC of 4.16 (95% confidence interval [CI]: 1.56—11.04); a trend per 0.1% increase in arachidonic acid of 1.77 in RR was observed (95% CI: 1.38—2.27). The fraction attributed the highest levels of arachidonic acid was 40.3%.

Conclusions.—Individuals with the highest relative concentrations of arachidonic acid in adipose tissue have a significantly greater risk of developing UC. Dietary modifications might therefore prevent UC or reduce disease symptoms.

▶ Arachidonic acid (AA) is a known component of cell membranes that can be converted to proinflammatory cytokines, resulting in cellular inflammation. High AA levels are found in red meats and certain dietary oils. High AA intake may be important in the pathogenesis of ulcerative colitis. Previous studies have suggested an increased risk for UC among those with high AA intake, but these studies were based on dietary questionnaires that are prone to recall bias. In this carefully conducted cohort study, AA levels were measured from gluteal fat samples at study entry among more than 57 000 unaffected subjects. Concentrations of AA were compared between those who later developed UC and controls. Those who developed UC within 18 months of study entry or had symptoms of UC at study entry were appropriately excluded. Findings were striking in that risk of UC was higher in a concentration (dose)-dependent fashion with higher AA concentrations. These findings are provocative and worthy of further study. The dose-dependent association, while suggestive, is certainly not causal, but there is certainly biologic plausibility to a link of AA intake with pathogenesis. Limitations, as pointed out by the investigators, include older subject age and the possibility of residual confounding (ie, increased AA intake was associated with some other dietary factor that was associated with UC). Despite these limitations, the authors present the results of an important epidemiologic study with careful measurement of AA that will hopefully inspire further interest in this area. AA intake may turn out to be an important risk factor for the development of ulcerative colitis.

M. F. Picco, MD, PhD

Treatment of Relapsing Mild-to-Moderate Ulcerative Colitis With the Probiotic VSL#3 as Adjunctive to a Standard Pharmaceutical Treatment: A Double-Blind, Randomized, Placebo-Controlled Study
Tursi A, Brandimarte G, Papa A, et al ("Lorenzo Bonomo" Hosp, Andria, Italy; "Cristo Re" Hosp, Roma, Italy; Catholic Univ, Roma, Italy; et al)
Am J Gastroenterol 105:2218-2227, 2010

Objectives.—VSL#3 is a high-potency probiotic mixture that has been used successfully in the treatment of pouchitis. The primary end point of the study was to assess the effects of supplementation with VSL#3 in patients affected by relapsing ulcerative colitis (UC) who are already under treatment with 5-aminosalicylic acid (ASA) and/or immunosuppressants at stable doses.

Methods.—A total of 144 consecutive patients were randomly treated for 8 weeks with VSL#3 at a dose of 3,600 billion CFU/day (71 patients) or with placebo (73 patients).

Results.—In all, 65 patients in the VSL#3 group and 66 patients in the placebo group completed the study. The decrease in ulcerative colitis disease activity index (UCDAI) scores of 50% or more was higher in the VSL#3 group than in the placebo group (63.1 vs. 40.8; per protocol (PP) $P = 0.010$, confidence interval $CI_{95\%}$ 0.51–0.74; intention to treat (ITT) $P = 0.031$, $CI_{95\%}$ 0.47–0.69). Significant results with VSL#3 were recorded in an improvement of three points or more in the UCDAI score (60.5% vs. 41.4%; PP $P = 0.017$, $CI_{95\%}$ 0.51–0.74; ITT $P = 0.046$, $CI_{95\%}$ 0.47–0.69) and in rectal bleeding (PP $P = 0.014$, $CI_{95\%}$ 0.46–0.70; ITT $P = 0.036$, $CI_{95\%}$ 0.41–0.65), whereas stool frequency (PP $P = 0.202$, $CI_{95\%}$ 0.39–0.63; ITT $P = 0.229$, $CI_{95\%}$ 0.35–0.57), physician's rate of disease activity (PP $P = 0.088$, $CI_{95\%}$ 0.34–0.58; ITT $P = 0.168$, $CI_{95\%}$ 0.31–0.53), and endoscopic scores (PP $P = 0.086$, $CI_{95\%}$ 0.74–0.92; ITT $P = 0.366$, $CI_{95\%}$ 0.66–0.86) did not show statistical differences. Remission was higher in the VSL#3 group than in the placebo group (47.7% vs. 32.4%; PP $P = 0.069$, $CI_{95\%}$ 0.36–0.60; ITT $P = 0.132$, $CI_{95\%}$ 0.33–0.56). Eight patients on VSL#3 (11.2%) and nine patients on placebo (12.3%) reported mild side effects.

Conclusions.—VSL#3 supplementation is safe and able to reduce UCDAI scores in patients affected by relapsing mild-to-moderate UC who are under treatment with 5-ASA and/or immunosuppressants. Moreover, VSL#3 improves rectal bleeding and seems to reinduce remission in relapsing UC patients after 8 weeks of treatment, although these parameters do not reach statistical significance.

▶ Probiotics have been touted as beneficial treatments in numerous digestive diseases and are readily available at health food stores and on the Internet. Despite claims of efficacy, definitive evidence is lacking, and use remains controversial. It is important to understand that all probiotics are not created equal and may not be effective despite claims from their manufacturers. VSL#3 is the most tested of the probiotics for the treatment of inflammatory bowel disease and has an established place in the prevention of recurrent pouchitis among patients who have an ileal pouch construction following colectomy for ulcerative colitis. In this study, the authors claim that VSL#3 is beneficial as an adjunctive treatment among patients with active mild to moderate ulcerative colitis (UC) on maintenance therapy. While this conclusion does have some merit, it must be interpreted in the context of the patients studied. While the authors claim that VSL#3 is effective for mild to moderate UC, the majority of the patients studied had mild disease as evident from their activity index. This may have been the reason that the outcome of a 50% drop in index score was met but a decrease in stool frequency or improvement in physician-rated disease activity could not be shown. Most were only taking low-dose mesalamine with only few receiving immunomodulator therapy, again suggesting that their disease was probably milder and would have responded to increasing the dose of mesalamine. Finally, there was no difference in the endoscopic improvement between the 2 groups, although this may have been because of the short duration of the trial. Remission rates between VSL#3 and placebo were not different, although there was a trend toward a benefit of the probiotic. Overall, while these results are encouraging, much more evidence is needed before VSL#3 should be adopted into routine clinical practice. The correct patient population for these agents needs to be defined, and a clear benefit over existing therapies must be proven.

M. F. Picco, MD, PhD

ABCB1 Single-Nucleotide Polymorphisms Determine Tacrolimus Response in Patients With Ulcerative Colitis

Herrlinger KR, Koc H, Winter S, et al (Robert-Bosch-Hosp, Stuttgart, Germany; Dr Margarete Fischer-Bosch Inst for Clinical Pharmacology, Stuttgart, Germany)
Clin Pharmacol Ther 89:422-428, 2011

Tacrolimus (Tac) is effective in the treatment of steroid-refractory ulcerative colitis (UC); however, nonresponse and unpredictable side effects are major limitations. Because Tac response in patients who have undergone solid-organ transplantation has been associated with the presence of variants in *CYP3A* and *ABCB1*, we elucidated the contributions of *CYP3A4*1B* and *CYP3A5*3* and of *ABCB1* 1236C>T, 2677G>T,A, and 3435C>T polymorphisms to Tac response in 89 patients with UC. Short-term remission and response were achieved in 61 and 14% of the patients, respectively, and were associated with colectomy-free survival. In a linear logistic regression model, patients with homozygous variants for one of the three *ABCB1* alleles showed significantly higher short-term remission rates as compared with those of other genotypes. The effects held true after multivariate analysis including multiple comparisons and were more pronounced after correction for dose-adjusted Tac blood trough levels. We suggest that *ABCB1*, but not *CYP3A5*, may predict short-term remission of Tac in steroid-refractory UC.

▶ Pharmacogenomics is a rapidly expanding field that studies patient-specific genetic factors that influence response and toxicity to drug therapies. The best example of this in inflammatory bowel disease (IBD) is with the metabolism of azathioprine and 6-mercaptopurine. Metabolism of these medications depends in part on thiopurine methyltransferase (TPMT). TPMT activity influences metabolism, and activity is genetically determined. TPMT measurement allows for more accurate dosing to maximize efficacy and minimize toxicity. Tacrolimus (TAC) has been studied in the treatment of IBD without consistent results and high rates of toxicity. In this article, the authors look at genetic factors that influence metabolism and response to TAC. TAC response has been associated with genetic factors in transplant populations. Variations in cytochrome P450 responsible for TAC metabolism and P-glycoprotein responsible for pumping TAC out of the cell (drug efflux) encoded by *ABCB1* gene have been associated with therapeutic response in transplant populations. The authors tested these genetic variants among a population with active ulcerative colitis (UC) treated with TAC. Unlike the transplant population, only *ABCB1* was associated with response in UC. This suggests that other factors such as the UC itself or concomitant therapies may also affect potential genetic influences. Overall, the study did have limitations, so the conclusions are limited. However, more pharmacogenomic research is coming and will likely improve our ability to match individual patients with specific therapies to maximize efficacy and minimize toxicity.

M. F. Picco, MD, PhD

E-health empowers patients with ulcerative colitis: a randomised controlled trial of the web-guided 'Constant-care' approach

Elkjaer M, Shuhaibar M, Burisch J, et al (Univ of Copenhagen, Denmark; Adelaide and Meath Hosp incorporating the Natl Children Hosp/Trinity College Dublin, Ireland; et al)
Gut 59:1652-1661, 2010

Background.—The natural history of ulcerative colitis requires continuous monitoring of medical treatment via frequent outpatient visits. The European health authorities' focus on e-health is increasing. Lack of easy access to inflammatory bowel disease (IBD) clinics, patients' education and understanding of the importance of early treatment at relapse is leading to poor compliance. To overcome these limitations a randomised control trial 'Constant-care' was undertaken in Denmark and Ireland.

Methods.—333 patients with mild/moderate ulcerative colitis and 5-aminosalicylate acid treatment were randomised to either a web-group receiving disease specific education and self-treatment via http://www.constant-care.dk or a control group continuing the usual care for 12 months. A historical control group was included to test the comparability with the control group. We investigated: feasibility of the approach, its influence on patients' compliance, knowledge, quality of life (QoL), disease outcomes, safety and health care costs.

Results.—88% of the web patients preferred using the new approach. Adherence to 4 weeks of acute treatment was increased by 31% in Denmark and 44% in Ireland compared to the control groups. In Denmark IBD knowledge and QoL were significantly improved in web patients. Median relapse duration was 18 days (95% CI 10 to 21) in the web versus 77 days (95% CI 46 to 108) in the control group. The number of acute and routine visits to the outpatient clinic was lower in the web than in the control group, resulting in a saving of 189 euro/patient/year. No difference in the relapse frequency, hospitalisation, surgery or adverse events was observed. The historical control group was comparable with the control group.

Conclusion.—The new web-guided approach on http://www.constant-care.dk is feasible, safe and cost effective. It empowers patients with ulcerative colitis without increasing their morbidity and depression. It has yet to be shown whether this strategy can change the natural disease course of ulcerative colitis in the long term.

▶ The prospect of harnessing the power of the Internet to assist in the management of patients with ulcerative colitis (UC) is very appealing. Most patients with this disorder are young and accustomed to using Web-based media in their daily lives. In this study, the authors have designed a Web-based program that empowers UC patients to participate in their own care, leading to better medication compliance and shorter duration of relapse. The results are exciting but only apply to a population with UC who have mild disease with exclusion of patients on immunomodulator or biologic therapy. However, this is still a large population of patients with UC. Simple interventions such as increasing mesalamine dosage in the event of a flare were successfully made by these patients with physician backup and, in cases of failure to respond, physician intervention. Outcomes were comparable to the usual care group but with fewer outpatient clinic visits. This led to happier patients, less resource utilization, and lower costs. The secret to their success was patient education about UC and the appropriate use of the Web-based system. In a motivated group of patients like this one where patient-directed decision choices are limited, such a system may have a role. While as the disease complexity increases, the role for independent patient decisions becomes more limited, Web-based systems can still improve access to care, enhance patient-physician communication, and likely lead to overall better patient outcomes. We need more studies like this one to unlock the power of the Web with its many applications.

M. F. Picco, MD, PhD

A Multicenter Experience With Infliximab for Ulcerative Colitis: Outcomes and Predictors of Response, Optimization, Colectomy, and Hospitalization

Oussalah A, Evesque L, Laharie D, et al (Univ Hosp of Nancy, France; Univ of Nice Sophia Antipolis, France; Haut-Lévêque Hosp, Pessac, France; et al)
Am J Gastroenterol 105:2617-2625, 2010

Objectives.—The objective of this study was to evaluate short- and long-term outcomes of infliximab in ulcerative colitis (UC), including infliximab optimization, colectomy, and hospitalization.

Methods.—This was a retrospective multicenter study. All adult patients who received at least one infliximab infusion for UC were included. Cumulative probabilities of event-free survival were estimated by the Kaplan—Meier method. Independent predictors were identified using binary logistic regression or Cox proportional-hazards regression, and results were expressed as odds ratios or hazard ratios (HRs), respectively.

Results.—Between January 2000 and August 2009, 191 UC patients received infliximab therapy. Median follow-up per patient was 18 months (interquartile range = 25−75th, 8−32 months). Primary nonresponse was noted in 42 patients (22.0%). "Hemoglobin at infliximab initiation ≤ 9.4 g/dl" (odds ratio = 4.35; 95% confidence interval (CI) = 1.81−10.42) was a positive predictor of non-response to infliximab. Infliximab optimization was required in 36 (45.0%) of 80 patients on scheduled infliximab therapy. The only predictor of infliximab optimization was "infliximab indication for acute severe colitis" (HR = 2.75; 95% CI = 1.23−6.12). Thirty-six patients (18.8%) underwent colectomy. Predictors of colectomy were: "no clinical response after infliximab induction" (HR = 7.06; 95% CI = 3.36−14.83), "C-reactive protein at infliximab initiation > 10 mg/l" (HR = 5.11; 95% CI = 1.77−14.76), "infliximab indication for acute severe colitis" (HR = 3.40; 95% CI = 1.48−7.81), and "previous treatment with cyclosporine" (HR = 2.53; 95% CI = 1.22−5.28). Sixty-nine patients (36.1%) were hospitalized at least one time and UC-related hospitalizations rate was 29 per 100 patient-years (95% CI = 24−35 per 100 patient-years). Predictors of first hospitalization were: "no clinical response after infliximab induction" (HR = 3.87; 95% CI = 2.29−6.53), "infliximab indication for acute severe colitis" (HR = 3.13, 95% CI = 1.65−5.94), "disease duration at infliximab initiation ≤ 50 months" (HR = 2.14, 95% CI = 1.25−3.66), "hemoglobin at infliximab initiation ≤ 11.8 g/dl" (HR = 1.77; 95% CI = 1.03−3.04), and "previous treatment with methotrexate" (HR = 0.30; 95% CI = 0.09−0.97).

Conclusions.—Primary non-response to infliximab was noted in one fifth of patients and increased by seven and four the risks of colectomy and hospitalization, respectively. Infliximab optimization, colectomy, and hospitalization were required in half, one fifth, and one third of patients, respectively. Infliximab indication for acute severe colitis increased by three the risks of infliximab optimization, colectomy, and UC-related hospitalization.

▶ This is a large real-world experience on the use of infliximab in ulcerative colitis. Patient outcomes are measured from how infliximab is typically used in practice outside clinical trials. Unfortunately, the trial was retrospective, and there were no objective criteria to measure clinical response or maintenance of clinical benefit. These outcomes were measured by physician judgment with only limited objective data on individual patients. While physician judgment is typically how treatment decisions are based in practice, practices may vary, especially with regard to assessment for treatment response.

Despite these limitations, the conclusions are important. Median follow-up of 18 months was adequate. The mix of patients included both hospitalized patients and outpatients. Nearly 20% were cyclosporine failures. The predictors of response, optimization, and colectomy made sense and fit with most clinicians' experience with the drug. Of particularly importance is that severe colitis (where infliximab is typically used in practice) resulted in a 3-fold risk of infliximab failure. The finding that concomitant use of immunomodulators did not affect infliximab optimization was surprising, especially in light of Crohn's disease favoring combined usage in treatment-naive patients and the reported risk of malignancy and infection with combined immunosuppression. It is not clear whether these patients were immunodulator failures or had these medications started at the time of first infliximab.

Ultimately, a randomized clinical trial is the only way to understand what are the true predictors of treatment response or failure. Unfortunately, such a trial is unlikely. This study validates what many clinicians have learned from experience. It does also raise important questions about the use of concomitant immunosuppression, which need to be answered.

M. F. Picco, MD, PhD

Prevalence of Colorectal Cancer Surveillance for Ulcerative Colitis in an Integrated Health Care Delivery System
Velayos FS, Liu L, Lewis JD, et al (Univ of California, San Francisco; Kaiser Permanente Northern California, Oakland, CA; Univ of Pennsylvania, Philadelphia; et al)
Gastroenterology 139:1511-1518, 2010

Background & Aims.—The absence of grade A supporting evidence for surveillance colonoscopy in patients with ulcerative colitis (UC) has led to controversy regarding its benefit, yet it is routinely recommended in practice guidelines. Limited data are available on rates of colonoscopy surveillance and factors associated with surveillance.

Methods.—A retrospective study of UC patients receiving care between 2006 and 2007 with ≥8 years history of UC was conducted. Primary outcome was the proportion of patients who underwent surveillance during this 2-year study period. Sociodemographic and disease factors were identified a priori from variables recorded electronically in the medical record; multivariable associations with surveillance were estimated using logistic regression.

Results.—Of 771 patients with ≥8 years history of UC, 24.6% of patients underwent at least 1 surveillance colonoscopy within the 2-year study period, with a maximum of 38.5% observed among patients with primary sclerosing cholangitis. In a multivariable analysis, gender, age, race, and education were not associated with surveillance. Factors associated with increasing surveillance included lack of significant comorbidity (Charlson-Deyo index 0 vs 1+: odds ratio [OR], 1.7; 95% confidence interval: 1.1−2.5), >3 inflammatory bowel disease-related outpatient visits (OR, 2.0; 95% CI: 1.4−3.0), and use of mesalamine (OR, 2.8; 95% CI: 1.7−4.4).

Conclusions.—Utilization of surveillance colonoscopy in a 2-year period was low, even among high-risk patients. Although specific factors recorded in computerized data were identified to be associated with surveillance, a greater understanding of how patients and physicians decide on surveillance is needed.

▶ The findings of this article are quite surprising. Rates of surveillance colonoscopy among a population derived from Kaiser Permanente Northern California with long-standing ulcerative colitis (UC) were very low. One would expect that the best rates of surveillance would come from such an integrated health system where patients receive all their health care within the plan and information on health care utilization would be complete. However, data acquisition was retrospective, and methods of identification of patients eligible for surveillance may have led to flawed estimates of surveillance rates. The first problem was that there is no code to identify surveillance procedures in UC. The authors relied on a computerized surveillance algorithm that identified surveillance colonoscopies. This resulted in a 20% false-negative level, suggesting that 20% of procedures classified as not for surveillance were in fact surveillance procedures. This may have contributed to a somewhat lower estimate of surveillance rates. In addition, the authors could not definitively separate patients based on extent of disease. The criteria used for identification and exclusion of proctitis patients were reasonable, but the authors could not separate left-sided colitis from pancolitis. Patients with left-sided colitis may undergo surveillance later than 8 years of disease, which may have led to a lower overall estimate of surveillance rates because they admit that 59% of their population had left-sided disease from a previous study. Despite these limitations, the findings are important. Even if case ascertainment was complete, surveillance rates would probably still be well below 100%. More work is needed to determine true patterns of surveillance among clinicians and reasons for disparities and barriers that interfere with compliance with current guidelines.

M. F. Picco, MD, PhD

Predicting the need for colectomy in severe ulcerative colitis: a critical appraisal of clinical parameters and currently available biomarkers
Travis S, Satsangi J, Lémann M (John Radcliffe Hosp, Oxford, UK; Univ of Edinburgh, UK; Université Paris 7 Diderot, France)
Gut 60:3-9, 2011

Background.—Acute severe ulcerative colitis is usually identified using the criteria of Truelove and Witts, specifically, having 6 or more bloody stools daily plus tachycardia (over 90 beats/min), temperature over 37.8°C, anemia (hemoglobin less than 10.5 g/dl), or elevated erythrocyte sedimentation rate (ESR) (over 30 mm/h). About 67% of patients respond to intensive treatment with hydrocortisone or methylprednisolone and 29% to betamethasone. However, clinicians must try to identify at an early stage who will likely fail intensive treatment and when to start rescue medical therapy so surgery will not be unduly delayed, carrying a poorer outcome. The clinical, laboratory, radiological, endoscopic, genetic, and composite factors that may predict colectomy were reviewed.

Clinical Criteria.—Most clinical markers depend on stool frequency, pulse, or temperature. The only validated index, the pediatric ulcerative colitis activity index (PUCAI), shows that number of daily stools on day 3 after admission to the hospital is linked to lack of response to intravenous steroids. No other clinical factors are as widely used. The number of Truelove and Witts' criteria present on admission is also associated with colectomy, with more symptoms present on admission predictive of colectomy.

Laboratory Criteria.—Biochemical markers such as C-reactive protein (CRP) and albumin measure the inflammatory response and can predict colectomy. CRP is included in the PUCAI and is the key biochemical marker in other indices. It is a useful, objective marker of predictive value for steroid failure. Rate of change in CRP during intensive treatment may also predict response. Low albumin levels in acute severe colitis are linked with colectomy in retrospective case studies, but albumin by itself is not an independent marker. Combining albumin with clinical and radiological data increases sensitivity. Fecal calprotectin, which correlates with severity of intestinal inflammation, may be significantly higher in patients who eventually require colectomy, with 97% specificity for a predictive threshold of 1922 µ/g, but low sensitivity (24%). It predicts nonresponse to steroids but not response to infliximab and is significantly less predictive than combining stool frequency and CRP. No other laboratory markers are validated.

Radiological Criteria.—Colonic dilatation over 5.5 cm and mucosal islands on a plain abdominal radiograph or single-stage colonic magnetic resonance imaging (MRI) are the primary radiological criteria predicting colectomy. Computed tomography and ultrasound have no predictive value but can assess the extent of colitis, measure colonic diameter, or detect complications such as intramural gas.

Endoscopic Criteria.—Surgery should be timed to avoid perforation, which can only occur after deep ulceration has developed. Endoscopy confirms the diagnosis of acute severe colitis and excludes confounding factors. Flexible sigmoidoscopy is preferred to colonoscopy to avoid perforation. Deep ulceration at the index examination is associated with an increased long-term risk of surgery.

Genetic Criteria.—Between 1% and 3% of the general population express HLA DRB1*103, but 16% of those who eventually require colectomy have this haplotype. Polymorphism in the gene for the multidrug resistance efflux pump is associated with steroid resistance, which leads to colectomy in patients with ulcerative colitis.

Composite Criteria.—The combination of CRP over 45 mg/l and stool frequency over 8 per day on day 3 after admission is the simplest composite index predicting the need for colectomy, with 85% of patients meeting these criteria needing the procedure. The Swedish index combines stool frequency per day and 0.14×CRP mg/l and has a 69% positive predictive value for colectomy within 90 days when a score of 8 occurs. A score of 180 or higher on the Seo index, which combines weighted components of stool frequency, pulse rate, albumin level, and hemoglobin, has a positive predictive value of 52% and a negative predictive value of 97% for predicting short-term colectomy. The combination of stool frequency, presence of colonic dilatation, and hypoalbuminemia (Edinburgh index) predicts colectomy in 85% of patients who achieve a score of 4 or more. The PUCAI most strongly predicts response compared to other measures. Sensitivity is important in early-stage disease. On day 3 a PUCAI exceeding 45 has a negative predictive value of 94% for patients likely to fail to respond to steroid therapy. On day 5 the specificity for needing rescue therapy is more important. The positive predictive value of a PUCAI score over 65 is 100%.

Conclusions.—The PUCAI and Oxford indices work better than the other methods for prospective validation in children, but there is no clearly preferred index. It is important to use an index to interject objectivity into the decision-making process. Numbers in the objective index should trigger contingency planning. Combining this with clinical judgment, which considers physician experience, patient age, previous pattern of colitis and therapy, radiographic appearance, endoscopic evidence of deep ulceration, and patient input, is the best way to reduce the mortality related to acute severe colitis.

▶ In this article, the authors critically review many of the published indices of severity for ulcerative colitis (UC). These indices attempt to reliably predict the need for colectomy or advanced therapy such as infliximab or cyclosporine among patients with UC. Typical clinical criteria rely on number of bowel movements and measurements of biochemical markers such as C-reactive protein (CRP), albumin, or fecal calprotectin. Purely clinical measures rely on subjective definitions such as to what constitutes as bowel movement or blood in the stool. CRP appears to be the best biomarker and most convenient, whereas fecal calprotectin, while promising, has not been validated, and erythrocyte sedimentation rate has not been shown to be useful. For the clinician, the simpler the index, the better. The timing of measurement of these indices of severity is also very important, especially with regard to responsiveness to steroid therapy and the eventual need for advanced medical therapy or colectomy. Clinical criteria at hospital admission are the basis for the Truelove and Witts criteria that can be predictive of colectomy. However, measurement after 3 to 5 days of steroid therapy appears to be the most important. Travis et al[1] had shown rates of colectomy of 85% among those with greater than 8 bowel movements per day after 3 days of corticosteroids or with stool frequency of 3 to 8 per day and a CRP of 45 mg/L or higher. Similarly, the pediatric ulcerative colitis index has also been validated at day 3 but relies only on clinical criteria of stool frequency, blood in stool, and abdominal pain.[2] Others have suggested radiographic and endoscopic criteria and genetic markers to predict outcome, but these do not seem to offer a greater advantage than simply measuring stool frequency and/or CRP. The measurement of CRP does provide a more objective measure compared with more subjective clinical measurements. While indices are important, they are not a substitution for good clinical judgment. They do allow the clinician and the patient to better understand the prognosis and provide evidence-based information on the decision to move to advanced medical therapy or colectomy.

M. F. Picco, MD, PhD

References

1. Travis SPL, Farrant JM, Ricketts C, et al. Predicting outcome in severe ulcerative colitis. *Gut.* 1996;38:905-910.
2. Turner D, Otley AR, Mack D, et al. Development, validation, and evaluation of a pediatric ulcerative colitis activity index: a prospective multicenter study. *Gastroenterology.* 2007;133:423-432.

Meta-analysis: the diagnostic yield of chromoendoscopy for detecting dysplasia in patients with colonic inflammatory bowel disease
Subramanian V, Mannath J, Ragunath K, et al (Nottingham Univ Hosp, UK)
Aliment Pharmacol Ther 33:304-312, 2011

Background.—Dysplasia in inflammatory bowel disease (IBD) is often multifocal and flat. Dye spraying is believed to enhance visualisation of subtle mucosal abnormalities.

Aim.—To perform a meta-analysis of the published studies to compare the diagnostic yield of dysplastic lesions in patients with IBD undergoing surveillance colonoscopy between chromoendoscopy and standard white light endoscopy.

Methods.—We searched electronic databases for full journal articles reporting on chromoendoscopy in patients with IBD. Pooled incremental yield of chromoendoscopy over white light endoscopy for dysplasia detection was determined. A fixed effects model was used unless there was significant heterogeneity. Publication bias was assessed using Funnel plots or Egger's test.

Results.—Six studies involving 1277 patients provided data on a number of dysplastic lesions detected. The difference in yield of dysplasia between chromoendoscopy and white light endoscopy was 7% (95% CI 3.2—11.3) on a per patient analysis with an NNT of 14.3. The difference in proportion of lesions detected by targeted biopsies was 44% (95% CI 28.6-59.1) and flat lesions was 27% (95% CI 11.2—41.9) in favour of chromoendoscopy.

Conclusions.—Chromoendoscopy is significantly better than white light endoscopy in detecting dysplasia in patients with colonic IBD. This holds true for all dysplastic lesions, proportion of targeted lesions and proportion of flat lesions detected.

▶ This article adds to the growing body of literature that supports the use of chromoendoscopy for the detection of colonic dysplasia in inflammatory bowel disease. In this meta-analysis, the authors pool the 6 important studies in this area. Only 1 study included patients with Crohn's colitis, but it is reasonable that conclusions regarding ulcerative colitis (UC) should also apply to

Crohn's colitis. The rate of detection of dysplasia during colonoscopy was higher for chromoendoscopy, especially for flat lesions, and added only about 11 minutes to the procedure. The authors do contend that random nontargeted biopsies, where there is no visible lesion present, should still be performed. Thus, they recommend that all patients still undergo the standard 32 random biopsies. They based this on the finding of dysplasia on nontargeted biopsies, but the yield was extremely low. In most studies, rate of dysplasia in random samples was 1 per 1000 biopsies. With such low yields, many advocate eliminating random biopsies, especially in the era of high-definition colonoscopy among patients having chromoendoscopy. This would serve to shorten the procedure time and significantly lower the overall expense of the procedure by decreasing pathology costs. This is another important advantage that chromoscopy has over standard colonoscopy. The acceptance of chromoendosocpy in UC has not, unfortunately, been universal. In recent practice guidelines from the American College of Gastroenterology, the authors did not advocate the procedure, while other organizations, such as the Crohn and Colitis Foundation of America, have endorsed it. The controversy is whether typically small lesions that are found with low-grade dysplasia are clinically important. We do need more longitudinal studies to show that the use of this technique truly leads to better patient outcomes. The lack of these studies is not reason to reject this technique in favor of random biopsy. Until such studies are published, our goal should be to identify dysplastic lesions by the best method possible, providing our patients the best chance to avoid colorectal cancer in inflammatory bowel disease. That method is chromoendoscopy.

M. F. Picco, MD, PhD

Randomised clinical trial: early assessment after 2 weeks of high-dose mesalazine for moderately active ulcerative colitis - new light on a familiar question
Orchard TR, van der Geest SAP, Travis SPL (St Mary's Hosp, London, UK; Warner Chilcott UK Ltd, Larne; John Radcliffe Hosp, Oxford, UK)
Aliment Pharmacol Ther 33:1028-1035, 2011

Background.—Rapid resolution of rectal bleeding and stool frequency are important goals for ulcerative colitis therapy and may help guide therapeutic decisions.

Aim.—To explore patient diary data from ASCEND I and II for their relevance to clinical decision making.

Methods.—Data from two randomised, double-blind, Phase III studies were combined. Patients received mesalazine (mesalamine) 4.8 g/day (Asacol 800 mg MR) or 2.4 g/day (Asacol 400 mg MR). Time to improvement or resolution of rectal bleeding and stool frequency was assessed and the proportion of patients experiencing symptom improvement or resolution at day 14 evaluated using survival analysis. Symptoms after 14 days were compared to week 6. A combination of prespecified and *post hoc* analyses were used.

Results.—Median times to resolution and improvement of both rectal bleeding and stool frequency were shorter with 4.8 g/day than 2.4 g/day (resolution, 19 vs. 29 days, $P = 0.020$; improvement, 7 vs. 9 days, $P = 0.024$). In total, 73% of patients experienced improvement in both rectal bleeding and stool frequency by day 14 with 4.8 g/day, compared to 61% with 2.4 g/day. More patients achieved symptom resolution by day 14 with 4.8 g/day than 2.4 g/day (43% vs. 30%; $P = 0.035$). Symptom relief after 14 days was associated with a high rate of symptom relief after 6 weeks.

Conclusions.—High-dose mesalazine 4.8 g/day provides rapid relief of the cardinal symptoms of moderately active ulcerative colitis. Symptom relief within 14 days was associated with symptom relief at 6 weeks in the majority of patients. Day 14 is a practical timepoint at which response to treatment may be assessed and decisions regarding therapy escalation made (Clinicaltrials.gov: NCT00577473, NCT00073021).

▶ The results of this study are not surprising, but they are reassuring. The finding of mesalamine treatment response at 14 days predicting response at 6 weeks confirms the validity of accepted clinical practice. The finding that 4.8 g/d is better than 2.4 g/d also fits with practice in that more mesalamine is better to treat mild to moderate ulcerative colitis (UC). Should we use the lack of response at 14 days to decide whether to escalate therapy? Although rates of response at 6 weeks were highest for those with response at 14 days, nearly half of those without symptom improvement in rectal bleeding at 14 days had symptom improvement at 6 weeks. Rates were lower for those without improvement in stool frequency at 14 days (25%). Should we abandon high-dose mesalamine for nonresponders at 14 days? The answer, not surprisingly, depends on the individual patient's clinical history and severity of symptoms. Patients who were receiving greater than 1.6 g/d of mesalamine were excluded from the study. This may have selected out a population more likely to respond and limited the applicability of the findings. Because most patients with UC are taking maintenance mesalamine at the time of a flare, this is an important exclusion. At best, assessment at 14 days of therapy provides a rough guide. Among patients with more severe symptoms or who worsen on treatment, changing therapy would be reasonable. It may be as simple as adding topical mesalamine or possibly topical or oral corticosteroids. For patients with mild symptoms who have an equivocal response or no response, adding topical mesalamine therapy or watchful waiting may be reasonable because many may respond and not require corticosteroids. Clinical judgment remains most important.

M. F. Picco, MD, PhD

Successive Treatment With Cyclosporine and Infliximab in Steroid-Refractory Ulcerative Colitis

Leblanc S, the GETAID (Université Paris-Diderot, France; et al)
Am J Gastroenterol 106:771-777, 2011

Objectives.—Rescue therapy with either cyclosporine (CYS) or infliximab (IFX) is an effective option in patients with intravenous steroid-refractory attacks of ulcerative colitis (UC). In patients who fail, colectomy is usually recommended, but a second-line rescue therapy with IFX or CYS is an alternative. The aims of this study were to investigate the efficacy and tolerance of IFX and CYS as a second-line rescue therapy in steroid-refractory UC or indeterminate colitis (IC) unsuccessfully treated with CYS or IFX.

Methods.—This was a retrospective survey of patients seen during the period 2000–2008 in the GETAID centers. Inclusion criteria included a delay of <1 month between CYS withdrawal (when used first) and IFX, or a delay of <2 months between IFX (when used first) and CYS, and a follow-up of at least 3 months after inclusion. Time-to-colectomy, clinical response, and occurrence of serious adverse events were analyzed.

Results.—A total of 86 patients (median age 34 years; 49 males; 71 UC and 15 IC) were successively treated with CYS and IFX. The median (±s.e.) follow-up time was 22.6 (7.0) months. During the study period, 49 patients failed to respond to the second-line rescue therapy and underwent a colectomy. The probability of colectomy-free survival (±s.e.) was 61.3 ± 5.3% at 3 months and 41.3 ± 5.6 % at 12 months. A case of fatal pulmonary embolism occurred at 1 day after surgery in a 45-year-old man. Also, nine infectious complications were observed during the second-line rescue therapy.

Conclusions.—In patients with intravenous steroid-refractory UC and who fail to respond to CYS or IFX, a second-line rescue therapy may be effective in carefully selected patients, avoiding colectomy within 2 months in two-thirds of them. The risk/benefit ratio should still be considered individually.

▶ Cyclosporine and infliximab are accepted treatments of severe ulcerative colitis (UC). They are typically prescribed after patients have not responded to parenteral steroids. Either of these agents (usually infliximab) is prescribed as a last-ditch effort to prevent colectomy. In this study, the authors take this strategy a step further. In their retrospective analysis, they look at patients who did not respond to infliximab and were given parenteral cyclosporine, or vice versa, for steroid-refractory UC. This is a most aggressive approach that should give clinicians pause. While either rescue approach did result in a significant number of patients avoiding colectomy, more than half did have colectomy at 1 year. Is this approach worth the risk in select patients? Arguably no, given the significant risk of dangerous opportunistic infections that result from either of these agents combined with corticosteroids and, in many cases, another immunomodulator. The number of patients in the study was small so that patient-specific variables that may have influenced response could not be examined. Immunosuppressive agents resulted in a longer colectomy-free survival, but this was a univariate analysis opening up the possibility of confounding. Furthermore, the study was retrospective, raising the possibility of patient selection bias. Treatment practices and definitions of treatment response were not standardized. Patient numbers were too small to determine if the delay in surgery that results from the addition of either agent led to worse postoperative outcomes. The emphasis of the authors' conclusions should be on "carefully selected patients" and not on 2-month data. For the majority of patients who do not respond to either infliximab or cyclosporine, colectomy remains the best alternative.

M. F. Picco, MD, PhD

Adalimumab induction and maintenance therapy for patients with ulcerative colitis previously treated with infliximab
Taxonera C, Estellés J, Fernández-Blanco I, et al (Hosp Clínico, Madrid, Spain; Hosp La Paz, Madrid, Spain; et al)
Aliment Pharmacol Ther 33:340-348, 2011

Background.—The long-term efficacy of adalimumab in patients with ulcerative colitis is not well known.

Aim.—To evaluate the short- and long-term outcomes of adalimumab in ulcerative colitis patients previously treated with infliximab.

Methods.—Patients with active ulcerative colitis were treated with adalimumab after failure of other therapies including infliximab. Short-term clinical response and remission were assessed at weeks 4 and 12. The proportion of patients who continued on adalimumab and the proportion of patients who remained colectomy free were assessed over the long term.

Results.—Clinical response at weeks 4 and 12 was achieved in 16 (53%) and 18 (60%) patients, respectively, and clinical remission was obtained in 3 (10%) and 8 (27%) patients, respectively. After a mean 48 weeks' follow-up, 15 patients (50%) continued on adalimumab. Six patients (20%) required colectomy. All patients who achieved clinical response at week 12 were colectomy free at long term.

Conclusions.—Adalimumab was well tolerated and induced durable clinical response in many patients with otherwise medically refractory ulcerative colitis. Patients achieving clinical response at week 12 avoided colectomy over the long term.

▶ Infliximab is the only approved anti—tumor necrosis factor biologic therapy for the treatment of ulcerative colitis in the United States. Typically, before patients receive this therapy, they either have not responded to or been able to wean off corticosteroid therapy. They have few options. In this study, the authors present uncontrolled data looking at adalimumab as a rescue therapy to prevent colectomy in these patients. Patients were chosen as part of a compassionate use program for adalimumab. While the criteria for selection were reasonable, the study methods were not standardized so that there was a potential for selection bias in favor of adalimumab. In addition, the decision to start or modify adalimumab therapy was also not standardized. Response rates, similar to those in Crohn's disease, were more impressive than remission rates. Remission was poorly defined and based only on clinical criteria. The number of patients was very small, with the majority (16 patients) having lost response to infliximab. The rest (12 patients) were intolerant to infliximab. Response rates were similar between these 2 groups, but because of the small sample size, further comparisons were difficult. Most of those who were intolerant had infusion reactions most likely related to the chimeric composition of infliximab. Of the entire patient group, only 2 were primary nonresponders, and, as one would expect, neither responded. This study suggests that ulcerative colitis patients who either are intolerant or have lost response to infliximab probably will respond to adalimumab, but few will attain remission. In this limited number of patients, the approach was safe. To definitively answer questions of efficacy and safety, a larger randomized clinical trial is needed. Until then, adalimumab therapy is reasonable in select patients with ulcerative colitis in an attempt to avoid colectomy.

M. F. Picco, MD, PhD

Perceived and Actual Quality of Life With Ulcerative Colitis: A Comparison of Medically and Surgically Treated Patients
Waljee AK, Higgins PDR, Waljee JF, et al (Univ of Michigan, Ann Arbor; et al)
Am J Gastroenterol 106:794-799, 2011

Objectives.—Patients with chronic ulcerative colitis (UC) often refuse colectomy, despite data indicating that it might improve quality of life. We hypothesized that perceived utility values are different for patients living with UC compared with UC patients after total proctocolectomy. Our aims were to compare the perceived utility assigned by UC patients with and without a colectomy to standardized chronic UC and post-colectomy scenarios, and to compare the utility of actual health states among groups.

Methods.—We surveyed patients in a tertiary referral center from three groups, including non-UC, UC patients without colectomy, and UC patients who were post-colectomy. We measured the Time-Trade-Off (TTO) utilities of subjects for standardized scenarios, describing moderate UC and a post-colectomy state. Among all UC patients (with and without colectomy), we measured TTO utility for their own health state.

Results.—Responses were obtained from 150 patients per group ($n = 450$). The non-UC patients considered UC and colectomy scenarios equally (0.92), which was similar to UC patients without colectomy (0.90 and 0.91). Post-colectomy patients strongly preferred the colectomy scenario to the UC scenario (0.86 vs. 0.92, $P < 0.001$). The median utility of UC patients without colectomy for their actual health state was higher than that of post-colectomy patients (0.96 and 0.92, $P < 0.05$). Patients with more social support were more likely to have undergone colectomy compared with patients with little social support (odds ratio = 1.20 per dependent/supporter).

Conclusions.—Patients living with UC prefer their actual health state to a perceived UC scenario or a post-colectomy scenario. Patients who have undergone colectomy equate the quality of life in their actual state with that in a post-colectomy scenario, and prefer each to a perceived chronic UC state. Given the variety of preferences and the importance of social support, opportunities to interact with UC patients who have previously undergone colectomy could help patients living with UC and their physicians to navigate these complex choices.

▶ Patient decisions regarding new therapies are like all decisions. They are based on individual point of view, experience, and often fear of the unknown. In this interesting study, the authors found that patients with ulcerative colitis (UC) perceived surgery outcomes as worse than their chronically active disease, whereas those who have had surgery prefer their actual postcolectomy state to their previous chronic colitis state. What does all this mean? As the authors point out, this suggests the need for education. If patients who require but resist surgery can interact with those who have had surgery, they may be able to make more informed decisions by better understanding what they can expect. The study assessed decision making by creating "standardized scenarios" to get at patient preferences. As the authors point out, these scenarios may not adequately reflect real life. Patients who have colectomy have experienced the final irreversible procedure and may be more likely to report a better quality of life because they have no other treatment alternatives. There is no easy way around this bias. Overall, the study is interesting but in the end emphasizes what we already should know: The need for education of patients not only through their health care provider but also through their peers suffering with ulcerative colitis is essential. It is through this and with good social support systems that patients become more confident in their choices and make good decisions.

M. F. Picco, MD, PhD

Randomised clinical trial: delayed-release oral mesalazine 4.8 g/day vs. 2.4 g/day in endoscopic mucosal healing - ASCEND I and II combined analysis

Lichtenstein GR, Ramsey D, Rubin DT (Hosp of the Univ of Pennsylvania, Philadelphia; Mason Business Ctr, Mason, OH; Univ of Chicago Inflammatory Bowel Diseases Ctr, IL)
Aliment Pharmacol Ther 33:672-678, 2011

Background.—Recent studies have focused on the importance of mucosal healing in ulcerative colitis (UC). However, it was still unclear whether higher doses of delayed-release mesalazine (mesalamine) could provide additional benefit.

Aim.—To examine how two doses of delayed-release mesalazine (4.8 g/day and 2.4 g/day) from ASCEND I and II compare in their relative ability to heal colonic mucosa over time.

Methods.—Primary data from two prospective 6-week, double-blind, randomised studies in patients with mildly to moderately active UC were pooled and analysed retrospectively. The mucosal healing analysis focuses on moderately active UC patients ($n = 391$), comprising a majority of patients (84%). Additional analyses examined the relationship between mucosal healing and dose, clinical response to therapy and patient quality of life (Inflammatory Bowel Disease Questionnaire, IBDQ).

Results.—At week 3, mucosal healing (endoscopy subscore of 0 or 1) was achieved in 65% of moderately active UC patients on 4.8 g/day and 58% of patients on 2.4 g/day ($P = 0.219$). At week 6, this increased to 80% for 4.8 g/day and 68% for 2.4 g/day ($P = 0.012$). Healing rates with the higher dose were also greater across all extents of disease and in patients with prior steroid use. At 6 weeks, clinical response to therapy and mucosal healing were found to be well correlated (kappa = 0.694). Likewise, the change in IBDQ at week 6 showed a significant relationship with mucosal healing ($P < 0.0001$).

Conclusion.—Mucosal healing rates in UC achieved at 6 weeks were statistically significantly higher with delayed-release mesalazine at 4.8 g/day vs. 2.4 g/day (Clinicaltrials.gov: NCT00577473, NCT00073021).

▶ The goals for treatment of inflammatory bowel disease have moved beyond induction and maintenance of clinical remission to the objective assessment of mucosal healing. Mucosal healing in Crohn's disease has led to better overall patient outcomes. In this study, the authors assess mucosal healing in the treatment of ulcerative colitis through analysis of the ASCEND studies. The ASCEND studies compared high-dose (4.8 g/d) with low-dose (2.4 g/d) mesalamine for the treatment of mild to moderate ulcerative colitis. High-dose mesalamine (4.8 g/d) was shown to be superior to low-dose mesalamine (2.4 g/d) for patients with moderate ulcerative colitis. In this article, the authors report their mucosal healing data. Patients on higher-dose mesalamine had higher mucosal healing rates, and mucosal healing also translated into better clinical outcomes. Although numerically 4.8 g/d was statistically superior, rates of mucosal healing were also high for the 2.4-g/d group. Unfortunately, the results are reported up to only 6 weeks of therapy. The authors contend that mucosal healing may result in a better overall prognosis, but the data are limited. There are many unanswered questions. It is not clear whether mucosal healing is maintained and if patients need high-dose mesalamine chronically. Can patients maintain mucosal healing once in remission with the common practice of lowering the mesalamine dose for maintenance therapy? Should patients in remission be assessed for mucosal healing after several months of therapy? If there is evidence of significant endoscopic findings at follow-up despite clinical remission, should the mesalamine dose be adjusted or alternative therapy considered? Longer-term follow-up studies are needed to answer these important questions.

M. F. Picco, MD, PhD

Miscellaneous

5-Aminosalicylate Is Not Chemoprophylactic for Colorectal Cancer in IBD: A Population Based Study

Bernstein CN, Nugent Z, Blanchard JF (Univ of Manitoba Inflammatory Bowel Disease Clinical and Res Centre, Winnipeg, Canada)
Am J Gastroenterol 106:731-736, 2011

Objectives.—We aimed to determine if use of 5-aminosalicylates (5-ASA) was associated with a reduced risk of colorectal cancer (CRC) in people with inflammatory bowel disease (IBD).

Methods.—We used the population-based University of Manitoba IBD Epidemiology Database that tracks all health-care visits from 1984 to 2008 of all Manitobans with IBD and all prescription medication use since 1995. In 2008, there were 8,744 subjects with IBD (ulcerative colitis 4,325, Crohn's disease 4,419, females 4,851, males 3,893). In study I, we assessed the incidence of CRC among 5-ASA users (≥ 1 year, ≥ 5 years of cumulative use) compared with nonusers. In study II, we assessed a cohort of those with CRC ($n = 101$) diagnosed in 1995–2008, matched to a control cohort by age, sex, disease duration, and disease diagnosis without CRC ($n = 303$), and logistic analysis was undertaken.

Results.—For study I, the hazard ratio for CRC among 5-ASA users was 1.04 (95% confidence interval (CI) 0.67–1.62, $P = 0.87$) at ≥ 1 year of use and 2.01 (95% CI 1.04–3.9, $P = 0.038$) at ≥ 5 years of use with no difference when assessing by diagnosis. Males, but not females, using 5-ASA for ≥ 5 years had an increased risk of CRC. In study II, CRC cases had similar use of any 5-ASA compared with controls for ≥ 1 year of use (1.02, 95% CI 0.60–1.74) or ≥ 5 years (1.96, 95% CI 0.84–4.55), and a similar mean number of 5-ASA prescriptions at 10 vs. 11 ($P = 0.8$) and a similar mean number of dose days at 330 vs. 410 ($P = 0.69$).

Conclusions.—Our results support the majority of studies to date that 5-ASA is not chemoprophylactic in IBD for CRC.

▶ Unfortunately, this study only adds to the controversy as to whether 5-aminosalicylates (5ASAs) are protective against cancer in inflammatory bowel disease (IBD). The study, although using a large population-based database, has significant methodological problems that limit the validity of its conclusions. These problems may have resulted in lack of a preventive effect of 5ASA on the development of colorectal cancer (CRC). First, the authors combined all IBD cases together. There was no way of knowing the distribution of colitis and, among the patients with Crohn's disease, whether they had colitis at all. Next, they had no way of looking at patterns of mesalamine usage. Increased use in some patients may have been a marker of more severe disease, putting a patient at higher risk for CRC. There was no marker for disease severity, such as hospitalization data or corticosteroid usage. In addition, the authors did not exclude incident CRC cases in the case-control portion of their study; that is, CRC cases diagnosed near the time of the IBD diagnosis.

If an individual was diagnosed with CRC within a year of diagnosis of IBD, 5-ASA may have appeared to increase the risk of CRC when it was unlikely to be a factor. Also, inclusion of these cases may have made longer duration of disease appear protective against CRC, which is at odds with accepted knowledge. This study, like many before it, suffers from the limitations of observational cohort studies. This is pointed out in the editorial that follows this article.[1] This area is clouded by studies having opposite conclusions. Each study is burdened by its limitations. What is a clinician to do? At this point, there is no definitive evidence as to whether 5ASAs are protective against CRC among patients with IBD. The practice of prescribing 5ASA will likely continue among clinicians because of the biologic plausibility of an effect and general lack of toxicity of these agents.

M. F. Picco, MD, PhD

Reference

1. Terdiman JP. The prevention of colitis-related cancer by 5-aminosalicylates: an appealing hypothesis that remains unproven. *Am J Gastroenterol.* 2011;106: 737-740.

Dietary Intake and Risk of Developing Inflammatory Bowel Disease: A Systematic Review of the Literature
Hou JK, Abraham B, El-Serag H (Baylor College of Med, Houston, TX)
Am J Gastroenterol 106:563-573, 2011

Objectives.—The incidence of inflammatory bowel disease (IBD) is increasing. Dietary factors such as the spread of the "Western" diet, high in fat and protein but low in fruits and vegetables, may be associated with the increase. Although many studies have evaluated the association between diet and IBD risk, there has been no systematic review.

Methods.—We performed a systematic review using guideline-recommended methodology to evaluate the association between pre-illness intake of nutrients (fats, carbohydrates, protein) and food groups (fruits, vegetables, meats) and the risk of subsequent IBD diagnosis. Eligible studies were identified via structured keyword searches in PubMed and Google Scholar and manual searches.

Results.—Nineteen studies were included, encompassing 2,609 IBD patients (1,269 Crohn's disease (CD) and 1,340 ulcerative colitis (UC) patients) and over 4,000 controls. Studies reported a positive association between high intake of saturated fats, monounsaturated fatty acids, total polyunsaturated fatty acids (PUFAs), total omega-3 fatty acids, omega-6 fatty acids, mono-and disaccharides, and meat and increased subsequent CD risk. Studies reported a negative association between dietary fiber and fruits and subsequent CD risk. High intakes of total fats, total PUFAs, omega-6 fatty acids, and meat were associated with an increased risk of UC. High vegetable intake was associated with a decreased risk of UC.

Conclusions.—High dietary intakes of total fats, PUFAs, omega-6 fatty acids, and meat were associated with an increased risk of CD and UC. High fiber and fruit intakes were associated with decreased CD risk, and high vegetable intake was associated with decreased UC risk.

▶ Diet has often been suggested as contributing to the development of inflammatory bowel disease (IBD). Proof of causality is extremely difficult because of problems in obtaining accurate dietary histories, the potential for recall bias, and the difficulties in conducting prospective studies. Histories are typically reported among those already affected with IBD because true population-based studies with prospective longitudinal follow-up are not feasible. In this article, the authors review 19 (18 case-control and 1 cohort) studies. The conclusions, while interesting, are open to the same criticism of the articles that they have reviewed. Five of the studies reported dietary intake in the year prior to the IBD diagnosis. While the authors show that the conclusions of these studies are similar to other studies, basing diet history on the year prior to diagnosis is a potential problem. Patients with early symptoms of IBD may have adjusted their diet away from fruits and vegetables in favor of protein and fat because of worsening bloating or diarrhea. It's not surprising that high intake of fat and meat was associated with development of IBD because they increase the risk of many diseases. This is widely known in most Western populations, but do they really increase the risk of IBD? The fact that most of the studies say so is not enough to demonstrate causality. The authors, unfortunately, provide little critical appraisal of the literature. They declare that pooling studies (meta-analysis) is not possible because of the heterogeneity of the studies presented. While this may be true, they should provide more of a discussion outlining the strengths and weaknesses of the individual studies that suggest dietary associations. The quality of the studies is most important. Just because it makes sense that high fat and meat intake increase the risk of IBD does not necessarily mean this is true.

M. F. Picco, MD, PhD

Managing symptoms of irritable bowel syndrome in patients with inflammatory bowel disease

Camilleri M (Mayo Clinic, Rochester, MN)
Gut 60:425-428, 2011

Background.—Symptoms common to irritable bowel syndrome (IBS) may occur in patients who have inflammatory bowel disease (IBD) that appears stable or in remission. They experience abdominal pain, bloating, diarrhea, and urgency but have no significant inflammation, constitutional symptoms, or rectal bleeding. Another disease may be present.

Initial Screening.—Symptom management requires, first, that the absence of infection be confirmed, then screening tests are done to discriminate between IBD and IBS. This includes tests of fecal calprotectin, lactoferrin and S100A12, which is a calcium-binding proinflammatory protein secreted by granulocytes. Magnetic resonance (MR) and computed tomography (CT) enterography are equally sensitive for detecting active small bowel inflammation, but MR enteroclysis involves no radiation exposure and better characterizes stenotic lesions. CT provides better temporal resolution, mesenteric imaging, and a shorter examination time. Bile acid malabsorption (BAM) may also cause steatorrhea. Its diagnosis is confirmed through tests of serum 7α-hydroxy-4-cholesten-3-one, 48-hr fecal bile acid excretion, or 23-selena-25-homotaurocholate retention on scintigraphy. A surrogate test of fasting serum fibroblast growth factor 19 or therapeutic trials of cholestyramine (4 g three times a day) or oral colesevelam (625 mg tablets with up to two tablets three times a day) can also be used to detect BAM.

Conditions To Exclude.—Symptomatic patients with IBD but no overt inflammation are further screened to detect other conditions that may be causing symptoms. Small bowel bacterial overgrowth (SBO) may be suspected if there are anatomical aberrations that result from Crohn's disease or bypass surgery. No sensitive, specific, and easily performed test is available for SBO, so a therapeutic trial using a poorly absorbed antibiotic such as neomycin, metronidazole, quinolone, or rifaximin is the most practical approach.

Chronic pancreatic insufficiency is rare in these patients. Little evidence indicates that visceral hypersensitivity occurs in patients with IBD, but further studies of afferent and pelvic floor function associated with IBD are needed.

IBS with IBD.—Some patients whose IBD is in remission but who have persistent abdominal discomfort and diarrhea may also have IBS. IBS-like symptoms impair the patient's quality of life and global well-being. Patients with IBD who have IBS-like symptoms tend to have higher levels of anxiety and depression, and studies have linked anxiety and duration of disease as significantly predictive of developing IBS-like symptoms. The IBS can be managed symptomatically, observing caution with anti-motility agents to avoid complications related to the IBD.

Conclusions.—Patients with IBD can also have IBS. Treatment of IBS is tailored to the symptoms, with measurements of gastrointestinal and colonic transit used to guide therapy for patients whose transit values are significantly accelerated.

▶ Clinicians are often faced with the problem of determining whether a patient with inflammatory bowel disease (IBD) presenting with gastrointestinal symptoms has active disease. Testing for active disease typically relies on invasive and potentially dangerous procedures. Invasive testing may not confirm disease activity, and an alternative diagnosis should be considered. In this article, Camilleri provides a comprehensive review of these mimickers of IBD, including common organic conditions of enteric infection, bacterial overgrowth, bile salt malabsorption, and short bowel syndrome along with the more rare conditions of celiac disease and pancreatic insufficiency. Irritable bowel syndrome is a very important functional cause along with pelvic floor dysfunction. The first step to diagnosing these conditions is awareness, and the majority can be diagnosed without the need for invasive testing. Among patients with IBD, recognition of typical symptoms of these common conditions along with a clinical judgment that an individual's IBD is in remission may avoid invasive testing. Stool marker studies such as calprotectin and lactoferrin, while advocated by the author as a noninvasive method of documenting disease activity, lack acceptable sensitivity and specificity to recommend as part of routine practice. It all comes down to clinical judgment and assessment of symptom severity. Patients without overt symptoms or signs of severe IBD but with findings of an associated condition—directed treatment can avoid needless invasive testing.

M. F. Picco, MD, PhD

Potential Association Between the Oral Tetracycline Class of Antimicrobials Used to Treat Acne and Inflammatory Bowel Disease
Margolis DJ, Fanelli M, Hoffstad O, et al (Univ of Pennsylvania School of Medicine, Philadelphia)
Am J Gastroenterol 105:2610-2616, 2010

Objectives.—Previous studies have shown an association between isotretinoin and inflammatory bowel disease (IBD). The majority of patients prescribed isotretinoin for their acne are previously on an extended course of antibiotics. Therefore, it is important to consider antibiotic use as a confounding variable for the development of IBD.

Methods.—We performed a retrospective cohort study using The Health Improvement Network database of the United Kingdom. We identified 94,487 individuals with acne who were followed up by a general practitioner for 406,294 person-years.

Results.—A prescription for minocycline was received by 24,085 individuals, for tetracycline/oxytetracycline by 38,603 individuals, and doxycycline by 15,032 individuals. IBD was noted in 41 individuals exposed to minocycline, 79 individuals exposed to tetracycline/oxytetracycline, 32 individuals exposed to doxycycline, and 55 (0.11%) individuals not exposed to any of these antibiotics. The hazard ratio (HR) for developing IBD for any exposure to a tetracycline antibiotic was 1.39 (1.02, 1.90). HRs for individual antibiotics were 1.19 (0.79, 1.79) for minocycline, 1.43 (1.02, 2.02) for tetracycline/oxytetracycline, and 1.63 (1.05, 2.52) for doxycycline. For ulcerative colitis, the associations (HR) were 1.10 (0.76, 1.82) for minocycline, 1.27 (0.78, 2.07) for tetracycline/oxytetracycline, and 1.06 (0.53, 2.13) for doxycycline. For Crohn's disease (CD), the associations (HR) were 1.28 (0.72, 2.30) for minocycline, 1.61 (0.995, 2.63) for tetracycline/oxytetracycline, and 2.25 (1.27, 4.00) for doxycycline.

Conclusions.—Tetracycline class antibiotics, and particularly doxycycline use may be associated with the development of IBD, particularly CD. Potential confounding by previous doxycycline exposure should be considered when assessing whether treatment with other acne medications increases the risk of IBD.

▶ The association of the use of isotretinoin for acne with the development of inflammatory bowel disease (IBD) is controversial. This study stokes the controversy further by suggesting that the tetracycline class of antibiotics is independently associated with development of IBD and may be an important confounding variable in the reported associations of IBD with isotretinoin. The authors base this conclusion from an analysis of a large outpatient database from the United Kingdom. They found that tetracycline antibiotics and specifically doxycycline were associated with developing IBD. This suggests that tetracycline antibiotics meet the true definition of a confounding variable. They are associated with acne (disease) and isotretinoin (exposure). This is important because nearly all patients who eventually are prescribed isotretinoin for acne have received long courses of tetracycline antibiotics. It would be highly unusual for a patient prescribed isotretinoin to not have received an antibiotic prior so that it would be very difficult to sort out any confounding without an extremely large number of subjects. Furthermore, because it is also unlikely for a patient without acne to receive isotretinoin or long-term tetracycline, it may be the acne itself that is responsible for the association. While the authors do point this out, they do not report risk of IBD in those with a history of acne compared with the overall population without acne. Furthermore, tetracycline antibiotics use may be a marker of more severe acne. IBD may then be associated with severe acne and not with tetracycline antibiotics. The importance of this study is not the antibiotic association but the potential for that association to cast doubt on reports that isotretinoin exposure increases the risk of IBD. This isotretinoin-IBD association has gained traction in recent years, and more study is needed to determine whether it is real or the result of confounding.

M. F. Picco, MD, PhD

Pregnancy outcome in patients with inflammatory bowel disease treated with thiopurines: cohort from the CESAME Study
Coelho J, for the CESAME pregancy study group (France) (Paris 7 Univ, France; et al)
Gut 60:198-203, 2011

Background and Aims.—Few studies have been conducted addressing the safety of thiopurine treatment in pregnant women with inflammatory bowel disease (IBD). The aim of this study was to evaluate the pregnancy outcome of women with IBD who have been exposed to thiopurines.

Methods.—215 pregnancies in 204 women were registered and documented in the CESAME cohort between May 2004 and October 2007. Physicians documented the following information from the women: last menstrual date, delivery term, details of pregnancy outcome, prematurity, birth weight and height, congenital abnormalities, medication history during each trimester, smoking history and alcohol ingestion. Data were compared between three groups: women exposed to thiopurines (group A), women receiving a drug other than thiopurines (group B) and women not receiving any medication (group C).

Results.—Mean age at pregnancy was 28.3 years. 75.7% of the women had Crohn's disease and 21.8% had ulcerative colitis, with a mean disease duration of 6.8 years at inclusion. Of the 215 pregnancies, there were 138 births (142 newborns), and the mean birth weight was 3135 g. There were 86 pregnancies in group A, 84 in group B and 45 in group C. Interrupted pregnancies occurred in 36% of patients enrolled in group A, 33% of patients enrolled in group B, and 40% of patients enrolled in group C; congenital abnormalities arose in 3.6% of group A cases and 7.1% of group B cases. No significant differences were found between the three groups in overall pregnancy outcome.

Conclusions.—The results obtained from this cohort indicate that thiopurine use during pregnancy is not associated with increased risks, including congenital abnormalities.

▶ Women with inflammatory bowel disease (IBD) are often diagnosed during or prior to their childbearing years. A woman's decision to become pregnant needs to be made with an understanding of the impact of IBD on pregnancy and the potential adverse effects of medications on fetal outcomes. Pregnancy outcomes are best among women in remission, but the decision on whether to continue medications that led to that remission may be difficult. The results of this article with regard to thiopurine use are encouraging. The CESAME cohort represents nearly 20 000 IBD patients followed in France over 3 years for cancer risk. Members of the cohort were invited to report pregnancies, and outcomes were followed. While 215 pregnancies in 204 women (86 had received thiopurines) do not seem like many, this represents one of the largest reported cohorts to date and demonstrates no increase in congenital anomalies. The first obvious criticism of this article is that the patient numbers are too small, and it does lack statistical power. This is true, as the authors concede, so that with number of pregnancies followed, only a 5-fold difference in anomalies from baseline 4% to 20% among those taking thiopurines could be detected. Furthermore, outcomes were patient reported and not verified by physicians. Overall, the conclusions from this study are severely limited. They are reassuring when taken along with the growing body of literature suggesting that thiopurines may be safe during pregnancy in doses used in IBD. The emphasis is on the "may," and a careful discussion should take place between patients and their physicians based on existing evidence well before pregnancy is contemplated. More information is needed in the form of larger studies or a meta-analysis. Many clinicians will continue these medications among their patients with IBD, but this must be an individual decision.

M. F. Picco, MD, PhD

Other Inflammatory Bowel Disease

Segmental Colitis Associated with Diverticulosis: Complication of Diverticular Disease or Autonomous Entity?

Tursi A (Servizio di Gastroenterologia Territoriale, Andria, Italy)
Dig Dis Sci 56:27-34, 2011

Segmental colitis associated with diverticulosis (SCAD) is a disease that affects colon harboring diverticula, mostly located in the sigmoid region. It has been considered a rare disease for many years, but new studies may contribute to easier recognition. Although its pathogenesis is not yet well defined, in the past SCAD has been considered a complication of diverticular disease, whilst new endoscopic, histological, and clinical data have encouraged the concept that SCAD includes pathogenetic and therapeutic aspects peculiar to inflammatory bowel diseases. We therefore describe herein current knowledge about this disease, and why it can be considered a truly autonomous entity instead of a complication of diverticular disease.

▶ In this article, the author presents a clear and concise review on an increasingly recognized condition of segmental colitis associated with diverticulosis (SCAD). Although the pathogenesis of this condition is not known, its clinical presentation is similar to inflammatory bowel disease (IBD), particularly Crohn's disease. It may be confused with IBD, but certain characteristics suggest the diagnosis. These include older presentation (after age 60 years) and mucosal inflammation in the region of diverticula only, with rectal sparing. Diverticulitis is usually more easily distinguished from SCAD because its presentation is more abrupt, and SCAD involves the interdiverticular mucosa where diverticulitis is confined to a diverticulum and peridiverticular area. The spectrum of severity of SCAD may vary from mild diarrhea or rectal bleeding to severe symptoms that mimic flares of ulcerative colitis or Crohn's disease. Unfortunately, knowledge of this disease is limited to small case series, and thus it is difficult to make definitive conclusions. The prognosis for mild disease is good, and most patients respond to mesalamine therapy. Antibiotics have also been used with some success. For mild disease, once a response has been achieved, most patients will enter a prolonged remission, and medications can be discontinued without a higher risk of recurrence. For more severe IBD-like cases, corticosteroids may be required, and these patients also tend to do well, rarely requiring chronic immunosuppressive therapy or surgery. Some may progress to overt IBD. Awareness of SCAD among clinicians is increasing, and although more studies are needed, it appears to have a better prognosis than IBD.

M. F. Picco, MD, PhD

6 Nutrition and Celiac Disease

Effect of *Helicobacter pylori* Infection on Symptoms of Gastroenteritis Due to Enteropathogenic *Escherichia coli* in Adults
Chang AH-M, Haggerty TD, de Martel C, et al (Stanford Univ, CA)
Dig Dis Sci 56:457-464, 2011

Background.—*Helicobacter pylori* can cause hypochlorhydria in some hosts and predispose to diarrheal infections.

Aims.—We tested the hypothesis that chronic *H. pylori* infection increases the risk of diarrheal illness due to an acid-sensitive organism: enteropathogenic *Escherichia coli* (EPEC).

Methods.—After testing healthy adult volunteers for *H. pylori*, 19 infected and 26 uninfected subjects had gastric pH probes placed and were given $5-10 \times 10^9$ EPEC organisms; six had previously received a proton pump inhibitor. We measured diarrhea and created a composite gastroenteritis severity score based on symptoms in the 48 h following exposure. Outcomes were compared using logistic regression and analysis of covariance.

Results.—More *H. pylori*-infected (36.8%) than *H. pylori*-uninfected subjects (7.7%) were hypochlorhydric ($P = 0.02$). Six (31.6%) *H. pylori*-infected and five *H. pylori*-uninfected subjects (19.2%) developed diarrhea ($P = 0.34$). Hypochlorhydria was a strong risk factor for diarrhea [odds ratio (OR) 6.25, confidence interval (CI): 1.29–30.35]. After adjusting for hypochlorhydria and EPEC dose, *H. pylori* was not associated with diarrhea (OR 0.89, CI: 0.17–4.58). Among those with symptoms, *H. pylori*-infected subjects had lower gastroenteritis severity score than did H. pylori-uninfected subjects (2.6, CI: 1.9–3.4 versus 1.5, CI: 1.1–1.9, $P = 0.01$), particularly if they were also hypochlorhydric (3.8, CI: 2.3–5.3 versus 1.9, CI: 1.3–2.5, $P = 0.02$).

Conclusions.—In adults, *H. pylori* infection was associated with hypochlorhydria but had no detectable effect on occurrence of diarrhea. Among symptomatic subjects, *H. pylori* infection decreased severity of gastroenteritis (Table 3).

▶ *Helicobacter* is one of the most common infections worldwide, and, while decreasing in prevalence in the United States, it continues to be frequent,

TABLE 3.—Odds Ratios for Diarrhea Following EPEC Ingestion for all 45 Study Subjects

Diarrhea	OR	Unadjusted 95% CI	P-Value	OR	Adjusted[a] 95% CI	P-Value
H. pylori infection	1.94	(0.49–7.66)	0.34	1.22	(0.19–7.69)	0.83
EPEC dose[b]	1.25	(0.93–1.68)	0.13	1.23	(0.87–1.73)	0.24
Hypochlorhydria	6.25	(1.29–30.35)	0.02	4.89	(0.85–28.19)	0.08
Hispanic versus other	1.08	(0.27–4.44)	0.91	0.50	(0.08–3.27)	0.47
PPI	3.88	(0.65–22.96)	0.14			

EPEC enteropathogenic *Escherichia coli*, PPI proton pump inhibitor.
[a]Multivariate logistic regression model including terms *H. pylori* infection, hypochlorhydria, race/ethnicity, and EPEC dose.
[b]Inoculation with 1×10^9 versus 5×10^8 EPEC organisms.

especially in older individuals and immigrants. *Helicobacter* can cause hypochlorhydria and is thought to predispose to diarrheal illnesses. The association with diarrhea has been based largely on observational studies. It is hypothesized that the hypochlorhydria makes the host more susceptible to acid-sensitive pathogens. It has been observed in epidemiologic studies that there may be an association between *Helicobacter pylori* and gastroenteritis, although the findings have been conflicting. It has even been suggested that *H pylori* can protect against gastroenteritis. This study was a direct challenge study, wherein individuals with and without *H pylori* infection were challenged with the acid-sensitive organisms enteropathogenic *Escherichia coli* (EPEC). This study was performed in healthy adults with and without *Helicobacter* infections in whom gastric pH was examined to identify hypochlorhydria. The results of this study indicated a not-surprising predisposition to *Helicobacter* infection in the Hispanic ethnicity. One-fifth of all patients were hypochlorhydric, a condition more common in those with *H pylori* infection than those without. The primary outcome was that there was no difference in the rate of diarrhea between *Helicobacter*-positive and *Helicobacter*-negative individuals. However, hypochlorhydria was a strong risk factor for diarrhea (Table 3). Interestingly, the severity of gastroenteritis was less in individuals who were *Helicobacter* positive than *Helicobacter* negative. Hypochlorhydria itself seemed to increase the severity of gastroenteritis.

Interestingly, *Helicobacter* was never isolated from the stool samples. EPEC, on the other hand, was recovered as early as 4 hours after ingestion, and there was a tendency for EPEC to be shed in the stool for longer in *Helicobacter*-infected individuals than not. All subjects were treated with antibiotic and ciprofloxacin, with eradication of the EPEC organism.

This study is important because it is the first direct challenge study with an acid-sensitive pathogen in individuals with *Helicobacter* infection or not. This study, performed without such a buffer, provides a closer–to–real world scenario and seems to support a role for hypochlorhydria in increasing risk and severity of gastroenteritis. *Helicobacter* itself, in the absence of hypochlorhydria, appears to have, if anything, a protective effect against the severity of gastroenteritis. There are some limitations in this study. The conclusions are based on a relatively mild pathogen. Whether these effects would be reproduced by a more virulent pathogen is uncertain. This study is carried out in a developed world; the developing world may be a different scenario in terms of host resistance to gastroenteritis and the severity of diarrhea that occurs. Nonetheless, this is an important study that points out weaknesses of observational studies. Of particular importance clinically is the role that hypochlorhydria plays in increasing risks of gastroenteritis and its clinical consequences. The far more common clinical scenario of iatrogenic hypochlorhydria induced by potent acid suppression may be of much greater importance to patients traveling from developed countries to locations where they would be at risk for acquisition of enteric pathogens. It raises the concern about travel-induced diarrhea in these individuals.

J. A. Murray, MD

Antibodies to the Wheat Storage Globulin Glo-3A in Children Before and at Diagnosis of Celiac Disease
Taplin CE, Mojibian M, Simpson M, et al (Univ of Colorado Denver, Aurora; Ottawa Hosp Res Inst, Ontario, Canada; Colorado School of Public Health, Aurora)
J Pediatr Gastroenterol Nutr 52:21-25, 2011

Objective.—Celiac disease (CD) is an autoimmune disease triggered by exposure to gluten-containing foods. IgA autoantibodies to tissue transglutaminase (TTG) are elevated in CD, but little is known about the gastrointestinal state before the appearance of TTG. Antibodies to wheat storage globulin Glo-3A have been studied in type 1 diabetes, and may be a marker of altered mucosal barrier and/or immune function. In the present study, we investigated antibody responses to Glo-3A in CD.

Patients and Methods.—In the Diabetes Autoimmunity Study in the Young, children were studied prospectively from birth for the appearance of TTG and CD. Fifty cases of CD were frequency matched with 50 controls on age (of TTG seroconversion in the case), sex, ethnicity, presence of a first-degree relative with type 1 diabetes mellitus, and human leukocyte antigen -DR3 genotype. In cases and controls, IgG antibodies to Glo-3A were analyzed in a blinded manner in the sample collected at the time of seroconversion to TTG positivity (or the matched sample in controls) and in all of the previous samples since birth (mean 4.5 samples). The association between Glo-3A antibody levels and CD case status was explored using t tests at the TTG-positive visit and when Glo-3A levels were highest, and mixed modeling to describe Glo-3A over time.

Results.—At the time of first elevated TTG (mean 4.9 years), patients with CD had higher Glo-3A antibody levels than controls (13.3 ± 17.2 vs 7.6 ± 11.7, $P = 0.005$). In both cases and controls, Glo-3A antibodies appear to peak at a mean age of 2.9 years, before mean age of initial TTG seroconversion. The peak Glo-3A antibody levels were higher in cases than controls (25.5 ± 21.8 vs 14.9 ± 18.3 $P = 0.0007$). Using mixed modeling to account for multiple visits per person, cases had higher levels of Glo-3A antibodies than controls at all ages from birth to TTG seroconversion ($\beta = 0.53$, $P = 0.002$).

Conclusions.—Compared with controls, CD cases have higher Glo-3A antibody responses in the beginning years, before initial detection of TTG.

▶ We know that celiac disease can start early in life and that breastfeeding and the timing and amount of gluten in the infant diet are important to trigger an early-onset celiac disease. Little is known about the other proteins in wheat. This study from Denver examines reactivity to a wheat storage globulin, and it demonstrates that children from a population-based birth cohort study who were followed up to the development of celiac disease developed antibodies against the storage globulin early in the process of disease transition. The control group was made up of children who did not undergo conversion to tissue transglutaminase antibodies. The study also showed that the antibodies to the globulin peaked earlier than the seroconversion to tissue transglutaminase antibodies. The significance of this finding may be that antibodies against the globulin, Glo-3A, may be a biomarker for impaired immune tolerance or increased gut permeability. It also indicated that the process occurs early within the first 2 to 3 years of life. Reaction to wheat proteins other than gluten may precede and even predict celiac disease.

J. A. Murray, MD

Albumin and C-reactive protein levels predict short-term mortality after percutaneous endoscopic gastrostomy in a prospective cohort study
Blomberg J, Lagergren P, Martin L, et al (Karolinska Institutet, Stockholm, Sweden)
Gastrointest Endosc 73:29-36, 2011

Background.—Percutaneous endoscopic gastrostomy (PEG) is a procedure with many complications that sometimes can be devastating. To give better advice to patients referred for PEG regarding risk of complications, important risk factors should be known.

Objective.—To evaluate whether age, body mass index, albumin levels, C-reactive protein (CRP) levels, indication for PEG, and comorbidity influence the risk of mortality or peristomal infection after PEG insertion.

Design.—Prospective cohort study from 2005 to 2009. Follow-up 14 days after PEG.

Setting.—University hospital.

Patients.—This study involved 484 patients referred for PEG.

Intervention.—PEG.

Main Outcome Measurements.—Mortality within 30 days and peristomal infection within 14 days after PEG insertion. All risk estimates were calculated with 95% CIs and adjusted for confounding.

Results.—Among 484 patients, 58 (12%) died within 30 days after PEG insertion. Albumin <30 g/L (hazard ratio [HR], 3.46; 95% CI, 1.75-6.88),

CRP ≥10 (HR, 3.47; 95% CI, 1.68-7.18), age ≥65 years (HR, 2.26; 95% CI, 1.20-4.25) and possibly body mass index <18.5 (HR, 2.04; 95% CI, 0.97-4.31) were associated with increased mortality. Patients with a combination of low albumin and high CRP levels had a mortality rate of 20.5% compared with 2.6% among patients with normal values, rendering an over 7-fold increased adjusted risk of mortality (HR, 7.45; 95% CI, 2.62-21.19).

Limitations.—Missing data in some study variables. Although the sample size was large, weaker associations could not be established.

Conclusion.—The combination of low albumin and high CRP levels indicates a substantially increased short-term mortality risk after PEG, which should be considered in decision making.

▶ Percutaneous endoscopic gastrostomy (PEG) can be associated with many complications. This study evaluated a number of factors to predict potential risk of mortality or peristomal infection following PEG insertion. This was a prospective, planned, follow-up study in a university hospital, undertaken 14 days after insertion of the PEG. A large number of patients were included (n = 484), and mortality was measured up to 30 days, and infection up to 14 days afterward. Overall, 12% of patients died within 30 days of placement. Low albumin (< 30 g/L), hazard ratio of 3.46, a C-reactive protein > 10. Age, and low body mass index were associated with a potential increased mortality. Indeed, patients who had low albumin and a high C-reactive protein had a mortality rate of 20% at 30 days, which calls into question whether patients with those parameters should undergo PEG in the first place. Peristomal infection developed in 11% of surviving subjects, but none of the risk factors reached statistical association with risk of infection. The high mortality of older patients, especially elderly patients who have low albumin and high C-reactive protein, would strongly suggest reconsideration of the advisability of PEG placement, and perhaps management or nutritional support by some less invasive means may be indicated in the short term.

J. A. Murray, MD

Natural history of celiac disease autoimmunity in a USA cohort followed since 1974

Catassi C, Kryszak D, Bhatti B, et al (Univ of Maryland School of Medicine, Baltimore)

Ann Med 42:530-538, 2010

Background.—The natural history and the possible changes of celiac disease (CD) prevalence over time are still unclear.

Objectives.—1) To establish whether loss of tolerance to gluten may occur at any age; 2) to investigate possible changes of CD prevalence over time; and 3) to investigate CD-related co-morbidities.

Methods.—We analyzed 3,511 subjects with matched samples from 1974 (CLUE I) and 1989 (CLUE II). To avoid a selection bias regarding survival, we also screened 840 CLUE I participants who deceased after the 1974 survey. Outcome measure. CD autoimmunity (positivity to auto-antibodies) over time.

Results.—CD autoimmunity was detected in seven subjects in 1974 (prevalence 1:501) and in an additional nine subjects in 1989 (prevalence 1:219). Two cases of CD autoimmunity were found among the 840 subjects deceased after CLUE I. Compared to controls, untreated CD subjects showed increased incidence of osteoporosis and associated auto-immune disorders, but they did not reach statistical significance.

Conclusions.—During a 15-year period CD prevalence increased 2-fold in the CLUE cohort and 5-fold overall in the US since 1974. The CLUE study demonstrated that this increase was due to an increasing number of subjects that lost the immunological tolerance to gluten in their adulthood.

▶ It has been shown previously that there has been an increase in prevalence of celiac disease in both the United States and European populations.[1,2] However, the previous US study was done in 2 cross-sectional cohorts, all of which constituted male patients. This study by Catassi et al has shown that celiac disease increased significantly in the United States between 1974 and 1989 in the same population of 3 511 subjects. The prevalence of celiac disease increased from 1:510 to 1:219. These previously undetected cases of celiac disease were associated with both osteoporosis and increased autoimmune disorder, although these were not statistically significant, probably limited by the cohort size. This study is important in that it documents a true increase in adults who previously had no evidence of celiac disease who subsequently developed celiac disease with a 15-year follow-up. This supports the contention that celiac disease can occur at any age, is frequently unrecognized, and can be associated with substantial consequences. Impact on survival could not be studied because of lack of power due to the relatively small size of the cohort. This study and others drive the impetus for trying to understand what in the environment is driving the increase in celiac disease in the adult population, as it cannot be explained by feeding practices in infants.[3]

J. A. Murray, MD

References

1. Rubio-Tapia A, Kyle RA, Kaplan EL, et al. Increased prevalence and mortality in undiagnosed celiac disease. *Gastroenterology*. 2009;137:88-93.
2. Lohi S, Mäki M, Rissanen H, Knekt P, Reunanen A, Kaukinen K. Prognosis of unrecognized coeliac disease as regards mortality: a population-based cohort study. *Ann Med*. 2009;41:508-515.
3. Vilppula A, Kaukinen K, Luostarinen L, et al. Increasing prevalence and high incidence of celiac disease in elderly people: a population-based study. *BMC Gastroenterol*. 2009;9:49.

Cow's-Milk Allergy is a Risk Factor for the Development of FGIDs in Children

Saps M, Lu P, Bonilla S (Northwestern Univ, Chicago, IL)
J Pediatr Gastroenterol Nutr 52:166-169, 2011

Objectives.—Functional gastrointestinal disorders (FGIDs) are common in children. Their pathogenesis remains unknown and is most likely multifactorial. We hypothesized that noninfectious causes of inflammation affecting the gastrointestinal (GI) tract early in life, such as cow's-milk allergy (CMA), can predispose to the development of FGIDs later in childhood.

Patients and Methods.—Case-control study. Subjects were patients between 4 and 18 years diagnosed with CMA in the first year of life at Children's Memorial Hospital in Chicago, IL, between January 2000 and June 2009. Diagnosis of CMA was based on history and clinical findings. Siblings 4 to 18 years of age without a history of CMA were selected as controls. Cases completed the parental form of the Pediatric Gastrointestinal Symptoms Rome III version questionnaire to assess for GI symptoms.

Results.—Fifty-two subjects (mean age 8.1 ± 4.48 years, 62% girls) and 53 controls (mean age 9.7 ± 4.20 years, 55% girls) participated in the study. Twenty-three of 52 subjects (44.2%) reported GI symptoms that included abdominal pain, constipation, or diarrhea compared with 11 of 53 controls (20.75%) (odds ratio 3.03, $P = 0.01$). Abdominal pain was significantly more common in cases (16/52, 30.8%) versus controls (5/53, 9.43%) (odds ratio 4.27 [1.43−12.7]) ($\chi^2 = 7.47$, $P = 0.01$). Abnormal stool habits were more common in cases (15/52, 28.8%) versus controls (7/53, 13.2%), but the difference was not statistically significant. Ten of 52 subjects (19.2%) met the Questionnaire on Pediatric Gastrointestinal Symptoms Rome III version criteria for diagnosis of an FGID (7 irritable bowel syndrome, 2 functional dyspepsia, 1 functional abdominal pain), whereas none in the control group did.

Conclusions.—CMA constitutes a risk factor for the development of FGIDs in children (Table 1).

▶ Functional gastrointestinal disorders (FGIDs) are common in both adults and children. The pathogenesis of these disorders remains obscure in the majority of patients. The role of mild or minimal inflammation as a trigger or as a contributor to the ongoing symptoms of FGIDs is increasingly recognized. Patients

TABLE 1.—Characteristics of the Sample

	Cases (N = 52)	Controls (N = 53)
Female, %	62	55
Age, mean ± SD, y	8.1 ± 4.48	9.7 ± 4.20
Gastrointestinal symptoms, % (n/N)	44.2 (23/52)	20.7 (11/53)
Abdominal pain	30.8 (16/52)	9.43 (5/53)
Abnormal stool habits	28.8 (15/52)	13.2 (7/53)
Rome II diagnosis, % (n/N)	13.4 (7/52)	—

frequently identified, or at least suspected, dietary factors as potential triggers for their symptoms. However, there are relatively few data to support specific food intolerances in the etiology of the symptoms of FGIDs. This study was a case-control study of children who had been identified with cow's milk allergy in the first year of life. These children were followed up between the ages of 4 and 18 years and compared with siblings who had not been affected by cow's milk allergy in infancy. Parents completed the ROME III pediatric gastrointestinal symptom questionnaire. The results illustrated a substantial excess of gastrointestinal symptoms, particularly abdominal pain, and abnormal stool habits in the patients but not in the controls. Almost 20% of the patients met criteria for an FGID, but none in the control group did. Infant cow's milk allergy seems to be a predictive risk factor for FGID symptoms. This is an important study because it illustrates the role of a common infant disorder, cow's milk allergy, affecting 2% to 5% of infants, in subsequent functional disease. Cow's milk allergy is considered to be of limited duration; however, in this circumstance, it leads to substantial long-term symptomatology. The mechanisms by which cow's milk allergy in infancy can lead to FGIDs later in childhood are not clear. This may be similar to other postinflammatory FGIDs, such as has been described after gastroenteritis or Henoch-Schönlein purpura. It is also possible that the injury to the intestine can change nerve function. By including a sibling control group, the strength of this study mimicked the environmental and family structure and used a robust document for detecting symptomatology in children. The authors speculated with regard to the role of increased intestinal or colonic permeability and eosinophils, which often permeate the bowel in cow's milk allergy, and their potential role in sensitizing their responses, that this could lead to long-term changes in sensation and motor function. It is also possible that the stress and painful stimuli of the gut in infancy could induce allodynia. A significant weakness in this study was the largely purely clinical nature of the diagnosis of cow's milk allergy in infants, based basically on the clinical scenario and response to avoidance of cow's milk protein. Because the majority of children with cow's milk allergy will reincorporate cow's milk protein into their diet after the age of 2, the role of an ongoing response to cow's milk protein in symptoms is also raised into question by this study. This study provides important documentation of the association of early infant cow's milk allergy with subsequent FGIDs. The treatment of cow's milk allergy in children may need to include a realization that future FGIDs are a possibility, and measures to limit inflammation and symptomatology in infants are likely worth investigation. The role of food avoidance in older children or young adults with FGIDs, particularly for cow's milk, may be worthy of investigation even at this late date in patients with an infant history.

J. A. Murray, MD

Effect of Hookworm Infection on Wheat Challenge in Celiac Disease — A Randomised Double-Blinded Placebo Controlled Trial

Daveson AJ, Jones DM, Gaze S, et al (Princess Alexandra Hosp, Brisbane, Australia; Queensland Inst of Med Res, Brisbane, Australia; et al)
PLoS One 6:e17366, 2011

Background and Aims.—The association between hygiene and prevalence of autoimmune disease has been attributed in part to enteric helminth infection. A pilot study of experimental infection with the hookworm *Necator americanus* was undertaken among a group of otherwise healthy people with celiac disease to test the potential of the helminth to suppress the immunopathology induced by gluten.

Methods.—In a 21-week, double-blinded, placebo-controlled study, we explored the effects of *N. americanus* infection in 20 healthy, helminth-naïve adults with celiac disease well controlled by diet. Staged cutaneous inoculations with 10 and 5 infective 3rd stage hookworm larvae or placebo were performed at week-0 and -12 respectively. At week-20, a five day oral wheat challenge equivalent to 16 grams of gluten per day was undertaken. Primary outcomes included duodenal Marsh score and quantification of the immunodominant α-gliadin peptide (QE65)-specific systemic interferon-γ-producing cells by ELISpot pre- and post-wheat challenge.

Results.—Enteric colonisation with hookworm established in all 10 cases, resulting in transiently painful enteritis in 5. Chronic infection was asymptomatic, with no effect on hemoglobin levels. Although some duodenal eosinophilia was apparent, hookworm-infected mucosa retained a healthy appearance. In both groups, wheat challenge caused deterioration in both primary and several secondary outcomes.

Conclusions.—Experimental *N. americanus* infection proved to be safe and enabled testing its effect on a range of measures of the human autoimmune response. Infection imposed no obvious benefit on pathology.

Trial Registration.—ClinicalTrials.gov NCT00671138

▶ The last decade has seen several attempts to treat celiac disease with alternatives to gluten-free diet. One goal has been an attempt to reestablish tolerance to gluten in patients with celiac disease. The role of parasite infections to treat other immune-based diseases, including inflammatory bowel disease, multiple sclerosis, and asthma, has been tested. This pilot study examines the effect of the safety and efficacy of an experimental infection with the hookworm in a group of patients with well-treated celiac disease. The outcome measures were safety, tolerability of the treatment, and if hookworm infection was able to suppress immune changes in response to a gluten challenge. In this double-blind placebo-controlled study, hookworm infection was induced with cutaneous inoculations with hookworm larvae or placebo. After infestation was established, a 5-day oral gluten rechallenge was undertaken, and the duodenal biopsies as well as immune responses of circulating lymphocytes to gliadin peptides were measured by ELISpot. Five individuals of the 10 infested with hookworms experienced painful enteritis, though no symptoms were experienced with chronic infestation. Some patients developed increased eosinophils in the duodenum. However, infestation did not protect against inflammatory changes in the intestine or immune responses to gluten challenge. In summary, this is a negative study that demonstrates that parasitic infection with hookworm does not protect against gluten-induced responses in patients with treated celiac disease. While parasitic infections have been suggested to be potentially beneficial in immune-based disorders, it is clear from this study that it clearly fails to benefit patients with celiac disease, and the further investigation of its use is not likely to be beneficial. This suggests that, while celiac disease has become much more common in the recent decades in developed countries, it is not likely to be the result of reduction of parasitic infections, and this negative study puts a damper on further studies of parasitic infections as a means of treating immune disorders.

J. A. Murray, MD

Morbidity and Mortality Among Older Individuals With Undiagnosed Celiac Disease
Godfrey JD, Brantner TL, Brinjikji W, et al (Mayo Clinic, Rochester, MN)
Gastroenterology 139:763-769, 2010

Background & Aims.—Outcomes of undiagnosed celiac disease (CD) are unclear. We evaluated the morbidity and mortality of undiagnosed CD in a population-based sample of individuals 50 years of age and older.

Methods.—Stored sera from a population-based sample of 16,886 Olmsted County, Minnesota, residents 50 years of age and older were tested for CD based on analysis of tissue transglutaminase and endomysial antibodies. A nested case-control study compared serologically defined subjects with CD with age- and sex-matched, seronegative controls. Medical records were reviewed for comorbid conditions.

Results.—We identified 129 (0.8%) subjects with undiagnosed CD in a cohort of 16,847 older adults. A total of 127 undiagnosed cases (49% men; median age, 63.0 y) and 254 matched controls were included in a systematic evaluation for more than 100 potentially coexisting conditions. Subjects with undiagnosed CD had increased rates of osteoporosis and hypothyroidism, as well as lower body mass index and levels of cholesterol and ferritin. Overall survival was not associated with CD status. During a median follow-up period of 10.3 years after serum samples were collected, 20 cases but no controls were diagnosed with CD (15.2% Kaplan–Meier estimate at 10 years).

Conclusions.—With the exception of reduced bone health, older adults with undiagnosed CD had limited comorbidity and no increase in mortality compared with controls. Some subjects were diagnosed with CD within a decade of serum collection, indicating that although most cases of undiagnosed CD are clinically silent, some result in symptoms. Undiagnosed CD can confer benefits and liabilities to older individuals.

▶ It is well known that there is increased morbidity and moderately increased mortality among patients with diagnosed celiac disease. The level of excess mortality varies depending on the studies. With regard to undiagnosed celiac disease, there have now been a number of studies that have suggested there may be increased mortality in individuals who have undiagnosed celiac disease;[1,2] however, not all studies suggest that there is increased mortality. A Finnish study showed no increase in mortality of these individuals. The study by Godfrey et al is important in that it studies a cohort of patients with undiagnosed celiac disease where serum had been saved in patients whose median age was 63 and whose follow-up was approximately 10 years. This study showed no excess mortality during this period of follow-up. There was some subtle morbidity in lower bone density and an increased propensity to hypothyroidism; however, there was no significant excess of gastrointestinal diagnoses or gastrointestinal procedures in this cohort. There was a trend toward lower body mass index and lower cholesterol in this cohort, suggesting some moderate nutritional impact of undiagnosed celiac disease. The conclusion of this study is that unrecognized celiac disease in patients first tested in their mid 60s followed for 10 years does not result in increased mortality. Interestingly, 16% of individuals were clinically recognized to have celiac disease by the end of the 10-year follow-up, suggesting that 1% of undiagnosed celiac disease will become symptomatic and will be diagnosed per year on average. What does this mean for practice? Routine screening of healthy people at an advanced age for celiac disease is probably not indicated; however, physicians should be aware that celiac disease seems to be quite common in people of this age group and may become symptomatic even at advanced ages. If there is no increased mortality over longer follow-ups than 10 years, then it is likely that patients who are found serendipitously without any symptoms may not necessarily vary greatly in terms of improved survival; however, it may prevent some morbidity.

J. A. Murray, MD

References

1. Rubio-Tapia A, Kyle RA, Kaplan EL, et al. Increased prevalence and mortality in undiagnosed celiac disease. *Gastroenterology.* 2009;137:88-93.
2. Metzger MH, Heier M, Mäki M, et al. Mortality excess in individuals with elevated IgA anti-transglutaminase antibodies: the KORA/MONICA Augsburg cohort study 1989-1998. *Eur J Epidemiol.* 2006;21:359-365.

A nationwide population-based study to determine whether coeliac disease is associated with infertility

Zugna D, Richiardi L, Akre O, et al (Univ of Turin, Italy; Karolinska Institutet, Sweden; et al)

Gut 59:1471-1475, 2010

Background and Objective.—Previous studies suggest that women with coeliac disease (CD) have reproductive difficulties but the data are often inconclusive and contradictory. Fertility in women with biopsy-verified CD was examined.

Methods.—Swedish population-based cohort study. Duodenal/jejunal biopsy data on CD (Marsh III; villous atrophy (VA); n=18 005 unique women) were collected from all (n=28) pathology departments in Sweden. From this dataset, 11 495 women with CD, aged 18−45 years, were identified at some point before the end of follow-up. Multinomial logistic regression and Cox regression were used to estimate fertility in these women compared with that in 51 109 age-matched reference women. Fertility was defined as the number of children according to the Swedish Multi-Generation Register.

Results.—During follow-up, 16 309 births occurred in women with CD and 69 245 in the reference women. The cumulative number of children slightly increased in women with CD compared with the reference group. Adjusting for age, calendar period and parity and stratifying by education, the overall fertility hazard ratio (HR) in CD was 1.03 (95% CI 1.01 to 1.05). Specifically, the fertility HR was 1.05 (95% CI 0.96 to 1.14) for CD diagnosed in women before 18 years, 1.04 (95% CI 1.01 to 1.07) for CD diagnosed in women between 18 and 45 years and 1.02 (95% CI 0.99 to 1.04) for CD diagnosed in women > 45 years of age. Taking date of CD diagnosis into account, fertility was decreased 0−2 years before time of diagnosis (HR=0.63; 95% CI 0.57 to 0.70), was identical to that of controls 0−5 years subsequent to diagnosis and increased to 1.12 (95% CI 1.03 to 1.21) thereafter.

Conclusion.—Overall, women with CD had a normal fertility, but their fertility was decreased in the last 2 years preceding CD diagnosis.

▶ Celiac disease has been associated with many consequences, both within and outside of the gastrointestinal tract. Of particular interest, especially to young women identified with celiac disease, is the potential association with impairment of fertility; however, the data on reproductive difficulties in celiac disease are both inconclusive and contradictory. This study used a unique cohort of more than 18 000 women in whom biopsy-proven celiac disease had been established throughout Sweden. Of these, 11 400 women between the ages of 18 and 45 years were followed, and their reproductive histories were compared with 51 000 age-matched reference women. Fertility was defined by the number of children, as recorded in the Swedish birth registries. Overall, there is slightly increased fertility in women who have been diagnosed with celiac disease between the ages of 18 and 45, but not so for women diagnosed when older than 45. Additionally, fertility was diminished between 0 and 2 years before the time of diagnosis of celiac disease, but rose to match that of controls in the first 5 years after diagnosis and indeed exceeded that in controls more than 5 years after diagnosis. With this extensive population-based study, we can conclude that overall fertility is normal in patients with celiac disease; however, fertility was likely diminished in the 2 years prior to diagnosis, but a compensatory increase in fertility occurred more than 5 years after diagnosis. This suggests that a minority of women with celiac disease have an impact on their reproductive capacity, most often prior to diagnosis. Women with a new diagnosis of celiac disease found at an early age can be counseled that their fertility should be normal, although awareness of undiagnosed celiac disease as a potential cause for impaired fertility would also be prudent for doctors looking after those patients.

J. A. Murray, MD

Weight Loss, Exercise, or Both and Physical Function in Obese Older Adults
Villareal DT, Chode S, Parimi N, et al (Washington Univ School of Medicine, St Louis, MO; et al)
N Engl J Med 364:1218-1229, 2011

Background.—Obesity exacerbates the age-related decline in physical function and causes frailty in older adults; however, the appropriate treatment for obese older adults is controversial.

Methods.—In this 1-year, randomized, controlled trial, we evaluated the independent and combined effects of weight loss and exercise in 107 adults who were 65 years of age or older and obese. Participants were randomly assigned to a control group, a weight-management (diet) group, an exercise group, or a weight-management-plus-exercise (diet-exercise) group. The primary outcome was the change in score on the modified Physical Performance Test. Secondary outcomes included other measures of frailty, body composition, bone mineral density, specific physical functions, and quality of life.

Results.—A total of 93 participants (87%) completed the study. In the intention-to-treat analysis, the score on the Physical Performance Test, in which higher scores indicate better physical status, increased more in the diet-exercise group than in the diet group or the exercise group (increases from baseline of 21% vs. 12% and 15%, respectively); the scores in all three of those groups increased more than the scores in the control group (in which the score increased by 1%) (P<0.001 for the between-group differences). Moreover, the peak oxygen consumption improved more in the diet-exercise group than in the diet group or the exercise group (increases of 17% vs. 10% and 8%, respectively; P<0.001); the score on the Functional Status Questionnaire, in which higher scores indicate better physical function, increased more in the diet-exercise group than in the diet group (increase of 10% vs. 4%, P<0.001). Body weight decreased by 10% in the diet group and by 9% in the diet-exercise group, but did not decrease in the exercise group or the control group (P<0.001). Lean body mass and bone mineral density at the hip decreased less in the diet-exercise group than in the diet group (reductions of 3% and 1%, respectively, in the diet-exercise group vs. reductions of 5% and 3%, respectively, in the diet group; P<0.05 for both comparisons). Strength, balance, and gait improved consistently in the diet-exercise group (P<0.05 for all comparisons). Adverse events included a small number of exercise-associated musculoskeletal injuries.

Conclusions.—These findings suggest that a combination of weight loss and exercise provides greater improvement in physical function than either intervention alone. (Funded by the National Institutes of Health; ClinicalTrials.gov number, NCT00146107.)

▶ Gastroenterologists are increasingly engaged in the management of obesity. Obesity is also increasing in the elderly US population. Obesity may contribute to the propensity for injury. The optimal approach to the management of obesity and frailty in the elderly is of increasing importance. Concerns regarding dietary interventions in obese elderly individuals have centered on increased risk of sarcopenia associated with successful weight loss. It has been a concern that reduction in muscle mass could lead to increased risk of fractures or frailty-associated injuries. Previous short-term studies have shown some benefit of a combination of weight loss and exercise in obesity. There have also been questions raised as to whether the elderly obese individual can change a lifetime of habits to successfully achieve weight loss.

The study by Villareal et al, undertaken in the US Midwest, examined the individual contributions of exercise and dietary intervention in elderly obese individuals. They compared the effects of combination diet and exercise as compared with diet alone or exercise alone versus no treatment in elderly adults. The primary outcome measure was the physical performance tests with secondary measures of frailty, body composition, bone density, physical functioning, and quality of life. The physical performance test is a study of common functions of daily living. Subjects were followed at 6 and 12 months. There was a high completion rate of 87% of subjects completing the study (Figure 1 in the original article). There was a predominance of women. The average body mass index was 37. Results indicated a superior impact of combination of diet and exercise on most parameters measured (Figure 2 in the original article). Weight loss was equivalent between those groups who received diet alone or diet and exercise together with a weight loss of approximately 10% achieved. Exercise alone improved many of the physical functioning parameters. This study demonstrates for the first time that in elderly obese individuals a combination of diet and exercise can achieve durable gains in both physical performance and nutritional outcomes without negatively affecting strength or stability or exacerbating frailty. This study supports widespread intervention for obese elderly individuals that incorporates changes in both dietary intervention coupled with exercise as the optimal approach to this epidemic of obesity in the elderly.

J. A. Murray, MD

Gluten sensitivity: from gut to brain

Hadjivassiliou M, Sanders DS, Grünewald RA, et al (Royal Hallamshire Hosp, Sheffield, UK; et al)
Lancet Neurol 9:318-330, 2010

Gluten sensitivity is a systemic autoimmune disease with diverse manifestations. This disorder is characterised by abnormal immunological responsiveness to ingested gluten in genetically susceptible individuals. Coeliac disease, or gluten-sensitive enteropathy, is only one aspect of a range of possible manifestations of gluten sensitivity. Although neurological manifestations in patients with established coeliac disease have been reported since 1966, it was not until 30 years later that, in some individuals, gluten sensitivity was shown to manifest solely with neurological dysfunction. Furthermore, the concept of extraintestinal presentations without enteropathy has only recently become accepted. In this Personal View, we review the range of neurological manifestations of gluten sensitivity and discuss recent advances in the diagnosis and understanding of the pathophysiological mechanisms underlying neurological dysfunction related to gluten sensitivity.

▶ It has long been recognized that celiac disease causes symptoms and consequences outside of the gastrointestinal tract. Particularly devastating to patients can be neurologic consequences of the disease; these include both central nervous system and peripheral nervous system effects, including ataxia, dementia,[1] and peripheral neuropathy. In recent years, the group from Sheffield, England, and colleagues have described neurologic associations of celiac disease and expanded this to include gluten sensitivity without the presence of celiac disease. In this personal view, they review in detail the neurologic associations of gluten sensitivity. They describe in detail the potential neurologic complications of the disease, specifically cerebellar ataxia or a form of ataxia similar to cerebellar ataxia, often associated with atrophy of the cerebellum, and circulating antibodies against native gliadin. This latter test is no longer routinely performed as part of the detection for celiac disease. In addition, they go on to describe the association with autoantibodies directed against transglutaminase 6. This is a close relative of tissue transglutaminase or TG2, which is the autoantibody recognized in celiac disease. This article is an important description and summary of the neurologic consequences that can occur as a result of gluten sensitivity, both with and without celiac disease. It raises the issue that, when considering this entity, tests directed against native gliadin may need to be resurrected as diagnostic tests, at least until more specific tests to detect autoantibodies directed against their target epitopes in the central nervous system are developed and widely disseminated. For gastroenterologists, it is important to recognize that these neurologic associations can occur even without the presence of celiac disease. It is also these authors' view that early intervention with gluten avoidance may reduce the ultimate impact of these neurologic syndromes on the patients. Controversy continues as to the initiating event: Is this a primary reaction against gluten, or are the autoantibodies directed against a primary antigen in the brain that in some way mimics the molecular structure or antigenic nature of gluten?[2]

J. A. Murray, MD

References

1. Hu WT, Murray JA, Greenaway MC, Parisi JE, Josephs KA. Cognitive impairment and celiac disease. *Arch Neurol.* 2006;63:1440-1446.
2. Rashtak S, Rashtak S, Snyder MR, et al. Serology of celiac disease in gluten-sensitive ataxia or neuropathy: role of deamidated gliadin antibody. *J Neuroimmunol.* 2011; 230:130-134.

A Biopsy is Not Always Necessary to Diagnose Celiac Disease
Mubarak A, Wolters VM, Gerritsen SAM, et al (Univ Med Ctr Utrecht, The Netherlands)
J Pediatr Gastroenterol Nutr 52:554-557, 2011

Objectives.—Small intestinal histology is the criterion standard for the diagnosis of celiac disease (CD). However, results of serological tests such as anti-endomysium antibodies and anti-tissue transglutaminase antibodies (tTGA) are becoming increasingly reliable. This raises the question of whether a small intestinal biopsy is always necessary. The aim of the present study was, therefore, to investigate whether a small intestinal biopsy can be avoided in a selected group of patients.

Patients and Methods.—Serology and histological slides obtained from 283 pediatric patients suspected of having CD were examined retrospectively. The response to a gluten-free diet (GFD) in patients with a tTGA level ≥100 U/mL was investigated.

Results.—A tTGA level ≥100 U/mL was found in 128 of the 283 patients. Upon microscopic examination of the small intestinal epithelium, villous atrophy was found in 124 of these patients, confirming the presence of CD. Three patients had crypt hyperplasia or an increased number of intraepithelial lymphocytes. In 1 patient no histological abnormalities were found. This patient did not respond to a GFD.

Conclusions.—Pediatric patients with a tTGA level ≥100 U/mL in whom symptoms improve upon consuming a GFD may not need a small intestinal biopsy to confirm CD.

▶ The diagnosis of celiac disease currently requires duodenal biopsies for confirmation. Mubarak et al have studied the necessity for biopsies in patients with high positive tissue transglutaminase antibodies. They performed a retrospective analysis of consecutive patients referred to the pediatric gastrointestinal department for endoscopy. They had 301 patients in whom both serologic testing and biopsies were available. They excluded patients with giardiasis and immunoglobulin A (IgA) deficiency. A total of 57.6% of patients ultimately had a biopsy-proven diagnosis of celiac disease. They demonstrated that the overall specificity for celiac disease using the tissue transglutaminase IgA test was 83% with a sensitivity of 96%. Interestingly, they found the sensitivity of the endomysial antibody IgA was 96%; the specificity was only 66%. They demonstrated that in those patients in whom the tissue transglutaminase antibody levels were very high (> 100), the specificity went up to 97% and indeed showed that just 1 subject had a completely normal biopsy result. In this setting, they make the case that extremely high positive tissue transglutaminase antibodies, in this case > 100, were highly predictive of celiac disease, and in the 1 patient, who was truly a false-positive, no response to diet occurred. This study demonstrates that extremely positive serology for celiac disease using the specific test of tissue transglutaminase IgA is highly predictive of celiac disease and may, in certain circumstances, permit the avoidance of biopsy in children. One cause for concern is the low specificity of endomysial antibodies, suggesting that perhaps endomysial antibody is such a specialized test that it should only be performed in high volume, which could help maintain the expertise and consistency of reporting. The other potential weakness is that major criteria for undertaking biopsies are positive serologic test results, leading to a common weakness in many such retrospective studies, that is, positive selection bias for serologically positive individuals undergoing biopsies. This phenomenon would lead to the overestimation of the accuracy of the tests. Nonetheless, when faced with a patient with very positive serology, the chance of celiac disease is extremely high with a positive predictive value in patients with suspicious symptoms for celiac disease of 97%. Lower positive predictive values may occur when populations with a lower pretest prevalence are studied. However, not all authors agree; Freeman reported a significant minority of patients with strongly positive tissue transglutaminase antibodies who have normal biopsy results.[1]

J. A. Murray, MD

Reference

1. Freeman HJ. Strongly positive tissue transglutaminase antibody assays without celiac disease. *Can J Gastroenterol.* 2004;18:25-28.

A New Intravenous Fat Emulsion Containing Soybean Oil, Medium-Chain Triglycerides, Olive Oil, and Fish Oil: A Single-Center, Double-Blind Randomized Study on Efficacy and Safety in Pediatric Patients Receiving Home Parenteral Nutrition

Goulet O, Antébi H, Wolf C, et al (Univ of Paris 5, René Descartes, France; Hôpital Saint Antoine, Paris, France)

JPEN J Parenter Enteral Nutr 34:485-495, 2010

Background.—SMOFlipid 20% is an intravenous lipid emulsion (ILE) containing soybean oil, medium-chain triglycerides, olive oil, and fish oil developed to provide energy, essential fatty acids (FAs), and long-chain ω-3 FAs as a mixed emulsion containing α-tocopherol. The aim was to assess the efficacy and safety of this new ILE in pediatric patients receiving home parenteral nutrition (HPN) compared with soybean oil emulsion (SOE).

Methods.—This single-center, randomized, double-blind study included 28 children on HPN allocated to receive either SMOFlipid 20% (n = 15) or a standard SOE (Intralipid 20%, n = 13). ILE was administered 4 to 5 times per week (goal dose, 2.0 g/kg/d) within a parenteral nutrition regimen. Assessments, including safety and efficacy parameters, were performed on day 0 and after the last study infusion (day 29). Lipid peroxidation was determined by measurement of thiobarbituric acid reactive substances (TBARS).

Results.—There were no significant differences in laboratory safety parameters, including liver enzymes, between the groups on day 29. The mean ± standard deviation changes in the total bilirubin concentration between the initial and final values (day 29 to day 0) were significantly different between groups: SMOFlipid group −1.5 ± 2.4 μmol/L vs SOE group 2.3 ± 3.5 μmol/L, $P < .01$; 95% confidence interval [CI], −6.2 to −1.4). In plasma and red blood cell (RBC) phospholipids, the ω-3 FAs C20:5ω-3 (eicosapentaenoic acid) and + C22:6ω-3 (docosahexaenoic acid) increased significantly in the SMOFlipid group on day 29. The ω-3:ω-6 FA ratio was significantly elevated with SMOFlipid 20% compared with SOE group (plasma, day 29: 0.15 ± 0.06 vs 0.07 ± 0.02, $P < .01$, 95% CI, 0.04–0.11; and RBC, day 29: 0.23 ± 0.07 vs 0.14 ± 0.04, $P < .01$, 95% CI, 0.04–0.13). Plasma α-tocopherol concentration increased significantly more with SMOFlipid 20% (15.7 ± 15.9 vs 5.4 ± 15.2 μmol/L, $P < .05$; 95% CI, −2.1 to 22.6). The low-density lipoprotein-TBARS concentrations were not significantly different between both groups, indicating that lipid peroxidation did not differ between groups.

Conclusions.—SMOFlipid 20%, which contains 15% fish oil, was safe and well tolerated, decreased plasma bilirubin, and increased ω-3 FA and α-tocopherol status without changing lipid peroxidation.

▶ One of the most feared complications of long-term parenteral nutrition is liver disease. It is a major cause of morbidity or even mortality in those who have long-term dependency on parenteral nutrition. Standard lipid solutions are based on soybean oil, which is suspected to be the major contributor to the liver abnormalities. Fish oil—based solutions have been developed, and this study is a short-term randomized controlled trial of the novel fish oil—based solution versus the standard soybean oil—based lipid solution in children with short bowel syndrome. The novel solution appeared safe and was associated with a lower bilirubin level than standard. The essential fatty acids EPA and DHA were higher in those treated with the novel lipid solution. Lipid peroxidation was not affected. Novel lipid solutions are safe and are associated with improved laboratory parameters of lipid nutrition and are likely to affect and possibly change the occurrence of liver dysfunction in patients on long-term parenteral nutrition.

J. A. Murray, MD

Detection of Celiac Disease and Lymphocytic Enteropathy by Parallel Serology and Histopathology in a Population-Based Study

Walker MM, Murray JA, Ronkainen J, et al (Imperial College London, UK; Mayo Clinic, Rochester, MN; Karolinska Institutet, Stockholm, Sweden; et al)
Gastroenterology 139:112-119, 2010

Background & Aims.—Although serologic analysis is used in diagnosis of celiac disease, histopathology is considered most reliable. We performed a prospective study to determine the clinical, pathologic, and serologic spectrum of celiac disease in a general population (Kalixanda study).

Methods.—A random sample of an adult general population (n = 1000) was analyzed by upper endoscopy, duodenal biopsy, and serologic analysis of tissue transglutaminase (tTg) levels; endomysial antibody (EMA) levels were analyzed in samples that were tTg+. The cut off values for diagnosis of celiac disease were villous atrophy with 40 intraepithelial lymphocytes (IELs)/100 enterocytes (ECs).

Results.—Samples from 33 subjects were tTg+, and 16 were EMA+. Histologic analysis identified 7 of 1000 subjects (0.7%) with celiac disease; all were tTg+, and 6 of 7 were EMA+. Another 26 subjects were tTg+ (7/26 EMA+). This was addressed by a second quantitative pathology study (nested case control design) using a threshold of 25 IELS/100 ECs. In this analysis, all 13 samples that were tTg+ and EMA+ had ≥25 IELs/100 ECs. In total, 16 subjects (1.6%) had serologic and histologic evidence of gluten-sensitive enteropathy. IELs were quantified in duodenal biopsy samples from seronegative individuals (n = 500); 19 (3.8%) had >25 IELs and lymphocytic duodenosis.

Conclusions.—Measurement of ≥25 IELs/100 ECs correlated with serologic indicators of celiac disease; a higher IEL threshold could miss 50% of cases. Quantification of tTg is a sensitive test for celiac disease; diagnosis can be confirmed by observation of ≥25 IELs/100ECs in duodenal biopsy specimens. Lymphocytic enteropathy (celiac disease and lymphocytic duodenosis) is common in the population (5.4%).

▶ Most patients with celiac disease in a community are not diagnosed. This has been substantiated by studies comparing the prevalence of known previously detected celiac disease with celiac disease detected by serology. However, up until this particular study, all these studies depended on or assumed that the sensitivity of serologic testing for celiac disease was quite high. This is the first study in which parallel endoscopically obtained duodenal biopsies and serology were undertaken in a general population sample. This was done in an adult population from northern Sweden. The study documented a high prevalence of undiagnosed celiac disease, comprising 1.6% of this adult population; when combined with the 2 patients of this 1000-population sample, a prevalence of 1.8% of the adult population had celiac disease. Serology, in this case using antibodies against tissue transglutaminase immunoglobulin A confirmed by endomysial antibody, was highly predictive of the histologic features of celiac disease. In addition, there was substantial proportion, 3.8%, of the population that had increased intraepithelial lymphocytosis in the absence of positive serology for celiac disease. The strongest association of this entity, called lymphocytic duodenosis, was *Helicobacter* infection on the gastric biopsies taken simultaneously. This study is important because it validates for the first time the sensitivity of the serologic testing in a general population sample and does so with parallel endoscopy in all subjects tested, not just those that are seropositive. It validates a very high specificity of the testing and also illustrates the high frequency of lymphocytic duodenosis. This entity has also been called increased intraepithelial lymphocytosis with normal villous architecture, or sometimes has been called Marsh![1]

The take-home message is that serologic testing for celiac disease is highly sensitive and quite specific. In addition, minimal infiltration of the duodenal epithelium with lymphocytes is most often not associated with celiac disease but frequently can be associated with other disorders that inflame the intestine, including *Helicobacter*-related gastritis.

J. A. Murray, MD

Reference

1. Marsh MN. Gluten, major histocompatibility complex, and the small intestine. A molecular and immunobiologic approach to the spectrum of gluten sensitivity ('celiac sprue'). *Gastroenterology.* 1992;102:330-354.

7 Gastrointestinal Surgery

Esophageal Dysmotility Disorders After Laparoscopic Gastric Banding—An Underestimated Complication
Naef M, Mouton WG, Naef U, et al (Spital STS AG Thun, Switzerland; et al)
Ann Surg 253:285-290, 2011

Objective.—To evaluate the effects of laparoscopic adjustable gastric banding (LAGB) on esophageal dysfunction over the long term in a prospective study, based on a 12-year experience.

Background.—Esophageal motility disorders and dilatation after LAGB have been reported. However, only a few studies present long-term follow-up data.

Methods.—Between June 1998 and June 2009, all patients with implantation of a LAGB were enrolled in a prospective clinical trial including a yearly barium swallow. Esophageal motility disorders were recorded and classified over the period. An esophageal diameter of 35 mm or greater was considered dilated.

Results.—Laparoscopic adjustable gastric banding was performed in 167 patients (120 females and 47males) with a mean age of 40.1 ± 5.2 years. Overall patient follow-up was 94%. Esophageal dysmotility disorders were found in 108 patients (68.8% of patients followed). Esophageal dilatation occurred in 40 patients (25.5%) with a mean esophageal diameter of 47.3 ± 6.9 mm (35.0−94.6) after a follow-up of 73.8 ± 6.8 months (36−120) compared with 26.2 ± 2.8 mm (18.3−34.2) in patients without dilatation (diameter of <35 mm) ($P < 0.01$). Thirty-four patients suffered from stage III dilatation (band deflation necessary) and 6 from stage IV (major achalasia-like dilatation, band removal mandatory). In 29 patients, upper endoscopy was carried out because of heartburn/dysphagia. In 18 patients, the endoscopy was normal; 9 patients suffered from gastroesophageal reflux disease, 1 from a stenosis, and 1 from a hiatus hernia.

Conclusions.—This study demonstrates that esophageal motility disorders after LAGB are frequent, poorly appreciated complications. Despite adequate excess weight loss, LAGB should probably not be considered the procedure of first choice and should be performed only in selected cases until reliable criteria for patients with a low risk for the procedure's long-term complications are developed.

▶ Debate has continued as to whether chronically obstructing the proximal stomach through gastric banding for obesity leads to esophageal dysfunction. There have been multiple reports of severe dysphagia with and without pseudoachalasia after laparoscopic adjustable gastric banding (LAGB). To date, LAGB is the most common weight loss operation performed in the United States, and with the US Food and Drug Administration's (FDA) recent approval of LAGB for use in patients whose body mass index (BMI) is 30 or higher (prior to this expanded criteria determination by the FDA, the band was only appropriate if the BMI was greater than 35), this makes the concern about the long-term effect of the LAGB on esophageal function even more important.

In this series, the authors found two-thirds of the patients with esophageal motility disorders at long-term follow-up and 25.5% with significant dilatation of the esophagus. This is a significant finding and one that needs to be addressed. The good news is that in 87% of patients with band deflation, esophageal dilatation was reversible. However, in 13% of the cases, the patients did not recover after band deflation, with persistent stage IV dilatation (major achalasia-like dilatation). Interestingly, in this series, stages III and IV dilatations occurred 3 to 10 years after surgery after a median follow-up of 74 months, emphasizing the need for long-term follow-up to detect these late complications.

LAGB has the potential for long-term irreversible esophageal dysfunction in more than 10% of patients, with significant numbers of patients experiencing reversible dysfunction. This potential complication and adverse outcome needs to be discussed openly with patients and considered when a patient presents with dysphagia at any time after this operation.

C. D. Smith, MD

Clinical Outcomes and Prognostic Factors of Metastatic Gastric Carcinoma Patients Who Experience Gastrointestinal Perforation During Palliative Chemotherapy

Kang MH, Kim SN, Kim NK, et al (Natl Cancer Ctr, Goyang, Gyeonggi, Republic of Korea)
Ann Surg Oncol 17:3163-3172, 2010

Background.—We conducted the current study to investigate the clinical outcomes of metastatic gastric carcinoma (MGC) patients who experienced gastrointestinal (GI) perforation during palliative chemotherapy and to examine the prognostic factors associated with survival after perforation.

Methods.—We reviewed the medical records of patients at the Center for Gastric Cancer of the National Cancer Center, Korea who developed GI perforation during palliative chemotherapy between January 2001 and December 2008.

Results.—Of the 1,856 patients who received palliative chemotherapy for MGC, 32 patients (1.7%) developed GI perforation during chemotherapy.

Patients with perforation at the primary gastric site were more likely to have ulcerative gastric cancer lesion (90.5 vs. 40.0%, $P = 0.034$) or gastric tumor bleeding (28.6 vs. 0%, $P = 0.298$), and less likely to have Bormann type IV (14.3 vs. 60.0%, $P = 0.062$), than patients with perforation at nongastric sites. In 14 patients (43.8%) who resumed chemotherapy after perforation, the disease control rate was 57.1%, and median overall survival (OS) after perforation was 7.5 months [95% confidence interval (CI), 6.0−9.0 months]. In all patients, median OS following perforation was 4.0 months (95% CI, 1.5−6.6 months), and multivariate analysis revealed that differentiated tumor histology, response to chemotherapy before perforation, and absence of septic shock at time of perforation were significantly associated with favorable OS after perforation.

Conclusions.—As patients experiencing GI perforation during palliative chemotherapy have heterogeneous clinical presentation, we need to adopt different approaches in the management of the patients that are compatible with the favorable prognostic factors.

▶ This article from Korea analyzes the outcomes in patients who are undergoing palliative chemotherapy for surgically unresectable or recurrent cancer resection and experience a gastrointestinal (GI) perforation. Granted, this is from Asia, and it is beyond this review to tackle the well-known debate about whether gastric cancer in Asia is the same as gastric cancer in North America, but suffice it to say that this large experience with advanced gastric cancer can give everyone some insight into the natural history of GI perforation during palliative care for gastric cancer.

The authors offer 2 important concepts in support of pursuing and publishing these data. First, they highlight that many physicians or surgeons view GI perforation during palliative chemotherapy for gastric cancer as a much more serious situation than it actually is and are frequently not willing to aggressively treat patients who present with this condition. Second, although chemotherapy itself does not seem to increase the risk of developing GI perforation, chemotherapy may complicate the management of patients with GI perforation, and understanding the natural history of perforation in these patients should facilitate establishing prognosis and appropriate management.

From a large registry of patients with gastric cancer, the authors identified 1856 patients who received palliative chemotherapy for gastric cancer over a 7-year period (2001-2008). Of these patients, 32 developed GI perforation (1.7%). Most presented with sudden onset of severe abdominal pain (87%), and all had CT findings of either pneumoperitoneum, free fluid, or contained fluid collection. Perforation occurred at the known primary tumor (69%), metastasis to the colon (25%), or an uninvolved other site in the GI tract (6%). Nineteen percent of the patients presented in septic shock. Most patients were receiving first-line combination chemotherapy and perforated soon after beginning chemotherapy (median 2 months) and a median of 8 days after the last dose. However, those that perforated at their primary tumor site presented sooner after initiation of chemotherapy than those with a noncancer perforation (1 month vs 33 months).

More than half of the patients underwent surgery to manage the perforation. The reasons to withhold surgery included advanced disease with carcinomatosis, poor functional status, patient refusal, or self-limited perforation. Almost half of the patients were able to resume chemotherapy (44%) after management of perforation, and the median overall survival after perforation was 7.5 months. Poorer overall survival was seen in patients with undifferentiated cancer, no response to chemotherapy, or septic shock at the time of perforation.

The authors conclude that GI perforation during palliative chemotherapy for gastric cancer is heterogeneous but not universally and immediately terminal. Select patients can resume palliative chemotherapy and gain additional time in overall survival. This experience provides some basis for decisions about if and how to intervene in this setting and what to tell patients and their families about what to expect.

C. D. Smith, MD

Esophagectomy Outcomes at Low-Volume Hospitals: The Association Between Systems Characteristics and Mortality

Funk LM, Gawande AA, Semel ME, et al (Harvard School of Public Health, Boston, MA; et al)
Ann Surg 253:912-917, 2011

Objective.—To evaluate the association between systems characteristics and esophagectomy mortality at low-volume hospitals.

Background.—High-volume hospitals have lower esophagectomy mortality rates, but receiving care at such centers is not always feasible. We examined low-volume hospitals and sought to identify characteristics of those with better outcomes.

Methods.—Using national data from Medicare and the American Hospital Association, we studied 4498 elderly patients who underwent an esophagectomy from 2004 to 2007. We divided hospitals into terciles based on esophagectomy volume and examined characteristics of patients and hospitals (size, nurse ratios, and presence of advanced medical, surgical, and radiological services). Our primary outcome was mortality. We identified 5 potentially beneficial systems characteristics in our data set and used multivariable logistic regression to determine whether these characteristics were associated with lower mortality rates at low-volume hospitals.

Results.—Of the 874 hospitals that performed esophagectomies, 83% (723) were low-volume hospitals whereas only 3% (25) were high-volume. Low-volume hospitals performed a median of 1 esophagectomy during the 4-year study period and cared for patients that were older, more likely to be minority, and more likely to have multiple comorbidities compared with high-volume centers. Low-volume hospitals that had at least 3 of 5 characteristics (high nurse ratios, lung transplantation services, complex medical oncology services, bariatric surgery services, and positron emission tomography scanners) had markedly lower mortality rates compared with low-volume hospitals with none of these characteristics (12.5% vs. 5.0%; P value = 0.042).

Conclusions.—Low-volume hospitals with certain systems characteristics seem to achieve better esophagectomy outcomes. A more comprehensive study of the beneficial characteristics of low-volume hospitals is warranted because high-volume hospitals are difficult to access for many patients.

▶ There has been a long-held belief that centers that do higher volumes of particular cases have better procedure-specific outcomes than those centers where smaller volumes are performed. Johns Hopkins was the first to extend this concept through their multiple publications regarding outcomes with pancreatic surgery at Johns Hopkins (a high-volume pancreatic resection center) when compared with other centers' outcomes with the same operation(s). Others have replicated similar data for other complex operations. Esophagectomy has been right alongside pancreatic resection as a procedure where the outcomes are better at high-volume centers.

That said, there have been exceptions, and "low-volume centers" point out these exceptions. The idea that certain procedures need to be referred to high-volume centers raises concerns about the balance of health care resource use: better value at high-volume centers versus the increased expense (both financial and human costs) of transporting people away from their local hospitals and support systems.

This article takes a more detailed look at the role the institution plays in these outcomes rather than the absolute number of the procedures performed. The concept is simple: Are there characteristics of a hospital's system that affect outcomes, even if the number of particular cases is "low volume"?

The take-home message from this study is simply that outcomes after esophagectomy are related to the hospital's ability to care for complex patients (eg, lung transplant, bariatric surgery, complex medical oncology), not simply the volume of esophagectomies performed. As health care reform emphasizes value (outcomes/cost), we will see more of these types of studies trying to unearth exactly what can help the numerator of the value equation improve.

C. D. Smith, MD

Small Bowel Obstruction: Outcome and Cost Implications of Admitting Service
Oyasiji T, Angelo S, Kyriakides TC, et al (Hosp of Saint Raphael, New Haven, CT)
Am Surg 76:687-691, 2010

We compared patients with small bowel obstruction (SBO) admitted through the emergency department to the surgical service (SS) with those admitted to the medical service (MS) with respect to outcomes and health-care cost. We conducted a retrospective analysis of our SBO database comparing 482 patients admitted to SS and 153 patients admitted to MS at a single institution over a 5-year period (January 2003 to December 2007). Study outcomes included length of hospital stay (LOS), time to surgery (TTS), hospital charges, incidence of bowel resection, and mortality. Both groups were comparable for age, gender, and race. The SS group had a shorter LOS (6.1 *vs* 7.5 days; $P = 0.01$), less hospital charges ($29,549 *vs* $35,789; $P = 0.06$), shorter TTS (log rank comparison; $P = 0.006$), and less mortality (eight [1.66%] *vs* six [3.92]; $P = 0.11$). The SS group had more bowel resections (13.1 *vs* 5.2%; $P = 0.007$). Coronary artery disease (CAD), acute renal failure (ARF), admission to SS, and female gender were significant predictors of bowel resection. CAD and ARF were significant predictors of mortality. Two hundred forty-four patients required operative intervention (surgery operative subgroup [SOS] 210 [43.6%], medicine operative subgroup [MOS] 34 [22.2%]). SOS and MOS were comparable for gender and race. SOS had shorter LOS (9.1 *vs* 12.3 days; $P = 0.02$), less hospital charges ($46,258 *vs* $62,778, $P = 0.05$), and less mortality (eight [3.81%] *vs* four [11.76%]; $P = 0.07$). Bowel resection was comparable (SOS 30% *vs* MOS 23%; $P = 0.44$). CAD and congestive heart failure (CHF) were significant predictors of bowel resection, whereas CAD was the only significant predictor of mortality in this subgroup. We recommend that patients with SBO be admitted to SS because this might translate to shorter LOS, earlier operative intervention, and reduced healthcare use direct cost. Bowel resection and death are more likely to occur in patients with comorbidities like CHF, CAD, diabetes mellitus, and ARF.

▶ In this very interesting article, the authors looked at the outcomes and cost of managing small bowel obstruction (SBO) based on the hospital's admitting service: surgical service (SS) versus medical service (MS). They found that the outcomes and cost are best when patients with bowel obstruction are managed on the SS. Additionally, those patients who ultimately required surgical intervention fared better when they had been admitted to the SS rather than the MS.

The study was a retrospective review of all patients with bowel obstruction admitted to a northeastern teaching hospital. This involved comparing 482 patients admitted to SS and 153 patients admitted to MS over a 5-year period (January 2003 to December 2007). Study outcomes included length of hospital stay (LOS), time to surgery (TTS), hospital charges, incidence of bowel resection, and mortality. The SS group had a shorter LOS (6.1 vs 7.5 days), lower hospital charges ($29 549 vs $35 789), shorter TTS, and less mortality. The authors recommend that patients with SBO be admitted to SS because this might translate to shorter LOS, earlier operative intervention, and reduced health care use direct cost.

The study suffers from being retrospective, with many important variables not controlled or even mentioned. I like the article for this review because it tackles an age-old question facing hospitals across the country: Should all patients with bowel obstruction be admitted to SS even though most can be managed nonoperatively, or should all but the patients who obviously will need surgery be admitted to MS with surgical consultation and assumed care if there is progression to surgical management? The pros and cons are well known. Surgeons are expensive resources and should be operating or caring for clearly surgical patients as much as possible versus the decision to operate, and perioperative management of bowel obstruction is best understood and managed by surgeons, if surgery is not inevitable.

The study has clearly answered this question for the hospital that was the subject of this study: Bowel obstruction is best managed with the SS providing the best value for this diagnosis (value = outcome/cost). However, I do not believe one can extend these results beyond this single hospital without repeating the study for your own hospital, or controlling for all of the other variables that can affect outcome and cost (eg, who makes the decision about which service gets the admission, communication and collaboration between the SS and MS during the care, or standardized protocols for management of these patients regardless of service).

C. D. Smith, MD

Demographically associated variations in outcomes after bariatric surgery
Turner PL, Oyetunji TA, Gantt G, et al (Univ of Maryland Med Ctr, Baltimore; Howard-Hopkins Surgical Outcomes Res Ctr, Washington, DC; et al)
Am J Surg 201:475-480, 2011

Background.—The incidence of morbid obesity and the use of bariatric surgery as a weight loss tool have increased significantly over the past decade. Despite this increase, there has been limited large-scale database evaluation of the effects of demographics on postoperative occurrences.

Methods.—An analysis of the American College of Surgeons National Surgical Quality Improvement Program database from 2005 to 2007 was performed. The bariatric procedures identified were open Roux-en-Y gastric bypass, laparoscopic Roux-en-Y gastric bypass, adjustable gastric banding, vertical banded gastroplasty, restrictive procedures other than vertical banded gastroplasty, and biliopancreatic diversion/duodenal switch. Outcomes examined were 30-day mortality and American College of Surgeons National Surgical Quality Improvement Program–defined morbidities. Multivariate analysis was performed.

Results.—A total of 18,682 bariatric procedures were identified. Increased body mass index, age, and undergoing open Roux-en-Y gastric bypass were associated with increased rates of postoperative complications. Hispanic and African American patients were noted to have increased rates of certain postoperative complications.

Conclusions.—Demographic factors may influence the postoperative course of patients undergoing bariatric surgery. Prospective studies may further elucidate the associations between demographic factors and specific postoperative complications.

▶ Over the past decade, several databases have been accumulating data from patients undergoing weight loss surgeries. One of the more substantial efforts to quantify and standardize our understanding of the use and outcomes of bariatric surgery is the National Surgical Quality Improvement Program (NSQIP) administered by the American College of Surgeons. This study mined the database looking specifically for demographic factors that might predict outcomes of bariatric surgery. It is well recognized that whereas most patients undergoing bariatric surgery realize good results in terms of weight loss and comorbidity resolution, there are subsets of patients who fail. Subgroups have been too small to identify which patients are more likely to fail surgical intervention, especially when considering demographic factors.

This is a retrospective analysis of the National Surgical Quality Improvement Program database from 2005 to 2007. A total of 18 682 bariatric procedures were identified. The bariatric procedures identified were open Roux-en-Y gastric bypass, laparoscopic Roux-en-Y gastric bypass, adjustable gastric banding, vertical banded gastroplasty, restrictive procedures other than vertical banded gastroplasty, and biliopancreatic diversion/duodenal switch. Outcomes examined were 30-day mortality and NSQIP-defined morbidities. Multivariate analysis was performed, finding that Hispanic and African American patients were noted to have increased rates of certain postoperative complications.

Many of us who have been offering bariatric surgery for more than 10 years have anecdotally observed that the outcomes vary not simply with procedure, but by individual patient. No single database has been large enough to convert these observations into scientifically valid findings. The NSQIP database is now approaching the size that allows these questions to be answered. This article's conclusions are weak, but some concrete evidence is beginning to be provided that some populations experience more complications of bariatric operations than others.

C. D. Smith, MD

Doppler-Guided Hemorrhoidal Artery Ligation and Rectoanal Repair (HAL-RAR) for the Treatment of Grade IV Hemorrhoids: Long-Term Results in 100 Consecutive Patients

Faucheron J-L, Poncet G, Voirin D, et al (Univ Hosp, Grenoble Cedex, France; et al)
Dis Colon Rectum 54:226-231, 2011

Background.—Doppler-guided hemorrhoidal artery ligation is a minimally invasive technique for the treatment of symptomatic hemorrhoids that has been applied successfully for grade II and III hemorrhoids but is less effective for grade IV hemorrhoids. Development of a special proctoscope enabled the combination of hemorrhoidal artery ligation with transanal rectoanal repair (mucopexy), which serves to lift and then secure the protruding hemorrhoids in place.

Objective.—The purpose of this study was to describe our experience with this combined procedure in the treatment of grade IV hemorrhoids.

Design.—Prospective observational study.

Setting.—Outpatient colorectal surgery unit.

Patients.—Consecutive patients with grade IV hemorrhoids treated from April 2006 to December 2008.

Intervention.—Hemorrhoidal artery ligation—rectoanal repair.

Main Outcome Measures.—Operating time, number of ligations, number of mucopexies and associated procedures, and postoperative symptoms were recorded. Pain was graded on a visual analog scale. Follow-up was at 2, 6, and 12 months after surgery, and then annually.

Results.—A total of 100 consecutive patients (64 women, 36 men) with grade IV hemorrhoids were included. Preoperative symptoms were bleeding in 80 and pain in 71 patients; 19 patients had undergone previous surgical treatment for the disease. The mean operative time was 35 (range, 17–60) minutes, with a mean of 9 (range, 4–14) ligations placed per patient. Eighty-four patients were discharged on the day of the operation. Nine patients developed early postoperative complications: pain in 6, bleeding in 4, dyschezia in 1, and thrombosis of residual hemorrhoids in 3. Late complications occurred in 4 patients and were managed conservatively. Recurrence was observed in 9 patients (9%), with a mean follow-up of 34 (range, 14–42) months.

Limitations.—The 2 main weaknesses of the study were the lack of very long-term follow-up and the absence of a comparison with hemorrhoidectomy or hemorrhoidopexy.

Conclusion.—Doppler-guided hemorrhoidal artery ligation with rectoanal repair is safe, easy to perform, and should be considered as an effective option for the treatment of grade IV hemorrhoids.

▶ I chose this to include manuscript because it highlights the role of Doppler-guided hemorrhoid artery (HA) ligation in the management of hemorrhoids, and it expands its use to Grade IV hemorrhoids. Although not terribly robust from the standpoint of scientific merit, it is important to be aware of this technique and work.

Hemorrhoids remain a common and vexing problem, afflicting nearly 10 million Americans. When medical and topical management fail, surgery is the only alternative. Historically, hemorrhoid surgery can be extremely painful and debilitating, especially when dealing with grade II (protruding) or grade IV (strangulated) hemorrhoids. The newest technique for surgically managing hemorrhoids in a more minimally invasive manner is Doppler-guided HA ligation. With this directed approach, the inflow can be ligated, obviating the need for an extensive dissection.

Everyone who sees or manages patients with hemorrhoids should be aware of this new technique. If your area surgeon is not offering this technique, suggest that he or she explore the possibility of offering Doppler-guided HA ligation.

C. D. Smith, MD

Impact of Nonresective Operations for Complicated Peptic Ulcer Disease in a High-Risk Population

Smith BR, Wilson SE (Univ of California Irvine Med Ctr, Long Beach; VA Long Beach Healthcare System, CA)
Am Surg 76:1143-1146, 2010

Over the past two decades, surgery for complicated peptic ulcer disease has evolved to a "less-is-more" approach due predominately to improved medical therapy. This study sought to determine whether a nonresective operative strategy has been an effective and prudent approach. A 20-year retrospective evaluation was conducted to compare outcomes of patients from the first decade (1990–1999) with those from the more recent decade (2000–2009). In all, 50 patients underwent surgery for complications of peptic ulcer disease, 36 in the early period and 14 in the later period, with 94 per cent being urgent or emergent. Acid-reducing procedures (vagotomy) decreased significantly from 29 to 7 over the two periods ($P = 0.04$), as did gastric resections from 23 to 3 ($P = 0.01$). The prevalence of *H. pylori* and use of NSAIDs both increased from 28 per cent to 36 per cent and 31 per cent to 43 per cent, respectively. Postoperative mortality remained unchanged, 22 per cent *vs* 7 per cent ($P = 0.41$) over the two periods. Resections and definitive acid-reducing procedures continue to decline with no increase in adverse outcomes. This more moderate operative approach to complicated peptic ulcer surgery is appropriate given the trend towards lower mortality and improved medical treatment. In our high-risk veteran population, overall perioperative mortality, length of stay, and reoperations have been reduced.

▶ This article provides some historic perspective to the surgical management of peptic ulcer disease. It is a retrospective analysis of a 20-year period at a single institution, looking at how peptic ulcer disease was managed operatively during the first 10 years versus the second 10 years. Perhaps not surprisingly, the authors found that in the 50 patients who underwent surgery for complications of peptic ulcer disease during the 20 years (36 in the early period and 14 in the later period), acid-reducing procedures (vagotomy) decreased significantly, as did gastric resections. The prevalence of *Helicobacter pylori* and the use of nonsteroidal antiinflammatory drugs both increased from the first 10 years to the second 10 years. Postoperative mortality remained unchanged.

This calls to mind a personal experience dating back to 1991, which is the beginning of the 20-year period of interest in this article. I was attending *Digestive Disease Week* (DDW) and standing in front of a poster detailing the technique and early outcomes of laparoscopic posterior truncal vagotomy and anterior highly selective vagotomy (Taylor procedure), including how this would be the cure for peptic ulcer disease and any surgeon who could offer this procedure would be overrun with referrals. As I was contemplating how to gain this new skill, a gastroenterologist friend tapped me on the shoulder and whispered, "don't bother; peptic ulcers will be cured with antisecretories and antibiotics," and off he went. I heeded the advice, and here we are today. I saw him at DDW last year and again thanked him for such good advice.

C. D. Smith, MD

Impaired Alcohol Metabolism after Gastric Bypass Surgery: A Case-Crossover Trial
Woodard GA, Downey J, Hernandez-Boussard T, et al (Stanford Univ School of Medicine, CA)
J Am Coll Surg 212:209-214, 2011

Background.—Severe obesity remains the leading public health crisis of the industrialized world, with bariatric surgery the only effective and enduring treatment. Poor psychological adjustment has been occasionally reported postoperatively. In addition, evidence suggests that patients can metabolize alcohol differently after gastric bypass.

Study Design.—Preoperatively and at 3 and 6 months postoperatively, 19 Roux-en-Y gastric bypass (RYGB) patients' breath alcohol content (BAC) was measured every 5 minutes after drinking 5 oz red wine to determine peak BAC and time until sober in a case-crossover design preoperatively and at 6 months postoperatively.

Results.—Patients reported symptoms experienced when intoxicated and answered a questionnaire of drinking habits. The peak BAC in patients after RYGB was considerably higher at 3 months (0.059%) and 6 months (0.088%) postoperatively than matched preoperative levels (0.024%). Patients also took considerably more time to return to sober at 3 months (61 minutes) and 6 months (88 minutes) than preoperatively (49 minutes). Postoperative intoxication was associated with lower levels of diaphoresis, flushing, and hyperactivity and higher levels of dizziness, warmth, and double vision. Postoperative patients reported drinking considerably less alcohol, fewer preferred beer, and more preferred wine than before surgery.

Conclusions.—This is the first study to match preoperative and postoperative alcohol metabolism in gastric bypass patients. Post-RYGB patients have much higher peak BAC after ingesting alcohol and require more time to become sober. Patients who drink alcohol after gastric bypass surgery should exercise caution.

▶ I thought this article should be reviewed because it provides some objective data that can be used by both patients and physicians. Specifically, this article evaluates alcohol metabolism in patients who have undergone Roux-en-Y gastric bypass for obesity.

Patients and many physicians have been under the impression that after any gastric reducing operation the absorption of alcohol is decreased (assumption has been that alcohol is absorbed mostly through the stomach). Those of us who take care of these patients know anecdotally that the post—gastric bypass patient can become intoxicated very quickly with alcohol ingestion and remain intoxicated for a longer-than-expected period. Most of this knowledge comes from patient stories of consuming a small amount of alcohol with subsequent unexpected results: stories of motor vehicle accidents, disturbing nights out, or acute illness.

Of course, we know that it is not just the stomach that absorbs alcohol, and the assumption that decreasing the size of the stomach would have no impact on alcohol absorption is unfounded. Additionally, there are other factors that might contribute to this phenomenon (eg, smaller capacity to consume anything, so alcohol consumption is not diluted by simultaneous ingestion of food).

The bottom line is that patients should be made aware of this occurrence and even see this article so that they understand and believe that they will get drunk much faster and require longer to sober up.

C. D. Smith, MD

Predictive value of procalcitonin for bowel ischemia and necrosis in bowel obstruction
Markogiannakis H, Memos N, Messaris E, et al (Univ of Athens, Greece)
Surgery 149:394-403, 2011

Background.—To our knowledge, the predictive value of procalcitonin for bowel strangulation has been evaluated in only 2 experimental studies that had conflicting results. The objective of this study was to evaluate the value of procalcitonin for early diagnosis of intestinal ischemia and necrosis in acute bowel obstruction.

Methods.—We performed a prospective study of 242 patients with small- or large-bowel obstructions in 2005. A total of 100 patients who underwent operation were divided into groups according to the presence of ischemia (reversible and irreversible) and necrosis, respectively, as follows: ischemia ($n = 35$) and nonischemia groups ($n = 65$) and necrosis ($n = 22$) and nonnecrosis groups ($n = 78$). Data analyzed included age, sex, vital signs, symptoms, clinical findings, white blood cell count, base deficit, metabolic acidosis, procalcitonin levels on presentation, the time between symptom onset and arrival at the emergency department and the time between arrival and operation, and the cause of the obstruction.

Results.—Procalcitonin levels were greater in the ischemia than the non-ischemia group (9.62 vs 0.30 ng/mL; $P = .0001$) and in the necrosis than the non-necrosis group (14.53 vs 0.32 ng/mL; $P = .0001$). Multivariate analysis identified procalcitonin as an independent predictor of ischemia ($P = .009$; odds ratio, 2.252; 95% confidence interval, 1.225-4.140) and necrosis ($P = .005$; odds ratio, 2.762; 95% confidence interval, 1.356-5.627). Using receiver operating characteristic (ROC) curve analysis, the area under the curve (AUC) of procalcitonin for ischemia and necrosis was 0.77 and 0.87, respectively. A high negative predictive value for ischemia and necrosis of procalcitonin levels <0.25 ng/mL (83% and

95%, respectively) and a positive predictive value of procalcitonin >1 ng/mL were identified (95% and 90%, respectively).

Conclusion.—Procalcitonin on presentation is very useful for the diagnosis or exclusion of intestinal ischemia and necrosis in acute bowel obstruction and could serve as an additional diagnostic tool to improve clinical decision-making.

▶ Bowel obstruction with strangulation remains one of the most common surgical emergencies managed by physicians and surgeons. Early diagnosis of bowel ischemia increases the likelihood that bowel necrosis or perforation can be avoided. When the management of bowel obstruction requires a bowel resection or management of perforation, the likelihood of morbidity and mortality is significantly increased. Currently, the decision about timing of surgery relies on surgeon judgment and a constellation of clinical and physical findings. At times, it boils down to following the old adage, "the sun should not set on a bowel obstruction." This dogma aims squarely at minimizing the likelihood of ischemic/necrotic bowel.

This article prospectively analyzed the potential for using elevated procalcitonin (PCT) levels to predict intestinal ischemia. This was a well-conceived and designed study. PCT on presentation at the emergency department was markedly greater in patients with ischemia compared with those without ischemia and in patients with necrosis compared with those without necrosis. The difference in PCT levels between these groups was of strong statistical significance. In addition, PCT was an independent predictor of ischemia and necrosis in the multivariate analysis. The overall predictive power of PCT was not extremely high, implying that PCT should not be considered as a substitute for careful clinical examination but as a useful additional parameter that could improve its accuracy.

With this we have another tool in our management of bowel obstruction to help guide the timing of surgical intervention, something important to anyone managing gastrointestinal conditions.

C. D. Smith, MD

Laparoscopic Repair of Paraesophageal Hernia: Long-term Follow-up Reveals Good Clinical Outcome Despite High Radiological Recurrence Rate
Dallemagne B, Kohnen L, Perretta S, et al (Univ Hosp of Strasbourg, France; Les Cliniques Saint-Joseph, Liege, Belgium)
Ann Surg 253:291-296, 2011

Objective.—The purpose of this report is to evaluate and compare the long-term objective and subjective outcome after laparoscopic paraesophageal hernia repair (LPHR).

Background.—Short-term symptomatic results of LPHR are often excellent. However, a high recurrence rate is detected at objective radiographic follow-up.

Methods.—Retrospective review of a prospectively gathered database of consecutive patients undergoing LPHR with and without reinforced crural repair at a single institution. Subjective and objective outcomes were assessed by using a structured symptoms questionnaire, Gastrointestinal Quality-of-Life Index, satisfaction score, and barium esophagogram.

Results.—From September 1991 to September 2005, LPHR was performed in 85 patients (median age, 66 years) with (25 patients) and without (60 patients) reinforced crural repair. Two patients (3%) underwent laparoscopic reoperation, for severe dysphagia and for symptomatic recurrence, respectively. Subjective outcome, available for 64 patients (75%), improved significantly at median follow-up of 118 months with a postoperative median Gastrointestinal Quality-of-Life Index score of 116. Radiographic recurrence (median follow-up, 99 months) occurred in 23 (66%) of the 35 patients, independently of age at operation, type of paresophageal hiatal hernias, and crural reinforcement, and showed no impact on quality of life.

Conclusions.—Although providing excellent symptomatic results, long-term objective evaluation of LPHR reveals a high recurrence rate even with reinforced cruroplasty. A tailored, lengthening gastroplasty and reinforced cruroplasty based on objective intraoperative evaluation, and not only on surgeon's personal judgment, may be the answer to recurrences.

▶ The authors report their long-term results in performing laparoscopic hiatal hernia repair between 1991 and 2005. Eighty-five patients underwent repair during this time, with 60 patients (70%) undergoing primary suture—only repair. The other 25 patients (30%) had the following: reinforcement with pledgets (18 patients), nonabsorbable composite prosthesis (6 patients), or biologic mesh (1 patient). There was long-term subjective follow-up in 75% of patients and radiologic follow-up in 54%. Median follow-up was 118 months.

This study confirmed what others have shown: Anatomic recurrence is common (66% of patients had a barium swallow revealing recurrent hiatal hernia). This is in stark contrast to the functional outcome, with 90% of patients satisfied with their outcome and most patients returning high symptom scores. New onset of dysphagia was not correlated with the finding of recurrence.

There are a few take-home messages here. First, I think most would agree that most hiatal hernias do not need to be fixed; it is the symptomatic hernias that are considered for surgical repair. Put simply, we do typically offer surgical repair for an asymptomatic hiatal hernia. With that background, it is not surprising that even with a high rate of recurrence, most patients achieve good outcomes with regard to the resolution of preoperative symptoms. This article reinforces the concept that failure after hiatal hernia repair should not be anatomic recurrence, but rather, symptomatic recurrence. With that definition of failure, laparoscopic hiatal hernia repair is very successful.

Another important take-home message is the issue of using mesh to fix hiatal hernia. Many surgeons have zealously pursued the elimination of anatomic recurrence by using mesh in most repairs. This has had a high cost, with some patients having spectacular failures when mesh is used, and some needing esophagectomy to correct problems. Although this article does not directly address this issue, it further establishes the success of nonmesh repair in providing correction of the patients' symptoms, which is the more important outcome for these patients.

C. D. Smith, MD

Impact of Surgeon Experience on 5-Year Outcome of Laparoscopic Nissen Fundoplication

Broeders JAJL, Draaisma WA, Rijnhart—de Jong HG, et al (Univ Med Ctr Utrecht, the Netherlands; et al)
Arch Surg 146:340-346, 2011

Objective.—To investigate the 5-year effect of surgeon experience with laparoscopic Nissen fundoplication (LNF). In 2000, a randomized controlled trial (RCT) was prematurely terminated because LNF for gastroesophageal reflux disease was associated with a higher risk to develop dysphagia than conventional Nissen fundoplication (CNF). Criticism focused on alleged bias caused by the relative lack of experience with the laparoscopic approach of the participating surgeons.

Design.—Multicenter RCT and prospective cohort study.

Setting.—University medical centers and tertiary teaching hospitals.

Patients.—In the RCT, 74 patients underwent CNF and 93 patients underwent LNF (LNFI). The complete setup of the cohort study (LNFII) (n = 121) mirrored the RCT, except that surgeon experience increased from more than 5 to more than 30 LNFs per surgeon.

Interventions.—Conventional Nissen fundoplication, LNFI, and LNFII.

Main Outcome Measures.—Intraoperative and inhospital characteristics, objective reflux control, and clinical outcome.

Results.—In LNFII, operating time (110 vs 165 minutes; $P < .001$), dysphagia (2.5% vs 12.3%; $P = .008$), dilatations for dysphagia (0.8% vs 7.0%; $P = .02$), and conversions (3.5% vs 7.7%; $P = .19$) were reduced compared with LNFI. Moreover, in LNFII, hospitalization (4.2 vs 5.6 days; $P = .07$ and 4.2 vs 7.6 days; $P < .001$) and in-hospital complications (5.1% vs 13.5%; $P = .046$ and 5.1% vs 19.3%; $P = .005$) were reduced compared with LNFI and CNF, respectively. In LNFII, the 6-month reintervention rate was reduced compared with LNFI (0.8% vs 10.1%; $P = .002$). Esophagitis and esophageal acid exposure at 3 months and reflux symptoms, proton-pump inhibitor use, and quality of life at 5 years improved similarly.

Conclusions.—Operating time, complications, hospitalization, early dysphagia, dilatations for dysphagia, and reintervention rate after LNF improve significantly when surgeon experience increases from more than 5 to more than 30 LNFs. In contrast, short-term objective reflux control and 5-year clinical outcome do not improve with experience. In experienced hands, LNF reduces inhospital complications and hospitalization compared with CNF, with similar 5-year effectiveness and reoperation rate.

▶ Experience matters when performing antireflux surgery! Whereas those of us who have been offering antireflux surgery for the past 10 to 15 years have intuitively known this, studies with data to support it are scarce. This is one of those studies, and the authors nicely document that outcomes after laparoscopic Nissen fundoplication (LNF) are better when the surgeon has experience with more than 30 procedures.

This study is an extension of an earlier prospective randomized controlled trial (PRCT) comparing LNF with conventional (open) Nissen fundoplication (CNF). This earlier study was terminated early when findings revealed a higher rate of dysphagia after LNF than CNF. Concern regarding the experience of the surgeons performing LNF was proffered as the reason for the difference.

The authors nicely demonstrate that short-term outcomes are superior when an LNF is performed by a surgeon with experience of more than 30 LNFs. In nearly all measures, results were superior with the more experienced surgeons (operating time, complications, hospitalization, early dysphagia, dilatations for dysphagia, and reintervention rate after LNF improve significantly when surgeon experience increases from more than 5 to more than 30).

The commentary at the end of this article warrants reading. The commentator suggests that antireflux surgery should be centralized to centers where experienced surgeons can consistently deliver these good outcomes. This is in stark contrast to how LNF was initially introduced in the early 1990s. At that time, surgeons were trained in weekend courses and told that the procedure was simple to perform, and patients were told they would experience immediate and dramatic results (positive) from this new procedure. This, combined with the prospective randomized controlled trials of Nissen versus medical management showing that surgery was superior, resulted in a stampede of patients seeking this new procedure. It wasn't until nearly a decade later that long-term follow-up data and newer PRCTs (including the one in this study) raised significant doubts about LNF effectiveness. A long-standing dictum of surgery is nicely confirmed through this narrative: Outcome = patient selection and surgical technique. Extending that further, good surgical technique requires experience!

C. D. Smith, MD

Impact of endoscopic assessment and treatment on operative and non-operative management of acute oesophageal perforation
Kuppusamy MK, Felisky C, Kozarek RA, et al (Virginia Mason Med Ctr, Seattle, WA)
Br J Surg 98:818-824, 2011

Background.—Surgeons have not typically utilized an endoscopic approach for diagnosis and management of acute oesophageal perforation, mainly due to fears of increased mediastinal contamination. This study assessed the evolution of endoscopic approaches and their effect on outcomes over time in acute oesophageal perforation.

Methods.—All patients with documented acute oesophageal perforation between 1990 and 2009 were enrolled prospectively in an Institutional Review Board-approved database.

Results.—Of 81 patients who presented during the study period, 52 had upper gastrointestinal endoscopy for diagnosis alone (12 patients; 23 per cent) or as a component of acute management (40 patients; 77 per cent). Use of endoscopy increased from four of 13 patients in the first 5 years of the study to 20 of 24 patients in the final 5 years. Endoscopy was used in conjunction with surgery in 28 patients, of whom 21 underwent primary repair, three had resection, and one a diversion; 12 patients in this group had hybrid operations (combination of surgical and endoscopic management). Primary endoscopic treatment was used in 15 patients (29 per cent), most commonly involving stent placement (7). Of those having endoscopy, complication rates improved (from 3 of 4 to 8 of 20 patients), as did mean length of stay (from 21·8 to 13·4 days) between the initial and final 5 years of the study. There were two deaths (4 per cent). Of 21 patients who had both endoscopic assessment and management in the operating room, endoscopy identified additional pathology in ten, leading to a change in management plan in five patients.

Conclusion.—Endoscopy is a safe and important component of the management of acute oesophageal perforation. It provides additional information that modifies treatment, and its wider use should result in improved outcomes.

▶ I chose this article because it highlights the changing perspectives of surgeons regarding the use of endoscopy to manage what has been traditionally considered a surgical condition, acute esophageal perforation. Most of us who trained over 20 years ago saw many examples of esophageal perforation in which, even with immediate and aggressive surgical management, patients did not do well. Acute esophageal perforation was one of the most dreaded conditions seen in transfers from other hospitals, with patients typically not doing well or requiring extensive debridement and diversion, leading to long and complicated recovery.

This article looks at a nearly 20-year period at a single institution analyzing the management and outcomes of all patients with acute esophageal perforation. From 1990 through 2009, 81 patients underwent care for acute esophageal perforation. The authors found that the use of endoscopy increased during the period analyzed, as did the role of endoscopy, with little use seen early in the series, evolving into mostly diagnostic use, and eventually use in conjunction with surgery, both therapeutically and to help identify additional pathology unrecognized with surgery alone.

The data from this article nicely reflect the growth and maturation of flexible upper endoscopy, and also the convergence of gastrointestinal (GI) surgery and GI endoscopy to the joint management of upper GI conditions. It also outlines a nice algorithm for the management of acute GI perforation. Some techniques are described for doing concomitant surgery/endoscopy to evaluate the extent of injury and use combined therapeutic approaches.

The one criticism I feel compelled to reveal relates to these data having been published in 2 different journals.[1] The publication in this journal (*British Journal of Surgery*) is under the banner of "Original Article," yet it appears that these same data were presented before this publication at a meeting that subsequently resulted in another publication of these same data (eg, 81 patients are described in both publications along with the same decision tree). So, you can find the results from this work in either the publication referenced here or the reference below. I have reviewed both and would recommend either.

C. D. Smith, MD

Reference

1. Kuppusamy MK, Hubka M, Felisky CD, et al. Evolving management strategies in esophageal perforation: surgeons using nonoperative techniques to improve outcomes. *J Am Coll Surg.* 2011;213:164-171.

Total or Posterior Partial Fundoplication in the Treatment of GERD: Results of a Randomized Trial After 2 Decades of Follow-up
Mardani J, Lundell L, Engström C (Sahlgrenska Univ Hosp, Gothenburg, Sweden; Karolinska Univ Hosp, Stockholm, Sweden)
Ann Surg 253:875-878, 2011

Objective and Background.—We lack long-term data (>10 years) on the efficacy of antireflux surgery when evaluated within the framework of randomized clinical trials. Hereby we report the outcome of a randomized trial comparing open total (I) and a Toupet posterior partial fundoplication (II) performed between 1983 and 1991.

Methods.—One hundred and thirty-seven patients with gastroesophageal reflux disease and were enrolled into the study. The mean follow up has now reached 18 years. During these years 26% had died and 16% were unable to trace for follow up. Symptom outcomes were assessed by the use of validated self-reporting questionnaires.

Results.—Long-term control of heartburn and acid regurgitation (reported as no or mild symptoms) were reported by 80% and 82% after a total fundoplication (I) and corresponding figures were 87% and 90% after a partial posterior fundoplication (II), respectively (n.s.).

The dysphagia scores were low 4.6 ± 1.3 (SEM) in group I and 3.3 ± 0.9 (SEM) in group II (n.s). The point prevalences of rectal flatulence and gas distension related complaints were of similar magnitude in the 2 groups. Twenty-three percentage of the patients in the total fundoplication group noted some ability to vomit compared with 31% in the partial posterior fundoplication group.

Conclusions.—Both a total and a partial posterior fundoplication maintain a high level of reflux control after 2 decades of follow up. The previously reported differences in mechanical side effects, in favor of the partial wrap, seemed to disappear over time.

▶ This article from Sweden documents long-term (18 years) outcomes in patients who underwent either a total, 3600 fundoplication (Nissen), or partial, 2700 fundoplication (Toupet), as part of a randomized trial. From 1983 to 1991, 72 patients were randomized to 3600 fundoplication and 65 to 2700 fundoplication. Long-term follow-up data were available in 34 3600 fundoplication patients (47%) and 39 2700 fundoplication patients (60%). The authors found good reflux control in both groups (80% to 90%), regardless of the type of wrap, and similar side-effect patterns in both groups. Specifically, they note that any difference in side effects (dysphagia, gas bloat, ability to regurgitate) between the 2 procedures vanishes over time.

This work is important for a few reasons:

1. There has long been a debate as to which antireflux procedure is better: the Toupet partial fundoplication or the Nissen total fundoplication. Proponents of the Toupet claim good control of reflux with a lower rate of early dysphagia and an ability to belch and vomit, thereby minimizing the vexing side effects of gas bloat. Proponents of the Nissen claim superior control of reflux, and even quote failure rates for the Toupet of 25% to 30%, and acceptable rates of gas bloat as long as a "floppy" wrap is done. Each group can find data in the literature to support either position. This article puts the debate to rest. Both procedures produce good control of gastroesophageal reflux disease (GERD) with side-effect profiles that resolve over time. From the article itself, "The main messages from this prospective, randomized trial, with a unique duration of follow-up, are that a high level of GERD control can be maintained by both the total and posterior partial fundoplication operations. Moreover, the previously observed advantage of a Toupet posterior partial repair, in the form of fewer mechanical side effects, seemed to disappear over time."

2. These data are from a prospective randomized trial from a country known to achieve good long-term patient care and follow-up. We tend to put more credibility in studies from the Netherlands, where socialized medicine has been in place for decades, and good long-term population-based data can be obtained and analyzed.

3. There have been claims that antireflux procedures in the form of fundoplication fail at a high rate. In my own practice, I see patients with horrible GERD (esophagitis, Barrett and associated hiatal hernia) who are told to get a surgical opinion about management, but be aware that "50% will fail in just a few years." I wish I could say this was a rare exception, but regrettably, many patients are left with the impression that failure of surgery is inevitable. This article confirms much higher success rates with antireflux surgery.

All that said, there are some things to highlight. Mainly, these were open procedures. Prior to laparoscopy, the few antireflux operations being performed were done in centers with considerable experience, and the open techniques were fairly standardized and generally well executed. When laparoscopic antireflux procedures arrived, the number of patients undergoing surgery dramatically increased, as did the number of surgeons performing the procedures.

We saw a significant dilution in the quality and consistency of the procedures being performed, and therefore a decrease in the successful outcomes, likely a lower number than found in this study.

Fortunately, there has been a consolidation in the number of surgeons offering antireflux surgery, and a corresponding improvement in the quality and consistency of the outcomes. This article again clearly documents that patients can get good results from antireflux surgery. Choose your surgeon and patients carefully.

C. D. Smith, MD

8 Liver Disease

Viral Hepatitis

Noninvasive Tests for Fibrosis and Liver Stiffness Predict 5-Year Outcomes of Patients With Chronic Hepatitis C

Vergniol J, Foucher J, Terrebonne E, et al (Hôpital Haut-Lévêque, Pessac, France; et al)
Gastroenterology 140:1970-1979, 2011

Background & Aims.—Liver stiffness can be measured noninvasively to assess liver fibrosis in patients with chronic hepatitis C. In patients with chronic liver diseases, level of fibrosis predicts liver-related complications and survival. We evaluated the abilities of liver stiffness, results from noninvasive tests for fibrosis, and liver biopsy analyses to predict overall survival or survival without liver-related death with a 5-year period.

Methods.—In a consecutive cohort of 1457 patients with chronic hepatitis C, we assessed fibrosis and, on the same day, liver stiffness, performed noninvasive tests of fibrosis (FibroTest, the aspartate aminotransferase to platelet ratio index, FIB-4), and analyzed liver biopsy samples. We analyzed data on death, liver-related death, and liver transplantation collected during a 5-year follow-up period.

Results.—At 5 years, 77 patients had died (39 liver-related deaths) and 16 patients had undergone liver transplantation. Overall survival was 91.7% and survival without liver-related death was 94.4%. Survival was significantly decreased among patients diagnosed with severe fibrosis, regardless of the noninvasive method of analysis. All methods were able to predict shorter survival times in this large population; liver stiffness and results of FibroTest had higher predictive values. Patient outcomes worsened as liver stiffness and FibroTest values increased. Prognostic values of stiffness ($P < .0001$) and FibroTest results ($P < .0001$) remained after they were adjusted for treatment response, patient age, and estimates of necroinflammatory grade.

Conclusions.—Noninvasive tests for liver fibrosis (measurement of liver stiffness or FibroTest) can predict 5-year survival of patients with chronic hepatitis C. These tools might help physicians determine prognosis at earlier stages and discuss specific treatments, such as liver transplantation.

▶ The evaluation of extent of liver fibrosis is important in the management of patients with chronic liver disease. It is a deciding factor in consideration of

231

the need to screen patients for complications of significant fibrosis, such as hepatocellular cancer and complications of portal hypertension, such as varices. Until recently, the only measure of liver fibrosis was liver biopsy. Liver biopsy is invasive and carries significant risk of complications. In addition, there can be bias in sampling variability. For these reasons, a noninvasive measure of liver fibrosis would be beneficial in patient management.

Liver stiffness measurement using a FibroScan probe has been shown to have a high degree of accuracy and reproducibility in predicting significant fibrosis in patients with chronic liver disease. Noninvasive markers, such as FibroTest, have been shown to be a surrogate marker of fibrosis and show a correlation with survival in patients with chronic liver disease. The aim of this study was to evaluate the 5-year prognostic value of noninvasive markers of liver fibrosis for predicting survival and liver-related death in patients with chronic hepatitis C virus (HCV) infection.

The results of this study independently validated the prognostic value of FibroTest and showed that markers of liver stiffness and FibroTest both predicted survival in patients with chronic HCV infection.

D. M. Harnois, DO

Hepatitis B Virus Infection and Risk of Intrahepatic Cholangiocarcinoma and Non-Hodgkin Lymphoma: A Cohort Study of Parous Women in Taiwan
Fwu C-W, Chien Y-C, You S-L, et al (Johns Hopkins Univ Bloomberg School of Public Health, Baltimore, MD; Natl Taiwan Univ, Taipei; et al)
Hepatology 53:1217-1225, 2011

Few studies have evaluated the risk of cancers other than hepatocellular carcinoma associated with hepatitis B virus (HBV) infection. This study aimed to estimate incidence rates of intrahepatic cholangiocarcinoma (ICC) and non-Hodgkin lymphoma (NHL) and its major subtypes in a nationwide cohort of parous women and to assess their associations with chronic HBV infection. We conducted a cohort study including 1,782,401 pregnant Taiwanese women whose HBV serostatus was obtained from the National Hepatitis B Vaccination Registry. Newly diagnosed ICCs and NHLs were ascertained through data linkage with the National Cancer Registry. Risks of ICC and NHL were assessed using Cox proportional hazards regression models. After a mean of 6.91 years of follow-up, there were 18 cases of ICC and 192 cases of NHL, including 99 cases of diffuse large B-cell lymphoma (DLBCL). Incidence rates of ICC were 0.09 and 0.43 per 100,000 person-years, respectively, among women who were hepatitis B surface antigen (HBsAg)-seronegative and HBsAg-seropositive, showing an age-adjusted hazard ratio (HR_{adj}) (95% confidence interval [CI]) of 4.80 (1.88-12.20). The incidence rates of NHL overall for HBsAg-seronegative and HBsAg-seropositive women were 1.23 and 3.18 per 100,000 person-years, respectively, with an HR_{adj} (95% CI) of 2.63 (1.95-3.54). Among NHL subtypes, HBsAg-seropositive women had an increased risk of DLBCL compared with those who were HBsAg-seronegative (incidence rates: 1.81 and 0.60 per 100,000 person-years, respectively; HR_{adj} [95% CI]: 3.09 [2.06-4.64]). The significantly increased risk was not observed for other specific subtypes of NHL.

Conclusions.—Chronic HBV infection was associated with an increased risk of ICC and DLBCL in women. Our data suggested a possible etiological role of HBV in the development of ICC and specific subtypes of NHL.

▶ The association of hepatitis B virus (HBV) infection in the etiology of hepatocellular cancer (HCC) has been well described. Several epidemiology studies have proposed an association of cholangiocarcinoma (CCA) and HBV infection.

The population in this study, conducted in Taiwan, included only parous women screened in a national vaccination program for HBV. Investigators report that HBV infection was associated with an increased risk of intrahepatic CCA in women. In addition, there was an increased risk of non-Hodgkin lymphoma (NHL)/diffuse large B-cell lymphoma in patients infected with HBV.

Still larger population-based studies are necessary to understand the impact of HBV infection in CCA and NHL. There may be a benefit to vaccination programs for HBV in reducing the rate of future CCA.

D. M. Harnois, DO

Interleukin-28B Polymorphisms Are Associated With Histological Recurrence and Treatment Response Following Liver Transplantation in Patients With Hepatitis C Virus Infection

Charlton MR, Thompson A, Veldt BJ, et al (Mayo Clinic, Rochester, MN; Duke Univ Med Ctr, Durham, NC)
Hepatology 53:317-324, 2011

Polymorphism in the *interleukin-28B* (*IL28B*) gene region, encoding interferon (IFN)-λ3, is strongly predictive of response to antiviral treatment in the nontransplant setting. We sought to determine the prevalence and impact on clinical outcomes of donor and recipient *IL28B* genotypes among liver transplant recipients. The cohort study included 189 consecutive patients infected with hepatitis C virus (HCV) who underwent liver transplantation between January 1, 1995, and January 1, 2005, at the Mayo Clinic, Rochester, MN. Genotyping of the polymorphism rs12979860 was performed on DNA collected from all donors and recipients in the cohort. Sixty-five patients received IFN-based antiviral therapy. The CC *IL28B* variant was less common in the chronic HCV-infected recipients than in non-HCV donor livers (33% versus 47%, $P = 0.03$). *IL28B* recipient genotype was significantly predictive of fibrosis stage, with TT genotype being associated with more rapid fibrosis (Pearson chi-quare $P = 0.024$ for the comparison G versus A). Donor and recipient *IL28B* genotype were independently associated with sustained virologic response ($P < 0.005$). The presence of *IL28B* CC variant in either the recipient (R) or donor (D) liver was associated with increased rate of sustained virologic response (D-non-CC/R-non-CC = 3/19 [16%] versus D-CC/R-non-CC = 11/22 [50%] versus D-non-CC/R-CC = 5/12 [42%] versus R-CC/DCC = 6/7 [86%], $P = 0.0095$). *IL28B* genotype was not significantly associated with survival (overall/liver-related).

Conclusion.—Recipient *IL28B* TT genotype is associated with more severe histological recurrence of HCV. Recipient and donor liver *IL28B* genotype are strongly and independently associated with IFN-based treatment response in patients after orthotopic liver transplantation. The data suggest that CC donor livers might be preferentially allocated to patients with HCV infection.

▶ Chronic hepatitis C virus (HCV) infection is the most common indication for liver transplantation in the Western world. Recurrence of HCV infection is a common cause of graft loss following liver transplantation. Treatment response, as measured by sustained virologic response (SVR), to pegylated interferon and ribavirin is lower in patients treated after liver transplantation than in nontransplant patients.

The genetic variability in the region of the *IL28B* gene on chromosome 19 has been strongly associated with spontaneous viral clearance and treatment response (SVR) in patients with genotype 1 HCV infection treated with pegylated interferon and ribavirin. The 3 *IL28B* genotypes are CC, CT, and TT. The CC genotype has a more favorable treatment response rate in nontransplant patients chronically infected with HCV. The impact of *IL28B* polymorphism in HCV recurrence after liver transplantation has not been previously investigated.

Investigators in this study performed a retrospective analysis of liver transplant patients in which both the recipient and donor liver DNA were tested for *IL28B* genotype. Interestingly, both recipient and donor liver *IL28B* genotype were independently associated with interferon-based treatment response after the liver transplant. In addition, the data suggested that recipient *IL28B* TT genotype was associated with a more rapid histologic recurrence of HCV. These data suggest that recipient and donor HCV *IL28B* genotype should be considered in making decisions about donor allocation in patients with HCV.

D. M. Harnois, DO

Boceprevir for Previously Treated Chronic HCV Genotype 1 Infection
Bacon BR, for the HCV RESPOND-2 Investigators (Saint Louis Univ School of Medicine, MO; et al)
N Engl J Med 364:1207-1217, 2011

Background.—In patients with chronic infection with hepatitis C virus (HCV) genotype 1 who do not have a sustained response to therapy with peginterferon—ribavirin, outcomes after retreatment are suboptimal. Boceprevir, a protease inhibitor that binds to the HCV nonstructural 3 (NS3) active site, has been suggested as an additional treatment.

Methods.—To assess the effect of the combination of boceprevir and peginterferon—ribavirin for retreatment of patients with chronic HCV genotype 1 infection, we randomly assigned patients (in a 1:2:2 ratio) to one of three groups. In all three groups, peginterferon alfa-2b and ribavirin were administered for 4 weeks (the lead-in period). Subsequently, group 1 (control group) received placebo plus peginterferon—ribavirin for 44 weeks; group 2 received boceprevir plus peginterferon—ribavirin for 32 weeks, and patients with a detectable HCV RNA level at week 8 received placebo plus peginterferon—ribavirin for an additional 12 weeks; and group 3 received boceprevir plus peginterferon—ribavirin for 44 weeks.

Results.—A total of 403 patients were treated. The rate of sustained virologic response was significantly higher in the two boceprevir groups (group 2, 59%; group 3, 66%) than in the control group (21%, P<0.001). Among patients with an undetectable HCV RNA level at week 8, the rate of sustained virologic response was 86% after 32 weeks of triple therapy and 88% after 44 weeks of triple therapy. Among the 102 patients with a decrease in the HCV RNA level of less than 1 $\log_{10}$ IU per milliliter at treatment week 4, the rates of sustained virologic response were 0%, 33%, and 34% in groups 1, 2, and 3, respectively. Anemia was significantly more common in the boceprevir groups than in the control group, and erythropoietin was administered in 41 to 46% of boceprevir-treated patients and 21% of controls.

Conclusions.—The addition of boceprevir to peginterferon—ribavirin resulted in significantly higher rates of sustained virologic response in previously treated patients with chronic HCV genotype 1 infection, as compared with peginterferon—ribavirin alone. (Funded by Schering-Plough [now Merck]; HCV RESPOND-2 ClinicalTrials.gov number, NCT00708500.)

▶ Chronic hepatitis C virus (HCV) infection affects more than 170 million people worldwide. The current standard of treatment with pegylated interferon and ribavirin results in a rate of sustained virologic response of less than 50% among patients with HCV genotype 1. Recent efforts have focused on the development of a new group of orally administered drugs directly acting against HCV.

Boceprevir is a serine protease inhibitor that binds reversibly to the HCV nonstructural 3 active site. Boceprevir must be given in combination with pegylated interferon and ribavirin to minimize the emergence of viral resistance.

In this *New England Journal of Medicine* article, the results of the Retreatment with Serine Protease Inhibitor Boceprevir and Pegintron/Rebetol 2 trial are reported. This trial examined the addition of boceprevir to pegylated interferon and ribavirin in the retreatment of patients who are infected with HCV genotype 1.

The addition of boceprevir to standard therapy improved sustained virologic response (SVR) in previously treated patients infected with genotype 1 HCV. Those patients who relapsed after standard therapy had the most improvement in SVR as opposed to those that did not respond to therapy. Those patients responding to therapy with undetectable HCV RNA at treatment week 8 may even be treated with a shorter course of therapy (32 weeks rather than

44 weeks). The response rate was even improved in some groups of patients less likely to respond, such as black patients and those with more advanced liver disease.

The use of protease inhibitors in combination with standard therapy will now be the new standard of care for the treatment of people infected with HCV genotype 1, and many patients who previously failed pegylated interferon and ribavirin therapy may benefit from the addition of these newer therapies.

D. M. Harnois, DO

Management of hepatitis C virus genotype 4: Recommendations of An International Expert Panel

Khattab MA, Ferenci P, Hadziyannis SJ, et al (Univ of Minia, Egypt; Med Univ, Vienna, Austria; Henry Dunant Hosp, Athens, Greece; et al)
J Hepatol 54:1250-1262, 2011

HCV has been classified into no fewer than six major genotypes and a series of subtypes. Each HCV genotype is unique with respect to its nucleotide sequence, geographic distribution, and response to therapy. Genotypes 1, 2, and 3 are common throughout North America and Europe. HCV genotype 4 (HCV-4) is common in the Middle East and in Africa, where it is responsible for more than 80% of HCV infections. It has recently spread to several European countries. HCV-4 is considered a major cause of chronic hepatitis, cirrhosis, hepatocellular carcinoma, and liver transplantation in these regions. Although HCV-4 is the cause of approximately 20% of the 170 million cases of chronic hepatitis C in the world, it has not been the subject of widespread research. Therefore, this document, drafted by a panel of international experts, aimed to review current knowledge on the epidemiology, natural history, clinical, histological features, and treatment of HCV-4 infections.

▶ Hepatitis C virus (HCV) is classified into 6 major genotypes. Each genotype has a unique nucleotide sequence and response to therapy. Genotypes 1, 2, and 3 are common throughout North America and Europe, whereas genotype 4 is common in the Middle East and Africa. It is estimated that 34 million people are infected with HCV genotype 4. Although there is a large amount of literature on the HCV genotypes common in Europe and North America, there have been few studies looking specifically at genotype 4. This article is a comprehensive review of the studies conducted in genotype 4 HCV. The article reviews the results of treatment trials to date and provides recommendations for response-guided therapy and management. HCV genotype 4 is becoming common in Europe and will likely become more common in the United States as well. It is important for physicians to become aware of this genotype and its unique features and response to treatment.

D. M. Harnois, DO

Excess Mortality in Patients with Advanced Chronic Hepatitis C Treated with Long-Term Peginterferon
Di Bisceglie AM, for the HALT-C Trial Group (Saint Louis Univ School of Medicine, MO; et al)
Hepatology 53:1100-1108, 2011

Chronic hepatitis C virus infection can cause chronic liver disease, cirrhosis and liver cancer. The Hepatitis C Antiviral Long-term Treatment against Cirrhosis (HALT-C) Trial was a prospective, randomized controlled study of long-term, low-dose peginterferon therapy in patients with advanced chronic hepatitis C who failed to respond to a previous course of optimal antiviral therapy. The aim of this follow-up analysis is to describe the frequency and causes of death among this cohort of patients. Deaths occurring during and after the HALT-C Trial were reviewed by a committee of investigators to determine the cause of death and to categorize each death as liver- or nonliver-related and as related or not to complications of peginterferon. Rates of liver transplantation were also assessed. Over a median of 5.7 years, 122 deaths occurred among 1,050 randomized patients (12%), of which 76 were considered liver-related (62%) and 46 nonliver-related (38%); 74 patients (7%) underwent liver transplantation. At 7 years the cumulative mortality rate was higher in the treatment compared to the control group (20% versus 15%, $P = 0.049$); the primary difference in mortality was in patients in the fibrosis compared to the cirrhosis stratum (14% versus 7%, $P = 0.01$); comparable differences were observed when liver transplantation was included. Excess mortality, emerging after 3 years of treatment, was related largely to nonliver-related death; liver-related mortality was similar in the treatment and control groups. No specific cause of death accounted for the excess mortality and only one death was suspected to be a direct complication of peginterferon.

Conclusion.—Long-term maintenance peginterferon in patients with advanced chronic hepatitis C is associated with an excess overall mortality, which was primarily due to nonliver-related causes among patients with bridging fibrosis.

▶ Hepatitis C virus infection is an important cause of chronic liver disease. Beginning in 2000, the Hepatitis C Antiviral Long-term Treatment against Cirrhosis trial sought to answer the question of the benefit of low-dose maintenance therapy with peginterferon compared with no therapy in slowing progression of liver disease and preventing complications of end-stage liver disease. The trial ended in 2007 and failed to show a benefit of long-term interferon on clinical outcomes. In fact, an increase in mortality was seen in the group treated with interferon with advanced fibrosis but not cirrhosis. This study sought to more completely understand the explanation for that increased mortality rate.

The finding of higher mortality rates observed in the patients treated with pegylated interferon persisted when analyzed with a longer follow-up. The excess mortality did not begin to rise until after 3 years into the treatment and continued for several years after treatment was stopped. Nonetheless, a thorough review of the causes of death in these patients failed to identify a direct relationship as we currently understand it between the death rate and pegylated interferon therapy.

This study provides additional evidence that the use of long-term pegylated interferon therapy should be avoided or, at a minimum, be used cautiously.

D. M. Harnois, DO

Peginterferon plus Adefovir versus Either Drug Alone for Hepatitis Delta
Wedemeyer H, for the HIDIT Study Group (Hannover Med School, Germany; et al)
N Engl J Med 364:322-331, 2011

Background.—Chronic infection with hepatitis B virus and hepatitis delta virus (HDV) results in the most severe form of viral hepatitis. There is no currently approved treatment. We investigated the safety and efficacy of 48 weeks of treatment with peginterferon alfa-2a plus adefovir dipivoxil, peginterferon alfa-2a alone, and adefovir dipivoxil alone.

Methods.—We conducted a randomized trial in which 31 patients with HDV infection received treatment with 180 μg of peginterferon alfa-2a weekly plus 10 mg of adefovir daily, 29 received 180 μg of peginterferon alfa-2a weekly plus placebo, and 30 received 10 mg of adefovir alone weekly for 48 weeks. Follow-up was conducted for an additional 24 weeks. Efficacy end points included clearance of HDV RNA, normalization of alanine aminotransferase levels, and a decline in levels of hepatitis B surface antigen (HBsAg).

Results.—The primary end point — normalization of alanine aminotransferase levels and clearance of HDV RNA at week 48 — was achieved in two patients in the group receiving peginterferon alfa-2a plus adefovir and two patients in the group receiving peginterferon alfa-2a plus placebo but in none of the patients in the group receiving adefovir alone. At week 48, the test for HDV RNA was negative in 23% of patients in the first group, 24% of patients in the second, and none of those in the third (P = 0.006 for the comparison of the first and third groups; P = 0.004 for the comparison of the second and third). The efficacy of peginterferon alfa-2a was sustained for 24 weeks after treatment, with 28% of the patients receiving peginterferon alfa-2a plus adefovir or peginterferon alfa-2a alone having negative results on HDV-RNA tests; none of the patients receiving adefovir alone had negative results. A decline in HBsAg levels of more than 1 $\log_{10}$ IU per milliliter from baseline to week 48 was observed in 10 patients in the first group, 2 in the second, and none in the third (P<0.001 for the comparison of the first and third groups and P = 0.01 for the comparison of the first and second).

Conclusions.—Treatment with peginterferon alfa-2a for 48 weeks, with or without adefovir, resulted in sustained HDV RNA clearance in about one quarter of patients with HDV infection. (Funded by Hep-Net [the German Network of Excellence on Viral Hepatitis] and others; Current Controlled Trials number, ISRCTN83587695.)

▶ Hepatitis delta virus (HDV) is an RNA virus that requires coinfection with hepatitis B virus (HBV) to replicate. The HDV genome is encapsidated by the surface antigen of the HBV. In patients who carry HBV, HDV coinfection can result in a fulminant acute hepatitis or a severe chronic hepatitis. There are currently no approved therapies for HDV. Previously tested oral agents including lamivudine, ribavirin, and famcyclovir are ineffective.

Using a large German-based network of physicians treating patients with viral hepatitis, the investigators were able to perform a randomized trial of 31 patients with HDV infection. Treatment with peginterferon alfa-2a for 48 weeks, with or without adefovir, resulted in a sustained HDV RNA clearance in approximately 25% of patients. No patients treated with adefovir alone achieved clearance of the virus. Patients were treated for a total of 48 weeks. It is uncertain if patients who were slower to initially respond to therapy may have benefited from additional therapy. There was 1 patient in the trial who developed hepatic decompensation on therapy, and that was a patient with thrombocytopenia initially (baseline platelet count of 74 000 per cubic millimeter). For this reason, the authors recommend caution in the use of peginterferon alfa-2a therapy for patients with platelet counts below 90 000 per cubic millimeter.

D. M. Harnois, DO

Outcomes of Treatment for Hepatitis C Virus Infection by Primary Care Providers
Arora S, Thornton K, Murata G, et al (Univ of New Mexico, Albuquerque; et al)
N Engl J Med 364:2199-2207, 2011

Background.—The Extension for Community Healthcare Outcomes (ECHO) model was developed to improve access to care for underserved populations with complex health problems such as hepatitis C virus (HCV) infection. With the use of video-conferencing technology, the ECHO program trains primary care providers to treat complex diseases.

Methods.—We conducted a prospective cohort study comparing treatment for HCV infection at the University of New Mexico (UNM) HCV clinic with treatment by primary care clinicians at 21 ECHO sites in rural areas and prisons in New Mexico. A total of 407 patients with chronic HCV infection who had received no previous treatment for the infection were enrolled. The primary end point was a sustained virologic response.

Results.—A total of 57.5% of the patients treated at the UNM HCV clinic (84 of 146 patients) and 58.2% of those treated at ECHO sites (152 of 261 patients) had a sustained viral response (difference in rates between sites, 0.7 percentage points; 95% confidence interval, −9.2 to 10.7; P = 0.89). Among patients with HCV genotype 1 infection, the rate of sustained viral response was 45.8% (38 of 83 patients) at the UNM HCV clinic and 49.7% (73 of 147 patients) at ECHO sites (P = 0.57). Serious adverse events occurred in 13.7% of the patients at the UNM HCV clinic and in 6.9% of the patients at ECHO sites.

Conclusions.—The results of this study show that the ECHO model is an effective way to treat HCV infection in underserved communities. Implementation of this model would allow other states and nations to treat a greater number of patients infected with HCV than they are currently able to treat. (Funded by the Agency for Healthcare Research and Quality and others.)

▶ There is no question that, in the future, the structure of the medical system will look very different than it does today. Technology will provide a framework for greater data acquisition and potentially for sharing of information and expertise in ways never dreamed possible.

In the United States, there have been many articles written regarding the discrepancies in health care delivery among various populations. In particular, those people in underserved areas do not have access to many of the same treatments that are available in cities or in academic medical centers. Occasionally, this is an issue of technology, but sometimes it is simply a limitation of expertise and support for otherwise affordable treatments.

In the United States, it is estimated that a minimum of 3.2 million individuals are infected with the hepatitis C virus (HCV). Chronic hepatitis C accounts for 10 000 deaths per year in the United States and is the leading reason for liver transplantation. It is also clear that many patients who qualify for HCV treatment do not receive that treatment. There are many reasons why that is true, but in underserved areas, it is, in part, related to lack of specialty-care physicians in these communities.

In this article from *The New England Journal of* Medicine, a new model for health care delivery is reported. The ECHO model (Extension for Community Healthcare Outcomes) was developed to link the expertise of physicians at the University of New Mexico with patients at primary care clinics in rural areas and prisons in New Mexico. The target of treatment in this article was HCV infection. The results of this study show that the ECHO model was an effective way to treat HCV infection in underserved communities and may serve as a model to other states wishing to set up similar networks of care.

D. M. Harnois, DO

Boceprevir for Untreated Chronic HCV Genotype 1 Infection
Poordad F, for the SPRINT-2 Investigators (Cedars—Sinai Med Ctr, Los Angeles, CA)
N Engl J Med 364:1195-1206, 2011

Background.—Peginterferon—ribavirin therapy is the current standard of care for chronic infection with hepatitis C virus (HCV). The rate of sustained virologic response has been below 50% in cases of HCV genotype 1 infection. Boceprevir, a potent oral HCV-protease inhibitor, has been evaluated as an additional treatment in phase 1 and phase 2 studies.

Methods.—We conducted a double-blind study in which previously untreated adults with HCV genotype 1 infection were randomly assigned to one of three groups. In all three groups, peginterferon alfa-2b and ribavirin were administered for 4 weeks (the leadin period). Subsequently, group 1 (the control group) received placebo plus peginterferon—ribavirin for 44 weeks; group 2 received boceprevir plus peginterferon—ribavirin for 24 weeks, and those with a detectable HCV RNA level between weeks 8 and 24 received placebo plus peginterferon—ribavirin for an additional 20 weeks; and group 3 received boceprevir plus peginterferon—ribavirin for 44 weeks. Nonblack patients and black patients were enrolled and analyzed separately.

Results.—A total of 938 nonblack and 159 black patients were treated. In the nonblack cohort, a sustained virologic response was achieved in 125 of the 311 patients (40%) in group 1, in 211 of the 316 patients (67%) in group 2 (P<0.001), and in 213 of the 311 patients (68%) in group 3 (P<0.001). In the black cohort, a sustained virologic response was achieved in 12 of the 52 patients (23%) in group 1, in 22 of the 52 patients (42%) in group 2 (P=0.04), and in 29 of the 55 patients (53%) in group 3 (P=0.004). In group 2, a total of 44% of patients received peginterferon—ribavirin for 28 weeks. Anemia led to dose reductions in 13% of controls and 21% of boceprevir recipients, with discontinuations in 1% and 2%, respectively.

Conclusions.—The addition of boceprevir to standard therapy with peginterferon—ribavirin, as compared with standard therapy alone, significantly increased the rates of sustained virologic response in previously untreated adults with chronic HCV genotype 1 infection. The rates were similar with 24 weeks and 44 weeks of boceprevir. (Funded by Schering-Plough [now Merck]; SPRINT-2 ClinicalTrials.gov number, NCT00705432.)

▶ Chronic hepatitis C virus (HCV) infection affects more than 170 million people worldwide. The current standard of treatment with pegylated interferon and ribavirin results in a rate of sustained virologic response < 50% among patients with HCV genotype 1. Recent efforts have focused on the development of a new group of orally administered drugs directly acting against HCV.

Boceprevir is a serine protease inhibitor that binds reversibly to the HCV nonstructural 3 (NS3) active site. Boceprevir must be given in combination with pegylated interferon and ribavirin to minimize the emergence of viral resistance.

In this *New England Journal of Medicine* article, the results of the SPRINT_2 (Serine Protease Inhibitor Therapy 2) trial are reported. This trial examined if the addition of boceprevir to standard therapy could improve the rates of sustained virologic response in previously untreated patients infected with HCV genotype 1.

The addition of boceprevir to standard therapy improved sustained virologic response from 40% to 67% in previously untreated patients infected with genotype 1 HCV. The rates of treatment response were similar with 24 weeks and

44 weeks of boceprevir, implying that shorter duration of treatment may be possible.

The use of protease inhibitors in combination with standard therapy will now be the new standard of care for the treatment of people infected with HCV genotype 1.

D. M. Harnois, DO

Three-Year Efficacy and Safety of Tenofovir Disoproxil Fumarate Treatment for Chronic Hepatitis B

Heathcote EJ, Marcellin P, Buti M, et al (Univ of Toronto, Ontario, Canada; Hôpital Beaujon, Clichy, France; Hospital General Universitari Vall d'Hebron and Ciberehd, Barcelona, Spain; et al)

Gastroenterology 140:132-143, 2011

Background & Aims.—Tenofovir disoproxil fumarate (TDF), a nucleotide analogue and potent inhibitor of hepatitis B virus (HBV) polymerase, showed superior efficacy to adefovir dipivoxil in treatment of chronic hepatitis B through 48 weeks. We evaluated long-term efficacy and safety of TDF monotherapy in patients with chronic hepatitis B who were positive or negative for hepatitis B e antigen (HBeAg$^+$ or HBeAg$^-$).

Methods.—After 48 weeks of double-blind comparison of TDF to adefovir dipivoxil, patients who underwent liver biopsy were eligible to continue the study on open-label TDF for 7 additional years; data presented were collected up to 3 years (week 144) from 85% of participants. Primary efficacy end points at week 144 included levels of HBV DNA and alanine aminotransferase, development of resistance mutations, and presence of HBeAg or hepatitis B surface antigen (HBsAg).

Results.—At week 144, 87% of HBeAg$^-$ and 72% of HBeAg$^+$ patients treated with TDF had levels of HBV DNA <400 copies/mL. Among patients who had previously received adefovir dipivoxil and then received TDF, 88% of the HBeAg$^-$ and 71% of the HBeAg$^+$ patients had levels of HBV DNA <400 copies/mL; overall, 81% and 74%, respectively, maintained normalized levels of alanine aminotransferase and 34% had lost HBeAg. Amino acid substitutions in HBV DNA polymerase that are associated with resistance to tenofovir were not detected in any patient. Cumulatively, 8% of HBeAg$^+$ patients lost HBsAg. TDF maintained a favorable safety profile for up to 3 years.

Conclusions.—TDF was safe and effective in the long-term management of HBeAg$^+$ and HBeAg$^-$ patients with chronic hepatitis B.

▶ Chronic infection with hepatitis B virus (HBV) results in significant morbidity and mortality worldwide. Loss of detectable hepatitis B surface antigen (HBsAg) in serum correlates with improved long-term clinical outcomes. Oral antivirals have been demonstrated to effectively suppress viral replication; however, development of resistance limits efficacy. Therefore, oral antiviral therapies without the propensity to result in resistance are desirable. Safe and well-tolerated potent oral antivirals that are able to induce HBsAg loss would allow patients to be treated for a finite period of time.

Treatment with oral antivirals is response based, whereas treatment with interferon is for a set time. The up to 3-year post-interferon efficacy data (including HBsAg loss) have been published in 2 observational follow-up protocols and observed sustained virological response, defined as either HBV DNA less than 400 copies/mL or HBV DNA of less than 10 000 copies/mL, in 19.0% and 28.0%, and HBsAg loss in 11.0% and 8.7% of patients, respectively. There are obvious advantages to an oral agent over interferon therapy if the same efficacy could be safely achieved.

Tenofovir disoproxil fumarate (TDF), the oral prodrug of tenofovir, is a nucleotide analogue with potent activity against HBV DNA polymerase and was recently shown to be superior to adefovir dipivoxil (ADV) in HBeAg− and HBeAg+ patients with chronic HBV. After 48 weeks of double-blind treatment, HBV DNA was less than 400 copies/mL in 93% of HBeAg− and 76% of HBeAg+ patients on TDF. Importantly, no resistance mutations developed. In addition, 3% of HBeAg+ patients lost HBsAg, and by week 96, 6% of HBeAg+ patients lost HBsAg.

These studies were designed to continue assessing the safety and efficacy of TDF treatment through 8 years. This article presents results at 3 years of treatment and includes a description of patients initially randomized to ADV after they rolled over to TDF. These 3-year data show a durable 3-year viral suppression with TDF, effective viral suppression of TDF in both viremic and virologically controlled patients previously on ADV treatment, continued normalization of ALT, increasing HBeAg and HBsAg loss in HBeAg+ patients, and importantly, no resistance to tenofovir developed after up to 3 years of TDF therapy.

These data demonstrate that TDF treatment has durable efficacy and good tolerability with no development of resistance over 3 years.

D. M. Harnois, DO

Oral combination therapy with a nucleoside polymerase inhibitor (RG7128) and danoprevir for chronic hepatitis C genotype 1 infection (INFORM-1): a randomised, double-blind, placebo-controlled, dose-escalation trial

Gane EJ, Roberts SK, Stedman CAM, et al (Auckland Clinical Studies, New Zealand; The Alfred Hosp, Melbourne, Victoria, Australia; Christchurch Clinical Studies, New Zealand; et al)
Lancet 376:1467-1475, 2010

Background.—Present interferon-based standard of care treatment for chronic hepatitis C virus (HCV) infection is limited by both efficacy and tolerability. We assessed the safety, tolerability, and antiviral activity of an all-oral combination treatment with two experimental anti-HCV drugs—RG7128, a nucleoside polymerase inhibitor; and danoprevir, an NS3/4A protease inhibitor—in patients with chronic HCV infection.

Methods.—Patients from six centres in New Zealand and Australia who were chronically infected with HCV genotype 1 received up to 13 days oral combination treatment with RG7128 (500 mg or 1000 mg twice daily) and danoprevir (100 mg or 200 mg every 8 h or 600 mg or 900 mg twice daily) or placebo. Eligible patients were sequentially enrolled into one of seven treatment cohorts and were randomly assigned by interactive voice or web response system to either active treatment or placebo. Patients were separately randomly assigned within each cohort with a block size that reflected the number of patients in the cohort and the ratio of treatment to placebo. The random allocation schedule was computer generated. Dose escalation was started in HCV treatment-naive patients; standard of care treatment experienced patients, including previous null responders, were enrolled in higher-dose danoprevir cohorts. Investigators, personnel at the study centre, and patients were masked to treatment allocation. However, the pharmacist who prepared the doses, personnel involved in pharmacokinetic sample analyses, statisticians who prepared data summaries, and the clinical pharmacologists who reviewed the data before deciding to initiate dosing in the next cohort were not masked to treatment allocation. The primary outcome was change in HCV RNA concentration from baseline to day 14 in patients who received 13 days of combination treatment. All patients who completed treatment with the study drugs were included in the analyses. This study is registered with ClinicalTrials. gov, NCT00801255.

Findings.—88 patients were randomly assigned to a study drug treatment regimen (n=74 over seven treatment groups; 73 received at least one dose of study drug) or to placebo (n=14, all of whom received at least one dose). The median change in HCV RNA concentration from baseline to day 14 ranged from -3.7 to -5.2 $\log_{10}$ IU/mL in the cohorts that received 13 days of combination treatment. At the highest combination doses tested (1000 mg RG7128 and 900 mg danoprevir twice daily), the median change in HCV RNA concentration from baseline to day 14 was -5.1 $\log_{10}$ IU/mL (IQR -5.6 to -4.7) in treatment-naive patients and -4.9 $\log_{10}$ IU/mL in previous standard of care null responders (-5.2 to -4.5) compared with an increase of 0.1 $\log_{10}$ IU/mL in the placebo group. The combination of RG7128 and danoprevir was well tolerated with no treatment-related serious or severe adverse events, no grade 3 or 4 changes in laboratory parameters, and no safety-related treatment discontinuations.

Interpretation.—This oral combination of a nucleoside analogue polymerase inhibitor and protease inhibitor holds promise as an interferon-free treatment for chronic HCV.

▶ There are currently 170 million people worldwide and 3.2 million people in the United States infected with the hepatitis C virus (HCV). HCV-related liver disease is the most common reason for liver transplantation. HCV-related hepatocellular cancer has the fastest growing cancer-related mortality rate in the United States. Standard of care for the treatment of hepatitis C has been for more than a decade subcutaneous pegylated interferon alfa in combination with oral ribavirin.

Newer therapies in the treatment of HCV infection have included drugs developed directly against various HCV targets. Two recently approved HCV protease inhibitors improved treatment outcome in some patients with HCV infection but required administration with interferon and ribavirin. It is estimated that less than 50% of patients who meet criteria for HCV treatment are currently receiving or have previously received therapy. The successful development of an interferon-free treatment would greatly benefit a number of patients.

This study published in the *Lancet* provided proof of concept for an oral interferon-free approach to HCV treatment. It is important, however, to remember that this was only a short phase 1 study that showed that this combination interferon-free regimen could safely suppress viral replication but was not designed to show and did not show that an interferon-free regimen can eradicate HCV. In addition, the trial did not enroll any patients with cirrhosis. Nonetheless, this is an important first step in what will likely be the next era in HCV treatment.

D. M. Harnois, DO

Cholestatic Liver Disease

Bone Disease in Patients With Primary Sclerosing Cholangitis
Angulo P, Grandison GA, Fong DG, et al (Univ of Kentucky Med Ctr, Lexington, KY; Mayo Clinic, Rochester, MN; et al)
Gastroenterology 140:180-188, 2011

Background & Aims.—Osteopenic bone disease occurs frequently among patients with chronic liver disease but has not been well studied in those with primary sclerosing cholangitis (PSC). We investigated the prevalence, rate of progression, and independent predictors of bone disease in a large number of patients with all stages of PSC.

Methods.—Bone mineral density of the lumbar spine, hip, and total body was measured yearly for 10 years in 237 patients with PSC.

Results.—Osteoporosis (T-score less than −2.5) was found in 15% of patients and occurred 23.8-fold (95% confidence interval [CI], 4.6–122.8) more frequently in those with PSC than expected from a matched population. By multivariate analysis, age 54 years or older (odds ratio [OR], 7.8; 95% CI, 3.3–18.3), body mass index ≤24 kg/m^2 (OR, 4.9; 95% CI, 1.9–12.6), and inflammatory bowel disease for ≥19 years (OR, 3.6; 95% CI, 1.5–8.4) correlated with the presence of osteoporosis. Osteoporosis was present in 75% of patients with all 3 risk factors but in only 3.1% of those without all of them. Patients with PSC lost 1% of bone mass per year; this rate of bone loss was significantly associated with duration of inflammatory bowel disease.

Conclusions.—Osteoporosis occurs frequently among patients with PSC. Old age, low body mass index, and long duration of inflammatory bowel disease can be used to identify patients with PSC who might derive the most benefit from measurements of bone density and treatments for bone diseases.

▶ Primary sclerosing cholangitis (PSC) is a cholestatic liver disease predominantly affecting young males. Despite this cohort being at a generally reduced risk for bone disease, patients with PSC in previous smaller studies have shown an increased risk of osteoporosis. In this large series of 237 patients with PSC, investigators found that 15% of patients had established osteoporosis (T-score less than minus 2.5) at the time of their first visit with a 23.8-fold increased risk of osteoporosis. Fourteen percent had severe osteoporosis (Z-score less than minus 2.0) at the time of their first visit with a 6.1-fold increased risk of severe osteoporosis.

Factors that were shown to independently predict the presence of osteoporosis included advanced age, lower body mass index, and longer duration of inflammatory bowel disease (IBD). Patients with PSC lost bone mass at a rate of 1% per year; this rate of bone loss over time seemed to be greatly influenced by the duration of IBD.

There are no clear guidelines regarding when and how often bone density measurement (BMD) needs to be performed and repeated in patients with PSC. Investigators in this publication developed a set of recommendations that are helpful in clinical practice. Because more than half of patients with PSC in this study presented with a T-score in the range of osteopenia or osteoporosis, it seems reasonable, as the investigators propose, to recommend measurement of bone density in all patients at the time of diagnosis of PSC. For those patients with normal bone mass and short duration of IBD, repeating the BMD measurement every 2 to 3 years seems appropriate; however, repeating the BMD measurement at annual or semiannual intervals seems to be appropriate for those patients with bone mass in the range of osteopenia, particularly those with long-lasting IBD.

Again, there are no data on prevention and treatment of bone disease in patients with PSC; however, general recommendations, such as supportive measurements for bone health (ie, increased physical exercise, discontinued alcohol intake and smoking) and ensuring a diet with an appropriate content of calcium and vitamin D, or their supplementation if deficient, can be implemented in patients with PSC. Similarly, there are no data regarding the appropriate time to start treatment for bone disease in patients with PSC; however, investigators point out that it seems reasonable to consider treatment in patients with PSC and BMD below the threshold of T-score less than minus 1.5. Although no controlled trials have been reported in PSC, some medications, including bisphosphonates, hormone replacement therapy, and selective estrogen receptor modulators, have been evaluated for the treatment of bone disease in patients with another cholestatic liver disease: primary biliary cirrhosis. These medications appear relatively efficacious and safe and can be considered in PSC, but controlled trials are needed to further evaluate the most appropriate therapy.

D. M. Harnois, DO

Low Bone Mass and Severity of Cholestasis Affect Fracture Risk in Patients With Primary Biliary Cirrhosis

Guañabens N, Cerdá D, Monegal A, et al (Univ of Barcelona, Spain)
Gastroenterology 138:2348-2356, 2010

Background & Aims.—The influence of osteoporosis and liver disease on fracture risk is not well characterized in patients with primary biliary cirrhosis (PBC). We studied a large series of women with PBC to assess the prevalence and risk factors for fractures and the fracture threshold.

Methods.—In female patients with PBC (n = 185; age, 55.7 ± 0.7 years; range 28—79 years), age, duration of PBC, menopausal status, and histologic stage and severity of liver disease were assessed. Vertebral and nonvertebral fractures were recorded in 170 and 172 patients, respectively. Osteoporosis and osteopenia were diagnosed based on densitometry analysis.

Results.—The prevalences of vertebral, non-vertebral, and overall fractures were 11.2%, 12.2%, 20.8%, respectively. Osteoporosis was significantly more frequent in patients with PBC than in normal women. Osteoporosis was associated with age, weight, height, histologic stage, severity, and duration of liver damage; fractures were associated with osteoporosis, menopause, age, and height but not with severity of PBC. Osteoporosis was a risk factor for vertebral fracture (odds ratio [OR], 8.48; 95% confidence interval [CI]: 2.67—26.95). Lumbar T score <-1.5 (OR, 8.27; 95% CI: 1.84—37.08) and femoral neck T score <-1.5 (OR, 6.83; 95% CI: 1.48—31.63) were significant risk factors for vertebral fractures.

Conclusions.—Fractures, particularly vertebral fractures, are associated with osteoporosis, osteopenia, and T scores less than -1.5, whereas osteoporosis and osteopenia are associated with the severity of liver damage. Patients with T scores less than -1.5 might require additional monitoring and be considered for therapy to prevent fractures.

▶ Patients with primary biliary cirrhosis (PBC) are most often women and very often postmenopausal. It has long been recognized that these patients were at an increased risk for osteoporosis. Studies have demonstrated an increase of osteoporosis in women with PBC when compared with age-matched controls without liver disease. Low bone density has been established as a predictor of fracture risk, but there are other risks, including age, use of glucocorticoids, falls, or a history of previous fractures.

This study shows that osteoporosis in PBC as defined by bone density measurements is related to the severity and duration of liver disease. In addition, it demonstrates a strong association between low bone density and fractures. In addition, a T-score cutoff of less than −1.5 at the lumbar spine indicates a higher risk for vertebral fractures in patients with PBC. Therefore, patients with PBC and T scores less than −1.5 should be closely monitored and may be candidates for aggressive therapy targeted at preventing fractures.

D. M. Harnois, DO

Liver Transplantation

PHOENIX: A Randomized Controlled Trial of Peginterferon Alfa-2a Plus Ribavirin as a Prophylactic Treatment After Liver Transplantation for Hepatitis C Virus

Bzowej N, for the PHOENIX Study Group (California Pacific Med Ctr, San Francisco; et al)
Liver Transpl 17:528-538, 2011

The efficacy, tolerability, and safety of the prophylactic treatment of hepatitis C virus (HCV) after liver transplantation (LT) with peginterferon alfa-2a and ribavirin are not known. LT recipients with HCV were randomized to peginterferon alfa-2a/ribavirin treatment or observation 10 to 26 weeks post-LT. Prophylaxis patients received peginterferon alfa-2a (135 μg/week for 4 weeks and then 180 μg/week for 44 weeks) plus ribavirin (the initial dose of 400 mg/day was escalated to 1200 mg/day). Observation patients received the same regimen only upon significant HCV recurrence (histological activity index $\geq$ 3 and/ or fibrosis score $\geq$ 2). The primary endpoint was the proportion of patients with histological evidence of significant HCV recurrence 120 weeks after randomization. In all, 115 patients were randomized (prophylaxis arm, n = 55; observation arm, n = 60). Sustained virological response was achieved by 12 of 54 prophylaxis patients (22.2%) and by 3 of 14 observation patients who switched to treatment (21.4%). On an intent-to-treat basis, significant HCV recurrence at 120 weeks was similar in the prophylaxis (61.8%) and observation arms (65.0%, $P = 0.725$). The patient and graft survival rates and the rates of biopsy-proven acute cellular rejection were similar in the 2 study arms. Approximately 70% of the treated patients in both arms had at least one dose reduction for safety reasons. The most common adverse event leading to treatment withdrawal was anemia. Because of the safety profile of peginterferon alfa-2a/ribavirin and the lack of a clear benefit in terms of HCV recurrence and patient or graft survival, this study does not support the routine use of prophylactic antiviral therapy.

▶ End-stage liver disease caused by hepatitis C virus (HCV) is the most common indication for liver transplant (LT) in the United States. HCV recurrence is inevitable in the postoperative setting of LT. The natural history of HCV infection varies substantially in the posttransplant setting. The optimum approach to the treatment of recurrence of HCV after LT is uncertain.

The PHOENIX was a large randomized study designed to compare the efficacy, tolerability, and safety of an escalating-dose regimen of peginterferon alfa-2a plus ribavirin for 48 weeks initiated before histological recurrence within 26 weeks after LT and initiation on evidence of recurrence.

The histological recurrence of HCV after LT was the same at 120 weeks in both groups of patients, that is, those treated in the prophylaxis group and those in the observational group. Both groups had the same rate of acute cellular rejection. The most common event leading to dose reduction was anemia.

Because of the toxicity observed, the PHOENIX trial did not support the routine use of prophylactic antiviral therapy after LT in patients transplanted for HCV infection.

D. M. Harnois, DO

A Case-Controlled Study of the Safety and Efficacy of Transjugular Intrahepatic Portosystemic Shunts After Liver Transplantation

King A, Masterton G, Gunson B, et al (Univ of Birmingham, UK; Royal Infirmary, Edinburgh, UK; et al)
Liver Transpl 17:771-778, 2011

The role of transjugular intrahepatic portosystemic shunt (TIPS) insertion in managing the complications of portal hypertension is well established, but its utility in patients who have previously undergone liver transplantation is not well documented. Twenty-two orthotopic liver transplantation (OLT) patients and 44 nontransplant patients (matched controls) who underwent TIPS were analyzed. In the OLT patients, the TIPS procedure was performed at a median of 44.8 months (range = 0.3-143 months) after transplantation. Eight (36.4%) had variceal bleeding, and 14 (63.6%) had refractory ascites. The underlying liver disease was cholestatic in 10 (45.4%) and viral in 4 (18.2%). The mean pre-TIPS Model for End-Stage Liver Disease (MELD) score was 13.4 ± 5.1. There were no significant differences in age, sex, indication, etiology, or MELD score with respect to the control group. The mean initial portal pressure gradients (PPGs) were similar in the 2 groups (21.0 versus 22.4 mm Hg for the OLT patients and controls, respectively), but the final PPG was lower in the control group (9.9 versus 6.9 mm Hg, $P < 0.05$). The rates of both technical success and clinical success were higher in the control group versus the OLT group [95.5% versus 68.2% ($P < 0.05$) and 93.2% versus 77.2% ($P < 0.05$), respectively]. The rates of complications and post-TIPS encephalopathy were similar in the 2 groups, and there was a trend toward increased rates of shunt insufficiency in the OLT group. The mortality rate of the patients with a pre-TIPS MELD score > 15 was significantly higher in the OLT group [hazard ratio (HR) = 4.32, 95% confidence interval (CI) = 1.45-12.88, $P < 0.05$], but the mortality rates of the patients with a pre-TIPS MELD score < 15 were similar in the 2 groups. In the OLT group, the predictors of increased mortality were the pre-TIPS MELD score (HR = 1.161, 95% CI = 1.036-1.305, $P < 0.05$) and pre-TIPS MELD scores > 15 (HR = 5.846, 95% CI = 1.754-19.485, $P < 0.05$). In conclusion, TIPS insertion is feasible in transplant recipients, although its efficacy is lower in these patients versus control patients. Outcomes are poor for OLT recipients with a pre-TIPS MELD score > 15.

▶ Transjugular intrahepatic portosystemic shunts (TIPS) are a therapeutic option for the management of portal hypertension complications in cirrhosis.

TIPS, however, can precipitate hepatic encephalopathy in up to 30% of patients and accelerate the progression of hepatic failure. There are occasions in the posttransplant setting when TIPS is needed in the management of complications of increased portal pressure, such as ascites or bleeding.

This study demonstrates the importance of the Model for End-Stage Liver Disease (MELD) score to outcomes after TIPS in liver transplant recipients. A MELD score greater than 15 before TIPS was predictive of poor outcomes following TIPS placement in patients after liver transplantation (LT). Therefore, although TIPS can be used after LT, it should be done with caution. The MELD score can assist in predicting the likely outcomes in these patients.

D. M. Harnois, DO

Variants in *IL28B* in Liver Recipients and Donors Correlate With Response to Peg-Interferon and Ribavirin Therapy for Recurrent Hepatitis C

Fukuhara T, Taketomi A, Motomura T, et al (Kyushu Univ, Fukuoka, Japan; et al)
Gastroenterology 139:1577-1585, 2010

Background & Aims.—Patients with hepatitis C virus (HCV)—related liver disease frequently undergo orthotopic liver transplantation, but recurrent hepatitis C is still a major cause of morbidity. Patients are treated with peg-interferon and ribavirin (PEG-IFN/RBV), which has substantial side effects and is costly. We investigated genetic factors of host, liver donor, and virus that might predict sensitivity of patients with recurrent hepatitis C to PEG-IFN/RBV.

Methods.—Liver samples were analyzed from 67 HCV-infected recipients and 41 liver donors. Liver recipient and donor DNA samples were screened for single nucleotide polymorphisms near the *IL28B* genes (rs12980275 and rs8099917) that affect sensitivity to PEG-IFN/RBV. HCV RNA was isolated from patients and analyzed for mutations in the core, the IFN sensitivity-determining region, and IFN/RBV resistance-determining regions in nonstructural protein 5A.

Results.—In liver recipients and donors, the *IL28B* single nucleotide polymorphism rs8099917 was significantly associated with a sustained viral response (SVR; $P = 0.003$ and $P = .025$, respectively). Intrahepatic expression of *IL28* messenger RNA was significantly lower in recipients and donors that carried the minor alleles (T/G or T/T) in rs8099917 ($P = .010$ and .009, respectively). Genetic analyses of *IL28B* in patients and donors and of the core and nonstructural protein 5A regions encoded by HCV RNA predicted an SVR with 83% sensitivity and 82% specificity; this was more effective than analysis of any single genetic feature.

Conclusions.—In patients with recurrent HCV infection after orthotopic liver transplantation, combination analyses of single nucleotide polymorphisms of *IL28B* in recipient and donor tissues and mutations in HCV RNA allow prediction of SVR to PEG-IFN/RBV therapy.

▶ Chronic hepatitis C virus (HCV) infection is the most common indication for liver transplantation (LT) in the Western world. Recurrence of HCV infection is a common cause of graft loss following liver transplant. Treatment response, as measured by sustained virologic response (SVR), to pegylated interferon and ribavirin (PEG-IFN/RBV) is lower in patients treated after liver transplant than in patients who did not receive liver transplant.

The genetic variability in the region of the *IL28B* gene on chromosome 19 has been strongly associated with spontaneous viral clearance and treatment response (SVR) in patients with genotype 1 HCV infection treated with PEG-IFN/RBV. The 3 *IL28B* genotypes are CC, CT, and TT. The CC genotype has a more favorable treatment response rate in patients chronically infected with HCV who did not receive transplants. The impact of *IL28B* polymorphism in HCV treatment response after LT has not previously been investigated.

In this study, the investigators demonstrated that genetic variations in *IL28B* of both recipients and donors were significantly associated with interferon sensitivity, including SVR and early treatment response (ETR) after LT. These genetic variations were significantly associated with *IL28B* mRNA expression in both the resected liver derived from the recipients and in the donated liver. Furthermore, the combined genetic analysis of *IL28B* and HCV-RNA was useful to predict the response to PEG-IFN/RBV therapy in patients with recurrent HCV infection after LT.

D. M. Harnois, DO

Non-Alcoholic Fatty Liver Disease

Risk of Cardiovascular Disease in Patients with Nonalcoholic Fatty Liver Disease

Targher G, Day CP, Bonora E (Univ of Verona, Italy; Newcastle Univ, Newcastle upon Tyne, UK)
N Engl J Med 363:1341-1350, 2010

Background.—Nonalcoholic fatty liver disease has reached epidemic proportions in Western countries and constitutes a significant public health problem. It ranges from simple steatosis to nonalcoholic steatohepatitis and cirrhosis. Evidence now suggests that cardiovascular disease dictates the outcome for patients with nonalcoholic fatty liver disease more frequently and pervasively than progressive liver disease does. Cardiovascular disease is the leading cause of death in patients with advanced nonalcoholic fatty liver disease, and liver disease is associated with an increased risk of incident cardiovascular disease independent of the risk accompanying traditional risk factors and metabolic syndrome components. The link between nonalcoholic fatty liver disease and cardiovascular disease was explored.

Prevalence and Incidence of Cardiovascular Disease.—Ultrasonographically diagnosed nonalcoholic fatty liver disease and increased carotid-artery intimal medial thickness as well as increased prevalence of carotid atherosclerotic plaques are strongly related. Carotid-artery intimal medial thickness is greatest with nonalcoholic steatohepatitis, intermediate with simple steatosis, and lowest in healthy persons. Degree of carotid-artery intimal medial thickness relates to histologic severity of steatohepatitis independent of classic cardiovascular risk factors, insulin resistance, and metabolic syndrome factors. Young patients with nonalcoholic fatty liver disease who are not obese, diabetic, or hypertensive have early left ventricular dysfunction on echocardiograms and impaired left ventricular energy metabolism on cardiac phosphorus-31 magnetic resonance spectroscopy. Clinically manifest cardiovascular disease is also more common in patients with nonalcoholic fatty liver disease than in control subjects with steatosis.

Mortality in patients with nonalcoholic fatty liver disease is higher than in the general population, principally because of concomitant cardiovascular disease and liver dysfunction. Cardiovascular disease is a serious threat to patients with nonalcoholic steatohepatitis. Use of elevated serum liver enzyme levels to indicate nonalcoholic fatty liver disease shows an elevated risk of cardiovascular disease independent of alcohol consumption and other cardiovascular risk factors. High serum γ-glutamyltransferase levels are an independent, long-term predictor of incident cardiovascular events in both men and women. Ultrasonographically detected nonalcoholic fatty liver disease is related to an increased risk of nonfatal cardiovascular events independent of cardiometabolic risk factors. In patients with type 2 diabetes, nonalcoholic fatty liver disease is an independent predictor of incident cardiovascular events. Analyzing the liver ultrasonographically helps diagnose nonalcoholic fatty liver disease and better stratify cardiovascular risk in patients with high levels of γ-glutamyltransferase.

Mechanisms.—Nonalcoholic fatty liver disease, especially the necroinflammatory variant, nonalcoholic steatohepatitis, may not only indicate an increased risk of cardiovascular disease but also be involved in its pathogenesis. Systemic release of proatherogenic mediators from a steatotic and inflamed liver or the effect of the liver disease on insulin resistance and atherogenic dyslipidemia may be among the mechanisms involved.

Treatment.—The treatment approaches for nonalcoholic fatty liver disease and cardiovascular disease are similar and involve primarily reducing insulin resistance and modifying cardiovascular risk factors. It is recommended that pharmacotherapy for nonalcoholic fatty liver disease be reserved for those with nonalcoholic steatohepatitis at highest risk for disease progression. Weight reduction through diet and exercise and treatment of the individual components of the metabolic syndrome are recommended as well. Therapies of choice have beneficial hepatic effects, including bariatric surgery for obesity, insulin sensitizers for type 2 diabetes, and antihypertensive agents aimed at the renin-angiotensin-aldosterone system. Lipid-lowering agents such as statins may not be beneficial for nonalcoholic steatohepatitis but can be safely used for indications such as diabetes and high cardiovascular risk. Antioxidants, anticytokine agents, and hepatoprotectant agents may also be of benefit.

Conclusions.—It is not clear whether treating nonalcoholic fatty liver disease will prevent or retard the development or progression of cardiovascular disease. Whether nonalcoholic fatty liver disease is prognostic of cardiovascular risk stratification remains unclear. However, the strong association between nonalcoholic fatty liver disease and cardiovascular risk should influence efforts in screening and surveillance strategies used clinically. All patients with nonalcoholic fatty liver disease, especially if they have nonalcoholic steatohepatitis, need early treatment of the liver disease and early and aggressive treatment of associated cardiovascular risk factors.

▶ Nonalcoholic fatty liver disease (NAFLD) encompasses a spectrum of liver disease ranging from simple noninflammatory steatosis to nonalcoholic steatohepatitis and cirrhosis. It is estimated that in the Western world, 20% to 30% of adults have NAFLD.

There is a strong association between NAFLD and metabolic syndrome. Metabolic syndrome has, of course, also been strongly associated with risks for cardiovascular disease. There has been accumulating evidence of a putative role of NAFLD in cardiovascular disease. Similarly, there is mounting evidence that cardiovascular disease significantly impacts morbidity and mortality in NAFLD.

This article outlines research in the areas of NAFLD and cardiovascular disease and explores possible mechanisms of the pathogenesis involved in each of these diseases. The conclusion of this study and its impact on clinical practice is that there needs to be attention and screening in each of these populations for both the consequences of liver disease and cardiovascular disease and aggressive management of any risk factors.

D. M. Harnois, DO

Prevalence of Nonalcoholic Fatty Liver Disease and Nonalcoholic Steatohepatitis Among a Largely Middle-Aged Population Utilizing Ultrasound and Liver Biopsy: A Prospective Study

Williams CD, Stengel J, Asike MI, et al (Brooke Army Med Ctr, Fort Sam Houston, TX)
Gastroenterology 140:124-131, 2011

Background & Aims.—Prevalence of nonalcoholic fatty liver disease (NAFLD) has not been well established. The purpose of this study was to prospectively define the prevalence of both NAFLD and nonalcoholic steatohepatitis (NASH).

Methods.—Outpatients 18 to 70 years old were recruited from Brooke Army Medical Center. All patients completed a baseline questionnaire and ultrasound. If fatty liver was identified, then laboratory data and a liver biopsy were obtained.

Results.—Four hundred patients were enrolled. Three hundred and twenty-eight patients completed the questionnaire and ultrasound. Mean age (range, 28–70 years) was 54.6 years (7.35); 62.5% Caucasian, 22% Hispanic, and 11.3% African American; 50.9% female; mean body mass index (BMI) (calculated as kg/m^2) was 29.8 (5.64); and diabetes and hypertension prevalence 16.5% and 49.7%, respectively. Prevalence of NAFLD was 46%. NASH was confirmed in 40 patients (12.2% of total cohort, 29.9% of ultrasound positive patients). Hispanics had the highest prevalence of NAFLD (58.3%), then Caucasians (44.4%) and African Americans (35.1%). NAFLD patients were more likely to be male (58.9%), older ($P = .004$), hypertensive ($P < .00005$), and diabetic ($P < .00005$). They had a higher BMI ($P < .0005$), ate fast food more often ($P = .049$), and exercised less ($P = 0.02$) than their non-NAFLD counterparts. Hispanics had a higher prevalence of NASH compared with Caucasians (19.4% vs 9.8%; $P = .03$). Alanine aminotransferase, aspartate aminotransferase, BMI, insulin, Quantitative Insulin-Sensitivity Check Index, and cytokeratin-18 correlated with NASH. Among the 54 diabetic patients, NAFLD was found in 74% and NASH in 22.2%.

Conclusion.—Prevalence of NAFLD and NASH is higher than estimated previously. Hispanics and patients with diabetes are at greatest risk for both NAFLD and NASH.

▶ The health implications of the current epidemic of obesity are not fully understood. As the article points out, recent estimates suggest that obesity in adults has increased to 33.8%, and the prevalence of diabetes in adults ages 45 to 64 years has increased to 10.6% in the United States. One of the health consequences of obesity is metabolic syndrome and nonalcoholic fatty liver disease. Nonalcoholic fatty liver disease (NAFLD) encompasses a spectrum of liver disease ranging from simple noninflammatory steatosis to nonalcoholic steatohepatitis (NASH) and cirrhosis.

In this prospective study of outpatients 18 to 70 years of age recruited from Brooke Army Medical Center, the overall prevalence of NAFLD was 46%, and NASH was 12.2%. Hispanics had the highest prevalence followed by Caucasians and then African Americans. There was a prevalence of NAFLD and NASH in diabetic patients. In this study, the prevalence of NASH in an asymptomatic adult population enrolled without regard to liver enzyme abnormalities was higher than previously estimated. In addition, 2.7% of patients had significant fibrosis (stage 2-4) secondary to NASH, many of these asymptomatic.

This study provides additional evidence with regard to the health implications of the current trend of obesity in the United States and the importance of health screening in these patients.

D. M. Harnois, DO

The natural history of nonalcoholic fatty liver disease with advanced fibrosis or cirrhosis: An international collaborative study

Bhala N, Angulo P, van der Poorten D, et al (Univ of Oxford, UK; Univ of Kentucky Med Ctr, Lexington; Univ of Sydney, Westmead, New South Wales, Australia; et al)
Hepatology 2011 [Epub ahead of print]

Information on the long-term prognosis of nonalcoholic fatty liver disease (NAFLD) is limited. We sought to describe the long-term morbidity and mortality of patients with NAFLD with advanced fibrosis or cirrhosis. We conducted this prospective cohort study including 247 patients with NAFLD and 264 patients with HCV infection that were either naïve or non-responders to treatment. Both cohorts were Child-Pugh class A and had advanced (stage 3) fibrosis or cirrhosis (stage 4) confirmed by liver biopsy at enrolment. In the NAFLD cohort, followed-up for 85.6 months mean (range 6-297), there were 48 (19.4%) liver-related complications and 33 (13.4%) deaths or liver transplants. In the HCV cohort, followed-up for 74.9 months mean (range 6-238), there were 47 (16.7%) liver-related complications and 25 (9.4%) deaths or liver transplants. When adjusting for baseline differences in age and gender, the cumulative incidence of liver-related complications was lower in the NAFLD than the HCV cohort (p=0.03), including incident hepatocellular cancer (6 vs 18; p=0.03), but that of cardiovascular events (p=0.17) and overall mortality (p=0.6) was similar in both groups. In the NAFLD cohort, platelet count, stage 4 fibrosis, and serum levels of cholesterol and ALT were associated with liver-related complications; an AST/ALT ratio <1 and older age were associated with overall mortality; and higher serum bilirubin levels and stage 4 fibrosis were associated with liver-related mortality.

Conclusions.—Patients with NAFLD with advanced fibrosis or cirrhosis have lower rates of liver-related complications and hepatocellular cancer than corresponding patients with HCV infection, but similar overall mortality. Some clinical and laboratory features predict outcomes in patients with NAFLD.

▶ Nonalcoholic fatty liver disease (NAFLD) has become the most prevalent cause of chronic liver disease worldwide. Regarded as the hepatic manifestation of the metabolic syndrome, NAFLD represents a histological spectrum of disease that extends from simple steatosis to steatohepatitis. NAFLD may be associated with advanced fibrosis or cirrhosis that can result in complications and mortality. Despite its prevalence, the prognosis of NAFLD with advanced fibrosis or cirrhosis remains poorly studied, and important aspects of the prognosis of patients with NAFLD still remain unclear. Finally, it is unclear which, if any, risk factors can independently predict liver, vascular, and overall morbidity and mortality.

To answer these questions, the investigators carried out an international, multicenter prospective study to assess the natural history and outcomes of liver biopsy—confirmed NAFLD with advanced fibrosis or cirrhosis. In this study from 4 countries, the investigators report the natural history of the biopsy-proven NAFLD with advanced fibrosis or cirrhosis. The NAFLD patients had well-compensated liver disease and no overt hepatic synthetic dysfunction at presentation. When they were compared with patients with liver disease secondary to chronic hepatitis C virus (HCV) infection with advanced fibrosis or cirrhosis of the same functional status, there were long-term differences, notably less liver-related complications and less hepatocellular carcinoma risk in patients with NAFLD as compared with patients with HCV infection. Interestingly, however, there were also remarkable long-term similarities for vascular disease and overall mortality in both groups. Larger prospective studies will be necessary to shed further understanding on the impact of NAFLD on liver- and vascular-related morbidity and mortality.

D. M. Harnois, DO

Cirrhosis and Complications

Transjugular intrahepatic portosystemic shunt for portal vein thrombosis with symptomatic portal hypertension in liver cirrhosis
Han G, Qi X, He C, et al (Fourth Military Med Univ, Xi'an, China)
J Hepatol 54:78-88, 2011

Background & Aims.—Data on the management of portal vein thrombosis (PVT) in patients with decompensated cirrhosis are extremely limited, particularly in the cases of the transjugular intrahepatic portosystemic shunt (TIPS). We assessed the outcome of TIPS for PVT in patients with cirrhosis and symptomatic portal hypertension and determined the predictors of technical success and survival.

Methods.—In the retrospective study, 57 consecutive patients receiving TIPS were enrolled between December 2001 and September 2008. All were diagnosed with chronic PVT, and 30 had portal cavernoma. Indications for TIPS were variceal hemorrhage ($n = 56$) and refractory ascites ($n = 1$).

Results.—TIPS were successfully placed in 75% of patients (43/57). The independent predictors of technical success included portal cavernoma, and the degree of thrombosis within the main portal vein (MPV), the portal vein branches, and the superior mesenteric vein. Only one patient died of severe procedure-related complication. The cumulative 1-year shunt dysfunction and hepatic encephalopathy rates were 21% and 25%, respectively. The cumulative 1- and 5-year variceal re-bleeding rates differed significantly between the TIPS success and failure groups (10% and 28% versus 43% and 100%, respectively; $p = 0.0004$), while the cumulative 1- and 5-year survival rates were similar between the two groups (86% and 77% versus 78% and 62%, respectively; $p = 0.34$). The independent predictor of survival in PVT patients with decompensated cirrhosis was the degree of MPV occlusion (hazard ratio 0.189, 95% CI 0.042−0.848).

Conclusions.—TIPS should be considered a safe and feasible alternative therapy for chronic PVT in selected patients with decompensated cirrhosis.

Both technical success and survival were closely associated with the degree of MPV occlusion.

▶ Portal vein thrombosis (PVT) is a clot within the main portal vein (MPV), with or without extension into the portal branches, splenic vein, or mesenteric venous system. Cirrhotic patients develop PVT at a prevalence rate of approximately 10% to 25%. The development of PVT can be seen in patients with decompensated cirrhosis.

Practice guidelines were developed by the American Association for the Study of Liver Disease and published in *Hepatology* in 2009. However, the management of individual cases remains controversial and challenging. The aim of this study was to review retrospectively the outcomes of transjugular intrahepatic portosystemic shunt (TIPS) combined with transhepatic and transsplenic approaches for the management of PVT in 57 patients with cirrhosis and symptomatic portal hypertension.

In this series, a standard TIPS procedure was performed in patients with a partially occluded portal vein. In patients with a completely occluded portal vein, TIPS was combined with transhepatic or transsplenic approaches.

Based on the results of this review, the investigators recommend that TIPS be attempted in patients with the following conditions (listed in order of decreasing technical success and increasing risk): (1) partially occluded MPV; (2) completely occluded MPV, in which recanalization could be attempted by a combination of transjugular and transhepatic or transsplenic approaches; and (3) completely occluded MPV or obliterated MPV with a large-caliber collateral. The investigators recommended against TIPS in patients with a fibrotic cord or MPV obliteration with fine collaterals.

In this retrospective study, the only independent predictor of survival in PVT patients with cirrhosis was the degree of MPV occlusion rather than TIPS insertion. The role of anticoagulation in patients with PVT and cirrhosis was not explored in this article and will require future trials. In addition, it is important to remember there are potentially significant complications that may result from TIPS in patients with cirrhosis, which may include complications directly related to the procedure itself and encephalopathy, as well as the potential for hepatic decompensation after TIPS placement.

D. M. Harnois, DO

Rifaximin Improves Driving Simulator Performance in a Randomized Trial of Patients With Minimal Hepatic Encephalopathy
Bajaj JS, Heuman DM, Wade JB, et al (Virginia Commonwealth Univ and McGuire VA Med Ctr, Richmond; et al)
Gastroenterology 140:478-487, 2011

Background & Aims.—Patients with cirrhosis and minimal hepatic encephalopathy (MHE) have driving difficulties but the effects of therapy on driving performance is unclear. We evaluated whether performance on a driving simulator improves in patients with MHE after treatment with rifaximin.

Methods.—Patients with MHE who were current drivers were randomly assigned to placebo or rifaximin groups and followed up for 8 weeks (n = 42). Patients underwent driving simulation (driving and navigation tasks) at the start (baseline) and end of the study. We evaluated patients' cognitive abilities, quality of life (using the Sickness Impact Profile), serum levels of ammonia, levels of inflammatory cytokines, and model for end-stage-liver disease scores. The primary outcome was the percentage of patients who improved in driving performance, calculated as follows: total driving errors = speeding + illegal turns + collisions.

Results.—Over the 8-week study period, patients given rifaximin made significantly greater improvements than those given placebo in avoiding total driving errors (76% vs 31%; $P = .013$), speeding (81% vs 33%; $P = .005$), and illegal turns (62% vs 19%; $P = .01$). Of patients given rifaximin, 91% improved their cognitive performance, compared with 61% of patients given placebo ($P = .01$); they also made improvements in the psychosocial dimension of the Sickness Impact Profile compared with the placebo group ($P = .04$). Adherence to the assigned drug averaged 92%. Neither group had changes in ammonia levels or model for end-stage-liver disease scores, but patients in the rifaximin group had increased levels of the anti-inflammatory cytokine interleukin-10.

Conclusions.—Patients with MHE significantly improve driving simulator performance after treatment with rifaximin, compared with placebo.

▶ Patients with cirrhosis often have an underrecognized impairment in cognitive dysfunction known as minimal hepatic encephalopathy (MHE). These symptoms can significantly impact quality of life and ability to maintain job performance or life activities. Skills required to drive include balance, attention, and integration of various cognitive inputs. These are areas affected by MHE.

In this study, patients with cirrhosis who were not on treatment for encephalopathy and with no history of overt symptoms of encephalopathy were identified on testing as having MHE. These patients were randomized to treatment with rifaximin 550 mg twice daily versus placebo. Their driving skills were then tested. Patients treated with rifaximin had significant improvement in driving-simulator performance versus placebo.

Many patients with cirrhosis have unidentified symptoms of MHE that may significantly impact their life. It is important to diagnose these patients and consider therapy with lactulose and/or rifaximin.

D. M. Harnois, DO

Prognostic Importance of the Cause of Renal Failure in Patients With Cirrhosis

Martín-Llahí M, Guevara M, Torre A, et al (Univ of Barcelona, Spain; et al)

Gastroenterology 140:488-496, 2011

Background & Aims.—The prognostic value of the different causes of renal failure in cirrhosis is not well established. This study investigated the predictive value of the cause of renal failure in cirrhosis.

Methods.—Five hundred sixty-two consecutive patients with cirrhosis and renal failure (as defined by serum creatinine >1.5 mg/dL on 2 successive determinations within 48 hours) hospitalized over a 6-year period in a single institution were included in a prospective study. The cause of renal failure was classified into 4 groups: renal failure associated with bacterial infections, renal failure associated with volume depletion, hepatorenal syndrome (HRS), and parenchymal nephropathy. The primary end point was survival at 3 months.

Results.—Four hundred sixty-three patients (82.4%) had renal failure that could be classified in 1 of 4 groups. The most frequent was renal failure associated with infections (213 cases; 46%), followed by hypovolemia-associated renal failure (149; 32%), HRS (60; 13%), and parenchymal nephropathy (41; 9%). The remaining patients had a combination of causes or miscellaneous conditions. Prognosis was markedly different according to cause of renal failure, 3-month probability of survival being 73% for parenchymal nephropathy, 46% for hypovolemia-associated renal failure, 31% for renal failure associated with infections, and 15% for HRS ($P < .0005$). In a multivariate analysis adjusted for potentially confounding variables, cause of renal failure was independently associated with prognosis, together with MELD score, serum sodium, and hepatic encephalopathy at time of diagnosis of renal failure.

Conclusions.—A simple classification of patients with cirrhosis according to cause of renal failure is useful in assessment of prognosis and may help in decision making in liver transplantation.

▶ Patients with cirrhosis are at an increased risk for renal failure from several sources. It has been known for some time that patients with cirrhosis with renal failure have a reduced survival compared with patients without renal failure. However, although impairment in renal function is known to be relevant to prognosis, it has never been clearly established if prognosis is in any way related to the cause of renal disease.

Investigators conducted a single-center, prospective study to evaluate causes of renal failure in hospitalized patients with cirrhosis and the relevance of cause of renal dysfunction to prognosis. Interestingly, the most common etiology for renal failure in patients with cirrhosis was infection related. The main finding of the study was that characterization of renal failure into 4 groups based on the etiology of their renal failure (infection, hypovolemia related, hepatorenal syndrome, and parenchymal nephropathy) had prognostic relevance. Patients with the best survival were those with parenchymal nephropathy (73% at

3 months). In contrast, those with hepatorenal syndrome had only a 15% 3-month survival.

If validated in larger studies in the future, the Model for End-Stage Liver Disease score for prioritizing patients with liver disease for liver transplant may include etiology for renal disease, but at this time the benefit of this study may be in allowing clinicians to more appropriately manage and triage their patients with cirrhosis and renal failure.

D. M. Harnois, DO

Sub-clinical hepatic encephalopathy in cirrhotic patients is not aggravated by sedation with propofol compared to midazolam: A randomized controlled study

Khamaysi I, William N, Olga A, et al (Rambam Med Ctr, Haifa, Israel; Holy Family Hosp, Nazareth, Israel; Ziv Med Centre, Safed, Israel)
J Hepatol 54:72-77, 2011

Background & Aims.—The risk of exacerbating sub-clinical hepatic encephalopathy (HE) by propofol has not been established. The aim of this study is to determine whether the use of propofol, for upper endoscopy in patients with cirrhosis, precipitates subclinical HE.

Methods.—Sixty-one patients with compensated HCV and HBV cirrhosis (CP score 5—6) were randomly selected and divided into two groups (intent-to-treat population) matched for age, gender, and BMI. The first group received a single propofol sedation ($N = 31$, age 57 ± 12, dose range 70—100 mg/procedure) and the second group ($N = 30$, age 56 ± 12, dose 3—6 mg/procedure) received a single midazolam sedation, all done by an anesthesiologist. All patients completed number connection test (NCT), cognitive function score, time to recovery, time to discharge sheets, and hemodynamic parameters before sedation, and at discharge from the endoscopy unit, 1 h post-procedure. Thirty control subjects without cirrhosis were matched to the cirrhotic patients who received sedation with regard to age, gender, BMI, and education level.

Results.—A total of 58/61 cirrhotic patients (95%) had sub-clinical encephalopathy before the endoscopy (mean NCT 84.7 ± 77 s, normal <30 s). No patient developed overt HE after sedation. There were no differences between groups in the incidence of adverse effects, cognitive function, MELD score, CP score, oxygen saturation, or respiratory and heart rates before and after sedation. Propofol did not exacerbate minimal HE when compared to midazolam (NCT changed from 87.5 ± 62 s prior to sedation to 74.2 ± 58 s after sedation in the propofol group versus 72.8 ± 62 s before to 85.6 ± 72 s after sedation in the midazolam group; p <0.01). Time to recovery (4.1 ± 1.9 min vs. 11.5 ± 5.0 min, p <0.001), and time to discharge (38.0 ± 9 min vs. 110 ± 42 min, p <0.001) were significantly shorter with propofol than midazolam. Pre- and post-procedure NCT (from 25 ± 20 s to 24 ± 20 s), cognitive function score (from 25 to 26), time to recovery (3.5 ± 1.0 min), and time to discharge (35 ± 10 min) did not change in the healthy controls.

Conclusions.—Sedation with propofol has a shorter time recovery and a shorter time to discharge than midazolam and does not exacerbate sub-clinical hepatic encephalopathy in patients with compensated liver cirrhosis.

▶ Hepatic encephalopathy is a neurologic disorder associated with advanced liver disease. Many patients with cirrhosis can have subclinical hepatic encephalopathy. Endoscopies are routinely performed in patients with chronic liver disease to screen for gastric and esophageal varices and portal hypertension. The recommended sedation for patients with cirrhosis and hepatic encephalopathy undergoing endoscopy is uncertain.

This article outlines a randomized, controlled trial using propofol compared with midazolam in patients with subclinical hepatic encephalopathy undergoing endoscopy. Sedation with propofol appeared to be safe, and patients were discharged more quickly and without significant impact on hepatic encephalopathy than patients sedated with midazolam.

D. M. Harnois, DO

Primary prophylaxis of gastric variceal bleeding comparing cyanoacrylate injection and beta-blockers: A randomized controlled trial
Mishra SR, Sharma BC, Kumar A, et al (G B Pant Hosp, New Delhi, India; Inst of Liver & Biliary Sciences (ILBS), New Delhi, India)
J Hepatol 54:1161-1167, 2011

Background & Aims.—Gastric variceal bleeding is severe and is associated with high mortality. We compared the efficacy of cyanoacrylate injection and beta-blockers in primary prophylaxis of gastric variceal bleeding.

Methods.—Cirrhotics with large gastroesophageal varices type 2 with eradicated esophageal varices or large isolated gastric varix type 1, who had never bled from gastric varix, were randomised to cyanoacrylate injection (Group I, $n = 30$), beta-blockers (Group II, $n = 29$) or no treatment (Group III, $n = 30$). Primary end-points were bleeding from gastric varix or death.

Results.—The actuarial probability of bleeding from gastric varices over a median follow-up of 26 months was 13% in Group I, 28% in Group II ($p = 0.039$), and 45% in Group III ($p = 0.003$). The actuarial probability of survival was higher in the cyanoacrylate compared to the no-treatment group (90% vs. 72%, $p = 0.048$). The median hepatic venous pressure gradient (HVPG) was increased in Group I (14−15 mm Hg, $p = 0.001$) and III (14−16 mm Hg, $p = 0.001$) but decreased in Group II (14 to 12 mm Hg, $p = 0.001$) during follow-up. Size of gastric varix >20 mm, a MELD score ≥17, and presence of portal hypertensive gastropathy predicted 'high risk' of first bleeding from gastric varices.

Conclusions.—Primary prophylaxis is recommended in patients with large and high risk gastric varices to reduce the risk of first bleeding and mortality. Cyanoacrylate injection is more effective than beta-blocker therapy in preventing first gastric variceal bleeding.

▶ Gastric varices are found in 20% of patients with portal hypertension. The mortality rate from gastric variceal bleeding is higher than that from esophageal variceal bleeding. While studies have been performed that have analyzed the bleeding risk and best recommendations for prophylaxis secondary to esophageal varices, there are few data available on primary prophylaxis and secondary prophylaxis in rebleeding risk of gastric varices.

This article is a randomized prospective study of prophylaxis of gastric variceal bleeding.

Patients who received cyanoacrylate injection, in comparison to β-blocker or no treatment, had a lower rate of a primary bleed from gastric varices. In addition, patients who received cyanoacrylate injection, in comparison to β-blocker or no treatment, also had a lower rate of rebleeding from gastric varices. The question remaining is whether cyanoacrylate injection in combination with β-blockers would offer greater benefit than either treatment alone.

D. M. Harnois, DO

Liver Lesions

New Staging System and a Registry for Perihilar Cholangiocarcinoma
DeOliveira ML, Schulick RD, Nimura Y, et al (Univ Hosp Zurich, Switzerland; Johns Hopkins Med Ctr, Baltimore, MD; Aichi Cancer Ctr, Nagoya, Japan; et al)
Hepatology 53:1363-1371, 2011

Perihilar cholangiocarcinoma is one of the most challenging diseases with poor overall survival. The major problem for anyone trying to convincingly compare studies among centers or over time is the lack of a reliable staging system. The most commonly used system is the Bismuth-Corlette classification of bile duct involvement, which, however, does not include crucial information such as vascular encasement and distant metastases. Other systems are rarely used because they do not provide several key pieces of information guiding therapy. Therefore, we have designed a new system reporting the size of the tumor, the extent of the disease in the biliary system, the involvement of the hepatic artery and portal vein, the involvement of lymph nodes, distant metastases, and the volume of the putative remnant liver after resection. The aim of this system is the standardization of the reporting of perihilar cholangiocarcinoma so that relevant information regarding resectability, indications for liver transplantation, and prognosis can be provided. With this tool, we have created a new registry enabling every center to prospectively enter data on their patients with hilar cholangiocarcinoma (www.cholangioca.org). The availability of such standardized and multicenter data will enable us to identify the critical criteria guiding therapy.

▶ Cholangiocarcinoma (CCA) is a cancer arising from the biliary epithelium. It represents about 10% of all primary hepatobiliary cancers. The rate of CCA appears to be increasing for unclear reasons.

Currently, the most commonly accepted classification system is based on the location of the tumor, intrahepatic, perihilar, or what is often referred to as a Klatskin tumor, and distal CCA. Previous classification systems have reviewed the recommendations for intrahepatic lesions. The purpose of this article was to describe a recommended classification of perihilar CCA.

The proposed staging system provides information regarding anatomic location, involvement along the portal vein and hepatic artery, the volume of potential future remnant if surgical resection is considered, lymph node metastasis, and metastatic status. In addition, tumor size, form, and underlying disease also make up the staging system.

It is hopeful that this new classification system will provide a better framework for a discussion of management of these challenging patients.

D. M. Harnois, DO

Validation of a liver adenoma classification system in a tertiary referral centre: Implications for clinical practice
van Aalten SM, Verheij J, Terkivatan T, et al (Erasmus Univ Med Centre, Rotterdam, The Netherlands)
J Hepatol 55:120-125, 2011

Background & Aims.—A molecular and pathological classification system for hepatocellular adenomas (HCA) was recently introduced and four major subgroups were identified. We aimed to validate this adenoma classification system and to determine the clinical relevance of the subtypes for surgical management.

Methods.—Paraffin fixed liver tissue slides and resection specimens of patients radiologically diagnosed as HCA were retrieved from the department of pathology. Immunostainings included liver-fatty acid binding protein (L-FABP), serum amyloid A (SAA), C-reactive protein (CRP), glutamine synthetase (GS) and β-catenin.

Results.—From 2000 to 2010, 58 cases (71 lesions) were surgically resected. Fourteen lesions were diagnosed as focal nodular hyperplasia with a characteristic map-like staining pattern of GS. Inflammatory HCA expressing CRP and SAA was documented in 36 of 57 adenomas (63%). Three of these inflammatory adenomas were also β-catenin positive as well as GS positive and only one was CRP and SAA and GS positive. We identified eleven LFABP- negative HCA (19%) and four β-catenin positive HCA (7%), without expression of CRP and SAA and with normal L-FABP staining, one of which was also GS positive. Six HCA were unclassifiable (11%). In three patients multiple adenomas of different subtypes were found.

Conclusions.—Morphology and additional immunohistochemical markers can discriminate between different types of HCA in >90% of cases and this classification, including the identification of β-catenin positive adenomas may have important implications in the decision for surveillance or treatment. Interpretation of nuclear staining for β-catenin can be difficult due to uneven staining distribution or focal nuclear staining and additional molecular biology may be required.

▶ Hepatocellular adenoma (HCA) is a rare benign tumor of the liver that occurs predominantly in women in child-bearing age. The estimated incidence is about 1 to 1.3 per 1 000 000 in women who have never used oral contraceptives (OC), compared with a substantially higher incidence of 30 to 40 per 1 000 000 in long-term users.

Recently, a new molecular and pathological classification of HCA was introduced by Bioulac-Sage and colleagues who suggested that the identification of subtypes might be of great clinical importance. This study sought to validate this classification system by retrospectively looking at resected surgical specimens and clinical outcomes in trying to determine the relevance of the classification system to management. The study demonstrated that it was possible to differentiate the subclasses of HCAs in surgically resected specimens. Whether the immunohistochemical markers will also be useful on biopsies from liver tumors suspected of being HCA needs to be investigated.

Current recommendations from the investigators of this article for the management of HCA in female patients are as follows: (1) All female patients with HCA are advised to stop the use of OC and other hormone medication, including hormone replacement therapy, as regression of HCA may occur when estrogens are withdrawn; (2) observation should be the first choice of treatment for most patients with HCA. The management of solitary adenomas by conservative treatment or continuous surgical resection is still a matter of debate. Most authors believe that surgical resection should be considered if the diameter exceeds 5 cm after 6 months of follow-up, if the lesion does not show adequate regression after discontinuation of OC, or if bleeding occurs. Surgical resection is also indicated if there is any suspicion of malignancy. The role of ablation therapy in HCA is unclear.

D. M. Harnois, DO

Autoimmune Liver Disease

Comparability of Probable and Definite Autoimmune Hepatitis by International Diagnostic Scoring Criteria
Czaja AJ (Mayo Clinic College of Medicine, Rochester, MN)
Gastroenterology 140:1472-1480, 2011

Background & Aims.—The diagnostic scoring systems for autoimmune hepatitis categorize some patients as having probable disease; this designation can affect treatment strategies and recruitment to clinical studies. A retrospective study was performed to determine the bases for the classification of probable autoimmune hepatitis and its clinical importance.

Methods.—The study included 185 adult patients who had been assessed at presentation for findings common to both international diagnostic scoring systems.

Results.—Seventeen patients (9%) were graded as probable autoimmune hepatitis by the revised original scoring system, and 28 patients (15%) were similarly designated by the simplified scoring system. These patients were distinguished from those designated as definite autoimmune hepatitis by male sex, concurrent immune diseases, lower serum γ-globulin and immunoglobulin G levels, and lower titers of autoantibody. Patients with definite or probable designations by either scoring system responded similarly to conventional corticosteroid regimens during comparable intervals of treatment. Full, partial, or nonresponses and treatment dependence were evident in all diagnostic categories with similar frequencies. Twenty-seven patients designated as probable autoimmune hepatitis by one system were designated as definite autoimmune hepatitis by the other system.

Conclusions.—The designation of probable autoimmune hepatitis by the international scoring systems is based on differences in clinical manifestations and does not reflect differences in the validity of the diagnosis or its treatment response. Large multicenter prospective studies are necessary to establish these observations.

▶ In 2010, the American Association for the Study of Liver Diseases published guidelines for the management of patients with autoimmune hepatitis (AIH) in *Hepatology*. Establishing the diagnosis of AIH has been codified by an international panel, and scoring systems have been developed. These scoring systems have been incorporated into diagnostic algorithms in patient management. The revised original scoring system is a comprehensive incorporation of multiple clinical, pathological, and laboratory features. The simplified scoring system assesses a smaller number of features validated in a multivariate analysis.

However, each of these scoring systems classifies a group of patients as having probable disease. The goals of this retrospective study were to better define the phenotype of patients designated as having probable AIH and evaluate the response of these patients to conventional corticosteroid therapy.

The results of this analysis showed that the designation of a probable diagnosis of AIH was based on clinical manifestations of the disease. More importantly, patients with either a probable or definite designation of AIH responded similarly to conventional corticosteroid regimens during a comparable period of time.

D. M. Harnois, DO

Long-term Outcomes of Patients With Autoimmune Hepatitis Managed at a Nontransplant Center

Hoeroldt B, McFarlane E, Dube A, et al (Rotherham General Hosp, England; Sheffield Teaching Hosps, England; et al)
Gastroenterology 140:1980-1989, 2011

Background & Aims.—The long-term outcomes of patients treated for autoimmune hepatitis (AIH) are considered to be good. However, follow-up data beyond 10 years are limited and confined to tertiary referral centers. We assessed long-term outcomes and determinants of outcome in patients with AIH from a nontransplant center.

Methods.—We studied 245 patients (204 women; median age, 56 years; range, 2.5−87 years) with AIH (167 definite by International AIH Group criteria) managed at a single nontransplant center from 1971 to 2007.

Results.—229 patients (93%) achieved normal serum levels of alanine aminotransferase within 12 months after treatment. After a median follow-up period of 9.4 years (range, 0.01−36 years), 11 patients received liver transplants (2 subsequently died). Seventy other patients died (30 from liver disease), 15 were censored (moved away, defaulted, or developed primary biliary cirrhosis), and 149 were still being followed up on December 31, 2007. Survival rates from all-cause death or transplantation were 82% ± 3% and 48% ± 5% after 10 and 20 years, respectively, and from liver-related death or transplantation were 91% ± 2% and 70% ± 5%, respectively. The standardized mortality ratio was 1.63 for all-cause death (95% confidence interval [CI], 1.25−2.02), 1.86 also considering liver transplant as "death" (95% CI, 1.49−2.26), and 0.91 for non−liver-related death (95% CI, 0.62−1.19). By Cox regression analysis, liver decompensation, cirrhosis at any time, failure to normalize levels of alanine aminotransferase within 12 months, and >4 relapses per decade were significantly associated with liver-related death or transplant.

Conclusions.—Despite a good initial response to immunosuppression, long-term mortality of patients with AIH is greater than that of the general population.

▶ Autoimmune hepatitis (AIH) is a chronic liver disease with an estimated prevalence of 10 to 50 per 100 000 in a Western population. Our knowledge of the natural history of the disease is largely limited to the first decade after diagnosis. This is one of the very few trials to present data on follow-up mortality in the second decade.

In this trial, survival rates after 10 and 20 years were 82% and 48%, respectively. Overall mortality was increased, and this was related to an increase in liver-related mortality. Liver decompensation, cirrhosis at presentation, failure to achieve biochemical remission within 12 months of therapy, and high relapse rates were associated with a poor outcome.

In summary, on the basis of this trial, AIH may progress despite immunosuppression therapy, even in patients achieving a biochemical remission. The disease process seemed to accelerate in this patient population in the second decade. Patients with AIH have a chronic liver disease that requires continued monitoring, even if they have achieved a biochemical remission and remained stable for greater than 10 years.

D. M. Harnois, DO

Paris Criteria Are Effective in Diagnosis of Primary Biliary Cirrhosis and Autoimmune Hepatitis Overlap Syndrome
Kuiper EMM, Zondervan PE, van Buuren HR (Erasmus Univ Med Ctr, Rotterdam, The Netherlands)
Clin Gastroenterol Hepatol 8:530-534, 2010

Background & Aims.—Primary biliary cirrhosis (PBC) and autoimmune hepatitis (AIH) differ in clinical, laboratory, and histologic features as well as in response to therapy. A small subgroup of patients have an overlap syndrome with features of both diseases, although there is no consensus on its definition or diagnostic criteria. We evaluated the significance of the criteria used to diagnose PBC—AIH overlap syndrome.

Methods.—This retrospective, single-center study included all patients diagnosed with PBC, AIH, or PBC—AIH overlap syndrome, based on the Paris criteria, since January 1990 (n = 134); patients were followed up for 9.7 ± 3.7 years. The 3 groups were compared for their clinical, laboratory, and histologic features. Patients with overlap syndrome or PBC were graded by the revised and simplified AIH scoring systems to assess the ability of this system to identify AIH cases properly.

Results.—The sensitivity and specificity of the Paris criteria for diagnosing the overlap syndrome were 92% and 97%, respectively. The sensitivity and specificity of the AIH scoring systems were considerably lower. Among patients with the overlap syndrome, the 10-year, transplantation-free survival rate was 92%.

Conclusions.—The Paris diagnostic criteria detect overlap syndrome (PBC and AIH) with high levels of sensitivity and specificity. The clinical value of the revised and simplified AIH scoring system is not as reliable. Patients with PBC—AIH overlap syndrome have a 92% rate of 10-year, transplantation-free survival.

▶ Primary biliary cirrhosis (PBC) and autoimmune hepatitis (AIH) are immune-mediated chronic liver diseases. They have different clinical, laboratory, and histological features. They can occur independently, simultaneously, or consecutively. A standardized diagnostic criterion for overlap syndrome of PBC and AIH has not been clearly defined.

This retrospective study attempted to analyze data from patients diagnosed with PBC, AIH, and overlap syndrome and confirm the value of the diagnostic criteria previously proposed in 1998 known as the Paris criteria. The Paris criteria require the presence of at least 2 of the 3 accepted criteria for diagnosis of PBC and AIH. The diagnostic criteria for PBC are as follows: (1) serum alkaline phosphatase level 2-fold or greater the upper limit of normal (ULN), or serum γ-glutamyltransferase levels 5-fold or greater the ULN; (2) positive test for anti-mitochondrial antibodies; and (3) liver biopsy specimen showing florid bile duct lesions. The diagnostic criteria for AIH are as follows: (1) serum alanine amino-transferase levels 5-fold or greater the ULN; (2) immunoglobulin G levels 2-fold or greater the ULN, or a positive test for smooth muscle antibodies; and (3) liver biopsy showing moderate or severe periportal or periseptal lymphocytic piece-meal necrosis.

In this study, the Paris criteria for overlap patients with PBC and AIH were more useful than the numeric AIH scoring systems. The patients in this study were treated with ursodeoxycholic acid and immunosuppressive treatment. The 10-year survival in these patients was 92%. Previous studies have demon-strated a 10-year survival rate of 55% to 85% in patients with overlap syndrome.

D. M. Harnois, DO

Budesonide Induces Remission More Effectively Than Prednisone in a Controlled Trial of Patients With Autoimmune Hepatitis
Manns MP, for the European AIH-BUC-Study Group (Hannover Med School, Germany; et al)
Gastroenterology 139:1198-1206, 2010

Background & Aims.—Autoimmune hepatitis (AIH) is a chronic liver disease associated with cirrhosis and liver failure. Corticosteroid therapy induces long-term remission but has many side effects. We compared the effects of budesonide (a steroid that is rapidly metabolized, with low systemic exposure) and prednisone, both in combination with azathioprine.

Methods.—We performed a 6-month, prospective, double-blind, random-ized, active-controlled, multicenter, phase IIb trial of patients with AIH without evidence of cirrhosis who were given budesonide (3 mg, three times daily or twice daily) or prednisone (40 mg/d, tapered to 10 mg/d); patients also received azathioprine (1–2 mg/kg/d). Treatment was followed by a 6-month, open-label phase during which all patients received budeso-nide in addition to azathioprine. The primary end point was complete biochemical remission, defined as normal serum levels of aspartate amino-transferase and alanine aminotransferase, without predefined steroid-specific side effects, at 6 months.

Results.—The primary end point was achieved in 47/100 patients given budesonide (47.0%) and in 19/103 patients given prednisone (18.4%) ($P < .001$; 97.5% 1-side confidence interval [CI] = 16.2). At 6 months, complete biochemical remission occurred in 60% of the patients given budesonide versus 38.8% of those given prednisone ($P < .001$; CI: 7.7); 72.0% of those in the budesonide group did not develop steroid-specific side effects versus 46.6% in the prednisone group ($P < .001$; CI = 12.3). Among 87 patients who were initially given prednisone and then received budesonide after 6 months, steroid-specific side effects decreased from 44.8% to 26.4% at month 12 ($P < .002$).

Conclusions.—Oral budesonide, in combination with azathioprine, induces and maintains remission in patients with noncirrhotic AIH, with a low rate of steroid-specific side effects.

▶ Autoimmune hepatitis (AIH) is a chronic liver disease that may be associated with significant complications and disease progression. In 2010, long-awaited guidelines on the management and treatment of patients with AIH were published from the American Association for the Study of Liver Disease. The standard treatment of these patients includes prednisone alone or in combination with azathioprine, which will induce a remission in 80%. Withdrawal of therapy can lead to relapse in 85% of cases, but long-term use of prednisone and, to a lesser extent, azathioprine, can lead to adverse events and side effects.

Budesonide is a steroid with a 90% first-pass metabolism in the liver and low systemic side effects. It has been assessed as an alternative treatment to prednisone in a number of immune-mediated diseases. This article reports the results of a large double-blind, randomized, controlled, multicenter, phase IIb trial of budesonide versus prednisone in combination with azathioprine in the treatment of noncirrhotic patients with AIH. Oral budesonide in combination with azathioprine induced and maintained remission in noncirrhotic patients with AIH and had a low rate of steroid-related side effects, making it an alternative to prednisone therapy in some AIH patients.

D. M. Harnois, DO

Drugs and the Liver

Drug-Induced Cholestasis
Padda MS, Sanchez M, Akhtar AJ, et al (Centennial Hills Hosp Med Ctr, Las Vegas, NV; Yale Univ School of Medicine, New Haven, CT; Charles Drew Univ of Medicine and Science, Los Angeles, CA)
Hepatology 53:1377-1387, 2011

Recent progress in understanding the molecular mechanisms of bile formation and cholestasis have led to new insights into the pathogenesis of drug-induced cholestasis. This review summarizes their variable clinical presentations, examines the role of transport proteins in hepatic drug clearance and toxicity, and addresses the increasing importance of genetic determinants, as well as practical aspects of diagnosis and management.

▶ Hepatic drug toxicity is a common cause of both mild liver test abnormalities and acute liver failure. In a previous publication in the *New England Journal of Medicine* in 2003, drug toxicity represented the cause of 50% of the cases of acute fulminant liver failure. Cholestatic and mixed cholestatic and heptocellular injury are 2 of the most severe manifestations of drug-induced liver injury. Patients may be asymptomatic or may present with very dramatic clinical features of liver injury and jaundice.

This article reviews the pathogenesis of liver-induced injury in these patients. However, perhaps more important to clinicians, it also outlines recommendations regarding establishing the diagnosis and treatment of these patients.

Most cases of drug-induced cholestasis will resolve with withdrawal of the offending agent. Levels of aspartate aminotransferase and bilirubin are the most important predictors of death or liver transplant in drug-induced liver injury. Management recommendations for pruritus are also outlined in the article. There are currently no approved therapies for drug-induced cholestatic liver injury, but ursodeoxycholic acid therapy may have a theoretical benefit. In the future, gene expression profile information may help better predict those patients likely to develop drug-induced liver injury.

D. M. Harnois, DO

Hereditary Liver Disease

Zinc Monotherapy Is Not as Effective as Chelating Agents in Treatment of Wilson Disease

Weiss KH, Gotthardt DN, Klemm D, et al (Univ Hosp Heidelberg, Germany; et al)
Gastroenterology 140:1189-1198, 2011

Background & Aims.—Wilson disease is a genetic disorder that affects copper storage, leading to liver failure and neurologic deterioration. Patients are treated with copper chelators and zinc salts, but it is not clear what approach is optimal because there have been few studies of large cohorts. We assessed long-term outcomes of different treatments.

Methods.—Patients in tertiary care centers were retrospectively analyzed (n = 288; median follow-up time, 17.1 years) for adherence to therapy, survival, treatment failure, and adverse events from different treatment regimens (chelators, zinc, or a combination). Hepatic treatment failure was defined as an increase in activity of liver enzymes (aspartate aminotransferase, alanine aminotransferase, and γ-glutamyltransferase) >2-fold the upper limit of normal or >100% of baseline with an increase in urinary copper excretion.

Results.—The median age at onset of Wilson disease was 17.5 years. Hepatic and neuropsychiatric symptoms occurred in 196 (68.1%) and 99 (34.4%) patients, respectively. Hepatic treatment failure occurred more often from zinc therapy (14/88 treatments) than from chelator therapy (4/313 treatments; $P < .001$). Actuarial survival, without transplantation, showed an advantage for chelating agents ($P < .001$ vs zinc). Changes in treatment resulted mostly from adverse events, but the frequency did not differ between groups. Patients who did not respond to zinc therapy showed hepatic improvement after reintroduction of a chelating agent.

Conclusions.—Treatments with chelating agents or zinc salt are effective in most patients with Wilson disease; chelating agents are better at preventing hepatic deterioration. It is important to identify patients who do not respond to zinc therapy and have increased activities of liver enzymes, indicating that a chelating agent should be added to the therapeutic regimen.

▶ Wilson disease is a genetic disorder of copper storage that leads to hepatic and neurologic symptoms through impaired hepatocellular utilization and biliary excretion of copper. The goal of therapy in Wilson disease is to create a negative copper balance. The most recent guidelines propose treatment regimens that consist of chelating agents and/or the use of zinc salts. The 2 most commonly used chelating agents are D-penicillamine and trientine. Zinc salts have been used as primary therapy, but the efficacy of zinc monotherapy is unclear. In addition, there are, as the article points out, limited data on the use of zinc salts in maintenance therapy.

This is a large retrospective cohort analysis of 288 patients treated with Wilson disease at a university health system in Germany and Austria between 1954 and 2008. The results of this trial suggest that zinc monotherapy was in some cases associated with a risk for hepatic decompensation. There may be a role for monotherapy as a treatment for asymptomatic patients or those with neurologic sequelae only, but with careful monitoring for the development of new neurologic symptoms or hepatic deterioration that suggests an incomplete response to therapy. This can happen even as late as after 15 years of unchanged therapy. In cases where inadequate response to therapy is detected, the addition of chelating agents is recommended.

D. M. Harnois, DO

Miscellaneous

Association of caffeine intake and histological features of chronic hepatitis C

Costentin CE, Roudot-Thoraval F, Zafrani E-S, et al (Groupe Hospitalier Henri Mondor-Albert Chenevier, Créteil, France; INSERM, Créteil, France; et al)
J Hepatol 54:1123-1129, 2011

Background & Aims.—The severity of chronic hepatitis C (CHC) is modulated by host and environmental factors. Several reports suggest that caffeine intake exerts hepatoprotective effects in patients with chronic liver disease. The aim of this study was to evaluate the impact of caffeine consumption on activity grade and fibrosis stage in patients with CHC.

Methods.—A total of 238 treatment-naïve patients with histologically-proven CHC were included in the study. Demographic, epidemiological, environmental, virological, and metabolic data were collected, including daily consumption of alcohol, cannabis, tobacco, and caffeine during the six months preceding liver biopsy. Daily caffeine consumption was estimated as the sum of mean intakes of caffeinated coffee, tea, and caffeine-containing sodas. Histological activity grade and fibrosis stage were scored according to Metavir. Patients (154 men, 84 women, mean age: 45 ± 11 years) were categorized according to caffeine consumption quartiles: group 1 (<225 mg/day,

$n = 59$), group 2 (225–407 mg/day, $n = 57$), group 3 (408–678 mg/day, $n = 62$), and group 4 (>678 mg/day, $n = 60$).

Results.—There was a significant inverse relationship between activity grade and daily caffeine consumption: activity grade >A2 was present in 78%, 61%, 52%, and 48% of patients in group 1, 2, 3, and 4, respectively ($p < 0.001$). By multivariate analysis, daily caffeine consumption greater than 408 mg/day was associated with a lesser risk of activity grade >A2 (OR = 0.32 (0.12–0.85). Caffeine intake showed no relation with fibrosis stage.

Conclusions.—Caffeine consumption greater than 408 mg/day (3 cups or more) is associated with reduced histological activity in patients with CHC. These findings support potential hepatoprotective properties of caffeine in chronic liver diseases.

▶ Many environmental factors may affect the degree of inflammation present in chronic hepatitis C. Caffeine and, in particular, coffee may have anti-inflammatory or antioxidant effects. Caffeine intake may reduce or protect against liver injury in patients with chronic liver diseases. High coffee consumption has been associated with a reduced risk of hepatocellular carcinoma in patients with chronic liver disease.[1] This study examined caffeine consumption in the 6 months before untreated patients with chronic hepatitis C underwent a liver biopsy.

Patients with high intakes (> 3 cups) of coffee had significantly less inflammation but no difference in fibrosis score, which suggests that coffee ingestion is not of any harm in patients with chronic hepatitis C. The other factors, such as degree of steatosis and age, were associated with increased degree of inflammation. Some unrecognized association with high caffeine consumption may confound these results and prior studies in chronic liver diseases; however, caffeine appears to be somewhat protective in 2 such confounders, age and alcohol consumption, which are associated with high coffee consumption. Although this study estimated caffeine consumption, it may be some other component of the primary source of caffeine, coffee, that is the source of benefit. Further study is needed to identify how the apparent benefit occurs. In the meantime, at the very least heavy coffee drinkers with hepatitis C should be encouraged to continue drinking their brew.

J. A. Murray, MD

Reference

1. Gelatti U, Covolo L, Franceschini M, et al. Coffee consumption reduces the risk of hepatocellular carcinoma independently of its aetiology: a case-control study. *J Hepatol.* 2005;42:528-534.

Article Index

Chapter 1: Esophagus

Chapter 2: Gastrointestinal Motility Disorders/Neurogastroenterology

Chapter 3: Pancreaticobiliary Disease

Chapter 4: Gastrointestinal Cancers and Benign Polyps

Chapter 5: Inflammatory Bowel Disease

Chapter 6: Nutrition and Celiac Disease

Chapter 7: Gastrointestinal Surgery

Chapter 8: Liver Disease

Author Index

Printed and bound by CPI Group (UK) Ltd, Croydon, CR0 4YY

08/05/2025

01864677-0007